Basic and Applied Sciences for Sports Medicine

Edited by

R.J. Maughan, BSc PhD
Professor of Human Physiology
Department of Biomedical Sciences
University of Aberdeen
Scotland, UK

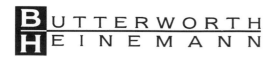

BUTTERWORTH HEINEMANN

OXFORD AUCKLAND BOSTON JOHANNESBURG MELBOURNE NEW DELHI

Butterworth-Heinemann
Linacre House, Jordan Hill, Oxford OX2 8DP
225 Wildwood Avenue, Woburn, MA 01801-2041
A division of Reed Educational and Professional Publishing Ltd

R A member of the Reed Elsevier plc group

First published 1999

British Library Cataloguing in Publication Data
Basic and applied sciences for sports medicine
  1. Sports medicine   2. Medical sciences
  I. Maughan, Ron J., 1951–
  617.1′027

Library of Congress Cataloguing in Publication Data
Basic and applied sciences for sports medicine/edited by R.J. Maughan.
    p. cm.
Includes bibliographical references and index.
ISBN 0 7506 3466 9
  1. Sports–Physiological aspects.   2. Sports medicine.   3. Sports
sciences.   I. Maughan, Ron J.
RC1235.B38

                    99–17155
                      CIP

ISBN 0 7506 3466 9

Typeset by Keyword Typesetting Services Ltd, Wallington, Surrey
Printed and bound in Great Britian by Biddles Ltd, Guildford and King's Lynn

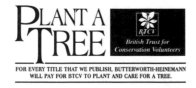

Contents

Foreword

'You must pray for a healthy mind in a healthy body'

The deserved and increasingly international recognition of sports sciences, sports medicine and the benefits of exercise has opened up exciting new fields of discovery, as well as opportunities for a wide range of integrated professional development. Publication of *Basic and Applied Sciences for Sports Medicine* highlights substantive fields of scientific endeavour as well as making a significant contribution to the continuing development of sport and exercise medicine as a recognized medical specialty.

The range and quality of the sports sciences, as demonstrated in this text, have helped to create the climate which, in July 1998, encouraged the Academy of Medical Royal Colleges and their Faculties in the United Kingdom and Ireland to support the development of the Intercollegiate Academic Board of Sport and Exercise Medicine. This Board is responsible for setting and appraising standards of education, training and clinical practice in this newly recognized specialty on behalf of the medical profession, with a view to benefiting society at large as well as individual patients.

Sports and exercise medicine is relevant to all aspects of medical practice – primary care, community and occupational health or specialist aspects of hospital medicine. Sports and exercise medicine, in conjunction with integration of the basic sciences as applied to sport, has the potential to fire the imagination of undergraduates and stimulate a life-long interest in the understanding of health and disability as well as disease prevention and management.

Exercise programmes designed to promote health should be risk-free but sport and competition invariably involve risk. Even the most gifted individuals when striving to improve their performance – whether against the clock, an opponent or the elements – need the support of an integrated medical and scientific team if they are to achieve success. Any lack of knowledge, failure of understanding or poor communication between members of the athlete's support team will increase the risk of injury, illness or even death. The medical and scientific support team must work with the athlete, the coach and the officials controlling the sport to promote the performance and health of the individual athlete as well as promoting safety. The support team must clearly understand the sports with which they are involved but this in itself is of little value if the individual team members do not have a solid grounding in the relevant basic sciences.

Publication of *Basic and Applied Sciences for Sports Medicine* will give a wide range of sports scientists, members of the professions allied to medicine, and doctors every opportunity to ensure that they are promoting exercise and sport from a position of strength based upon mutual professional respect. Professor Ron Maughan and his team of authors are to be congratulated on the major contribution they have made to the integration of sport and exercise medicine with the sports sciences by presenting a wealth of clinically relevant, performance-related basic science in a readily approachable and reader-friendly manner.

Doctors and the professions allied to medicine have traditionally concentrated their endeavours on the management of 'failure'. Practitioners in the field of sports and exercise medicine have always appreciated the importance of understanding why 'failure' occurs and endeavouring to prevent it, and the publication of *Basic and Applied Sciences for Sports Medicine* will help them achieve this ambition. It will also give a more logical approach to and a better understanding of any treatments offered and encourage a more scientific, evidence-based, approach to outcome measurement. This improved level of knowledge and understanding will help ensure that clinicians involved in sports and exercise medicine will be in a position to contribute to the development of athletes, patient care and academic progress in this specialty on the basis of sound scientific knowledge.

Professor Donald Macleod
Honorary Professor of Sports Medicine (Aberdeen University)
Chairman, Intercollegiate Academic Board of Sport and Exercise Medicine
President, British Association of Sport and Medicine
Edinburgh, 1999

Preface

Sports medicine is now being recognized as a distinct entity that is important in its own right. The subject encompasses the preparation of and care for the competitive athlete, from the weekend warrior whose participation may be largely for social reasons, to the elite athlete who aspires to Olympic victory. The discipline is much wider than this, however, and also embraces exercise as medicine, recognizing that many of the common diseases that afflict modern man are the consequences of a sedentary lifestyle: in many cases, progression of these illnesses can be slowed or reversed by physical activity.

The elite athlete is endowed with the genetic potential that provides the physiological and biochemical basis for success. The athlete must build on this foundation with intensive training, which requires motivation and mental toughness. Supporting an intensive training load requires good nutrition, and special nutritional strategies can improve performance in competition. Olympic success is open to only a few, but all can enjoy the benefits of exercise, both in terms of improved fitness and better health. There is compelling evidence that regular exercise reduces the risk and severity of many of the health problems that are common in modern industrialized societies, thus promoting both health and fitness.

This book explores the science that underpins the practice of sports medicine. It takes a broad approach to the sports sciences, but explores each in some detail. Each of the major scientific disciplines is covered in detail in the first part of the book, and chapters highlighting practical applications of this information are included in the later part of the book. One or more chapters are devoted to physiology, biochemistry, biomechanics, nutrition, psychology and immunology. Additional chapters cover training and the assessment of athletes.

This book has been written with two primary audiences in mind. The first consists of medical practitioners with an interest in sports medicine who wish to understand the scientific basis of the subject. The second is sports scientists who wish a single volume that gives a broad coverage of the whole field. Few scientists are experts in all of these fields, but the study of the whole human requires a familiarity with many different disciplines. The authors who have contributed chapters to this book are all internationally recognized as experts in their fields, and their depth of knowledge shows in their ability to make complex material understandable to the non-specialist. It has been a pleasure for me to work with them, and to them belongs the credit for all that is good in this book.

Ron Maughan

Contributors

Nicolette C. Bishop BSc
Lettie Claire Bishop is a research student working on the modifying influence of diet on immune responses to exercise. She obtained a first class honours degree in sport and exercise sciences at the University of Birmingham in 1997 and was awarded the C.T.M. Davies prize for outstanding academic achievement.

Elizabeth M. Broad BSc, DipNutr Diet, MAppSci
After graduating in dietetics in 1989, Liz worked in Launceston, Tasmania as a clinical dietitian then diabetes specialist before undertaking a Commonwealth Government Public Health Project. During the latter part of this time, Liz began specializing in sports nutrition, including consulting to the Tasmanian Institute of Sport. In 1994, Liz attained the Sports Nutrition Fellowship at the Australian Institute of Sport under the direction of Dr Louise Burke. She was then fortunate enough to obtain ongoing work at the AIS for the next 3 years, culminating in being in charge of the Sports Nutrition Department for most of 1997 while Dr Burke was on sabbatical. At the same time, Liz consulted to the ACT Academy of Sport, the ACT Brumbies Rugby Union Team, and undertook some tutoring and lecturing at the University of Canberra. In 1997 Liz also completed her Master of Applied Science (Sports Studies) in exercise science, with a thesis entitled 'The effects of heat on performance in wheelchair shooters'. Liz is currently the Sports Science Co-ordinator and Sports Dietitian for Australian Canoeing, looking after the national sprint and slalom canoe squads. Liz has written several papers for scientific publications, coaching journals and 'lay' magazines.

Louise M. Burke PhD, BSc (nutr) GDip Diet
Louise Burke has been the Head of the Department of Sports Nutrition at the Australian Institute of Sport since 1990. She has written a number of books on sports nutrition, and contributes articles to many sports magazines and coaching journals. Her research interests include post-exercise recovery, glycaemic index and sports performance, and nutritional ergogenic aids. She has been appointed as Adjunct Professor at Deakin

University in Victoria where she is involved in post-graduate education in sports nutrition. She serves on the executive board of Sports Dietitians Australia.

Jeff S. Coombes PhD

Jeff Coombes was born and raised in Tasmania, Australia. He graduated from the University of Tasmania with bachelor degrees in education and applied science and a masters degree in exercise physiology. Upon receiving his PhD from the University of Florida, he returned to the University of Tasmania where he is currently a faculty member in the Centre for Human Movement.

Haydar A. Demirel MD, PhD

Haydar A. Demirel was born in Turkey. He received his BS from the University of Gazi, his MD from the University of Ankara, and his PhD from the University of Florida. He is currently a faculty member in the School of Sport Sciences and Technology at the University of Hacetepe, Ankara, Turkey.

Michael Gleeson BSc PhD

Mike Gleeson is a senior lecturer in exercise biochemistry in the School of Sport and Exercise Sciences at the University of Birmingham. His first degree was in biochemistry at the same university. His PhD project concerned the effects of diet–exercise interactions on energy metabolism and was carried out at the University of Central Lancashire. Over the past 20 years he has published over 150 papers on exercise physiology and biochemistry. He is a member of the Physiological Society and Nutrition Society, and he is an accredited exercise physiologist of the British Association of Sport and Exercise Sciences. He is also a Fellow of the European College of Sport Science and is the physiology section editor for the *Journal of Sports Sciences*. His current research on the effects of exercise, muscle damage and overtraining on immune function is sponsored by the English Sports Council.

Paul L. Greenhaff BSc PhD

Paul Greenhaff is a Reader in Muscle Metabolism in the School of Biomedical Sciences at the University of Nottingham. His research group has an active interest in the regulation of energy metabolism and fatigue during exercise.

Karyn L. Hamilton MS, RD

After earning a BS in nutrition from Montana State University, USA, Karyn L. Hamilton worked in clinical nutrition at the University of California San Francisco Medical Center and the University of Washington Medical Centers, Harborview. Following completion of her

MS in exercise physiology, she began pursuing her PhD at the Center for Exercise Science at the University of Florida. Her specific area of interest is in the influence of exercise training, nutritional antioxidants, and heat shock proteins on myocardial ischemia reperfusion injury.

Adrianne E. Hardman MSc PhD
Adrianne Hardman is Reader in Human Exercise Metabolism at Loughborough University. Her research interests are in the influence of moderate-intensity exercise on fitness and on the metabolic risk factors for cardiovascular disease. She was a member of the Scientific Advisory Board for the 1992 Allied Dunbar National Fitness Survey and is presently a member of the International Relations Committee of the American College of Sports Medicine.

John A. Hawley BSc MA PhD FACSM
John Hawley is currently Professor of Human Biology and Movement Science at RMIT University, Melbourne, Australia. He obtained his BSc from Loughborough University, his MA from Ball State University, Indiana, and his PhD from the University of Cape Town Medical School. He has published extensively in the scientific literature and recently completed his first book on training and nutritional strategies for optimizing sport performance. He was the first New Zealand researcher to be elected a Fellow of the American College of Sports Medicine (FACSM) in 1994. His current research interests include the biochemistry and nutrition of exercise metabolism, adaptions to training in previously well-trained individuals, and laboratory testing to monitor and predict athletic performance. He has worked with many elite athletes from a wide variety of sports, and has been closely involved in the scientific and medical testing of many National teams in several continents.

Eric Hultman MD PhD
Eric Hultman is Professor of Clinical Chemistry in the Department of Clinical and Laboratory Sciences, Huddinge University Hospital, Karolinska Institute, Sweden. Professor Hultman has researched and published extensively on the topic of human muscle metabolism during exercise and he is an accepted world authority in this area. His work over the past 30 years has been responsible for some of the major new developments in exercise metabolism. His current research interests include the intergration of carbohydrate and fat oxidation during steady-state exercise and the role of creatine supplementation in sports nutrition.

Yiannis (John) Koutedakis BSc MA PhD
Yiannis Koutedakis has attended many national, international and world championships and Olympic Games as competitor, coach/trainer or physiologist. He was one of the main contributors to the initial setting-up of

the British Olympic Medical Centre (London), and he has been physical fitness and training advisor to Olympic squads, professional dance companies and professional soccer clubs. He is currently senior lecturer in sport and exercise physiology at Wolverhampton University, and visiting lecturer at the London Contemporary Dance School, the Northern School of Contemporary Dance (Leeds) and Thessaly University (Greece). His research focuses on aspects of physical fitness and training, and he has published numerous journal articles and book chapters, in English, Greek, Italian and French.

Henryk K. A. Lakomy BSc MA PhD
Henryk Lakomy is currently a lecturer in exercise physiology at Loughborough University. His first degree, in electronics at Sussex University, was followed by a Master's Degree in Sports Science at the University of California, Davis where he specialized in kinesiology. His doctorate, which was completed at Loughborough University, was in the measurement of external power output during high intensity exercise. In the course of this work he developed a number of unique ergometers capable of measuring human power output during activities being performed at maximum intensity.

R. J. Maughan BSc PhD
Ron Maughan is currently Professor of Human Physiology at the University Medical School, Aberdeen, Scotland. He obtained his BSc (Physiology) and PhD from the University of Aberdeen, and held a lecturing position in Liverpool before returning to Aberdeen where he is now based in the Department of Biomedical Sciences. His research interests are in the physiology, biochemistry and nutrition of exercise performance, with an interest in both the basic science of exercise and the applied aspects that relate to health and to performance in sport. He has published extensively in the scientific literature, and is on the editorial board of several international journals. Professor Maughan is a Fellow of the American College of Sports Medicine and a member of many scientific organizations, including the Physiological Society, the Nutrition Society, the Biochemical Society, the Medical Research Society and the New York Academy of Sciences. He chairs the Human and Exercise Physiology Group of the Physiological Society. He also chairs the Nutrition Steering Group of the British Olympic Association and played a leading role in the production of the acclimatization strategy that was employed by British and other competitors preparing for the 1996 Olympic Games held in Atlanta, Georgia. A former runner, he now leads a more sedentary life.

William P. Morgan EdD FACSM
William P. Morgan is Professor in the Department of Kinesiology and Director of the Sport Psychology Laboratory at the University of

Wisconsin-Madison. A fellow of the American Psychological Association, Society for Personality Assessment, American College of Sports Medicine, Society for Clinical and Experimental Hypnosis, and the American Academy of Kinesiology and Physical Education, his published research has dealt with personality, perception hypnosis, motivation, psychopathology, overtraining, panic behaviour in scuba divers, and the antidepressant and anxiolytic effects of physical activity. He has edited four books in exercise science and his most recent volume is entitled *Physical Activity and Mental Health* (Taylor and Francis, 1997).

Scott K. Powers PhD EdD FACSM
Scott Powers is currently a professor and the director of the Center for Exercise Science at the University of Florida. He also serves as an adjunct professor in the Department of Physiology. He earned a BS (Carson Newman College) and MEd (University of Georgia) in Physical Education. Later, he earned a doctoral degree from the University of Tennessee and a second PhD in Physiology from Louisiana State University. Dr. Powers has more than 20 years' experience in teaching and research in the field of exercise physiology. Early in his academic career he also directed an adult fitness programme and taught collegiate courses relating to cardiac rehabilitation. More recently, Dr. Powers' work has focused on the mechanisms responsible for cardiac and skeletal muscle adaptation to stress.

John S. Raglin PhD
John S. Raglin is currently an associate professor in the Department of Kinesiology at Indiana University, Bloomington. He is a fellow of the American College of Sports Medicine and the American Psychological Association. His research involves the psychological effects of physical activity, emotion in sport performance, and the psychobiological consequences of overtraining.

N.C. Craig Sharp BVMS MRCVS PhD FIBiol FBASES FPEA
Craig Sharp graduated in veterinary medicine from Glasgow University and worked in practice before joining the Physiology Department of the Glasgow Vet School, under Dr (later Sir) James Black, Nobel Laureate, later transferring to the Department of Experimental Medicine there. In 1971 he joined the Birmingham University Department of Physical Education and Sports Science, and was founder co-director of their human motor performance laboratory. He has been selected for four Olympic Games as coach or physiologist, and has been variously an international competitor, trainer, coach, team manager and team selector. He was co-founder of and director of physiological services at the British Olympic Medical Centre, and is currently Professor of Sports Science at Brunel University, and Adjunct Professor of Sports Science at the University of Limerick and at Stirling University.

N.C. Spurway MA PhD

Neil Spurway is Professor of Exercise Physiology in the University of Glasgow's Centre for Exercise Science and Medicine. After studying science and sport with about equal commitment at school, he was lured away from the intention of being a physicist by the exciting things going on in physiology. He graduated in this subject in 1960, and spent 3 years researching muscle membrane permeability. Muscle has been his scientific focus ever since, particular interests being the comparative quantitative histochemistry of vertebrate skeletal muscles and the effects of pH changes on the smooth muscles of blood vessels; his main current research now is in sporting and clinical aspects of human skeletal muscle training and metabolism. His main sports now are distance running and dinghy racing: in the latter he still competes at UK level, and was founding coach to the Scottish junior sailing squad. He played a leading role in setting up the University of Glasgow's degree in physiology and sports science (the first sports science degree in a traditional British university) in 1985, and has been course leader ever since. He has chaired the physiology section of the British Association of Sport and Exercise Sciences, sits on the Exercise Physiology Steering Group of the British Olympic Association as well as the Scottish Committee of the British Association of Sport and Medicine, and is a Fellow of the European College of Sport Science.

Muscle

N.C. Spurway

The attempt in this chapter is to review, quite briefly, material covered in most undergraduate medical courses, but to give more detail about sport-related aspects of muscle function which the reader is less likely to have met before.

The motor unit and the individual fibre

Skeletal muscle, unlike cardiac and smooth, can operate only under neural control. It is therefore appropriate to begin our consideration of it at the lower motoneurone – the 'final common path' (Sherrington, 1904) for neural signalling to muscle.

All working muscle fibres are innervated by motoneurones in the largest size-range (**α-motoneurones**), with large-diameter myelinated axons. Because it is large, each neurone is able to innervate not one but a family of muscle fibres; and the neurone plus its family is termed a **motor unit** (Figure 1.1). The family may be as few as 10 muscle fibres, in one of the smallest units of a small muscle (say an extraocular or laryngeal), or as many as 3000 in one of the largest units of a large muscle (e.g. quadriceps or latissimus dorsi).

In turn, the fibres themselves vary immensely in size. The smallest, in the very small muscles, may be 2–3 mm long and about 10 μm in diameter; the largest may be 20–30 cm × ~ 100 μm. All, however, are very large as cells go – too large for their cytoplasmic volume to be efficiently controlled by a single nucleus. Thus every skeletal muscle fibre is multinucleate, though the number of nuclei varies from ~ 10 to ~ 3000. In mature muscle these lie at the peripheries of fibres, just deep to the surface layer or **sarcolemma** – which is the name for the cell membrane plus its carbohydrate-rich external lamina and collagenous outer coat. Within this envelope lies the contractile cytoplasm, characterized under appropriate stains or optical contrast techniques by its **cross-striated** pattern of alternating A or dark bands and I or light ones. Other features of the structure are illustrated in Figure 1.2.

MOTOR UNIT

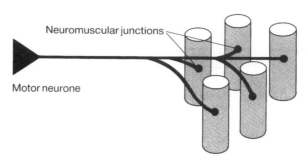

Figure 1.1. The motor unit. (From Vander, A. *et al.* (1994). *Human Physiology*, 6th Edn. reproduced by permission of The McGraw-Hill Companies.)

The individual fibre is the unit of growth, metabolism and force production – yet it is the motor unit which is the unit of control.

Types of motor unit

Within a given muscle, the smallest motor units (controlled by the smallest neurones within the α range) have the lowest thresholds for recruitment. That is, they are the easiest to call into play and the hardest to prevent from responding, so they are generally considered to be active (so far as they can be, within the constraints of fatigue or pathology) whenever the muscle is producing any force at all (Figure 1.3). By contrast, the largest units within the muscle have the highest thresholds, and so are recruited only for the maximum force. This is the **size principle** of motoneurone, and hence motor unit, recruitment (Henneman *et al.*, 1965). It applies in all circumstances where the muscle concerned is the prime mover in a shortening ('concentric') contraction; thus it dominates the muscle characteristics. There is some evidence that large units may be preferentially selected for 'eccentric' actions, i.e. those in which the muscle lengthens under load (Enoka, 1996); however, we shall see later that eccentric actions make minimal metabolic demands, so they have negligible influence on fibre biochemistry.

Since many of the highest forces are aimed at achieving very fast movements, it should be no surprise that the fibres composing the largest units in each muscle are capable of the fastest shortening. Conversely, low forces normally bring about slow movements, or none at all – they may instead maintain posture or hold an object steady. Predictably, therefore, the smaller motor units of each muscle have fibres which contract relatively slowly, even when they are shortening under zero load. Their velo-

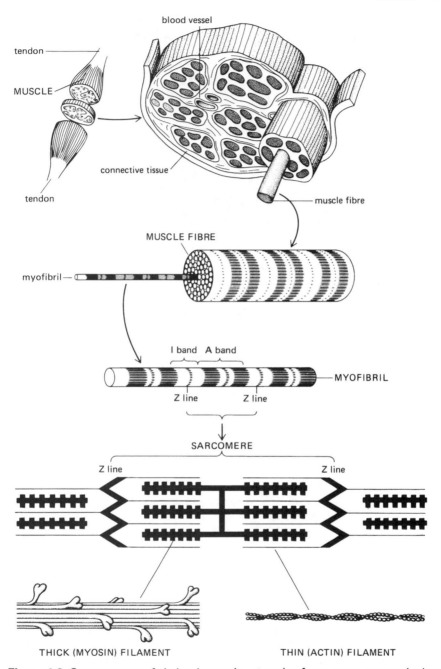

Figure 1.2. Components of skeletal muscle, at scales from gross anatomical to macromolecular. (From di Prampero, P.E. (1985). *Journal of Experimental Biology*, **115**, 319 reproduced by permission of Company of Biologist Ltd)

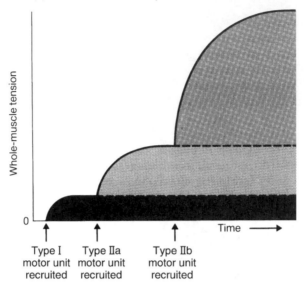

Figure 1.3. Tension elicited by increasing activation of motor units in an imaginary muscle consisting of only one unit of each type. Curved portions of plot indicate that each unit gives greater mean force as the frequency of action potentials in its motor nerve increases ('rate modulation'). Successive steps indicate that units are recruited in order: the one which comprises fewest fibres and is therefore weakest (a type I unit) is recruited first, the one comprising most fibres and which is therefore strongest (type IIb) is recruited last, while the IIa unit is between the others. (From Vander, A. *et al.* (1994). *Human Physiology*, 6th Edn. reproduced by permission of The McGraw-Hill Companies)

city under these conditions is one-quarter that of fast fibres (Bottinelli *et al.*, 1996).

However, these small units, though producing quite small forces and moving fairly slowly, are used very frequently. Their muscle fibres must therefore resist fatigue (Burke *et al.*, 1961). One contribution to this is made by the relative slowness of the contractile machinery: it follows from what is said later (see 'Cross-bridge mechanisms') that, other things being equal, a fibre which shortens at one-quarter the speed of another uses ATP about a quarter as fast. Even more crucial to fatigue resistance is that the supply of ATP should be capable of being maintained almost indefinitely. For this, it must operate in balance with oxygen (O_2) supply, i.e. **aerobically**; thus the fibres of small motor units have been described as 'pay as you go' fibres. The cytoplasmic machinery providing this property – a generous supply of mitochondria, plus myoglobin to facilitate O_2 diffusion – gives the fibres a red-brown colour. Fibres with these properties are termed **'slow red'** or **type I** fibres.

The largest fibres, being used only rarely, do not need this provision: indeed, they could rarely profit by it, for when large numbers of them are being used simultaneously, as happens whenever we have a major weight to lift or load to move, so much O_2 demand would arise that only a much larger chest could provide the cardio-respiratory capacity required – and the weight of this chest, the other 99.99 per cent of the time, would surely have been evolutionarily disadvantageous. Thus the largest fibres are essentially **anaerobic**; they have a smattering of mitochondria, to enable them to recover from one intensive effort before (if we are wise) we ask them to perform the next ('pull now, pay later' fibres), but during any vigorous activity they supply virtually all the ATP their contractile machinery needs by the glycolytic pathway. They are pale cream or pink-ish white in colour and fast fatiguing, and are known as **'fast white'** or **type IIb** fibres.

In between the two extremes comes a fibre type which is nearly as fast as the IIb, yet about as red as the type I – this is the **'fast red'** or **type IIa** fibre. (For comparisons between the three fibre types, see Figure 1.4.)

It is interesting that the fibres of any one motor unit are not grouped together but spread in a mosaic over the cross-section of the fasciculus to which they belong. Presumably this has the advantage of distributing both mechanical and metabolic loads.

In a mature limb muscle, under a stable pattern of use, only perhaps 2 per cent of fibres will not be classifiable into one of the three types just named. By contrast, when intensity of use has recently been stepped substantially up or down, perhaps 10 per cent of fibres are likely to dis-play intermediate forms. Such a form is usually interpreted as indicating that the fibre is in transition from one main type to another. The IIc fibre, intermediate between types I and IIa, is prominent in such circumstances. It is also frequently seen in the muscles of endurance athletes subjecting themselves to very strenuous training regimes, such as runners covering over 100 miles every week. In this case it seems likely that, though the regime is stable, individual fibres are not and frequently alternate between suffering and recovering from overuse damage.

Biochemical differences between different types of fibre

The chief protein of the contractile system, myosin, comes in a variety of forms. Since they all do the same category of job they are called **isoen-zymes**. The main components of the myosin molecule, the **heavy chains**, show the greatest variety. The heavy chains of type I fibres differ from those of type IIa, which in turn differ from those of type IIb. In a number of reactions, some of which are used in identification, type IIa myosin is at an extreme of the three types (Brooke and Kaiser, 1970 and cf. Figure 1.5b) – an early guess that it might be an intermediate or even hybrid between types I and IIb is thus not correct. However, **type IIc** fibres do contain a mixture of type I and type IIa myosins; and a hybrid between types IIa and IIb, called simply **type IIab**, is even more common in many circum-stances (Billeter *et al.*, 1980).

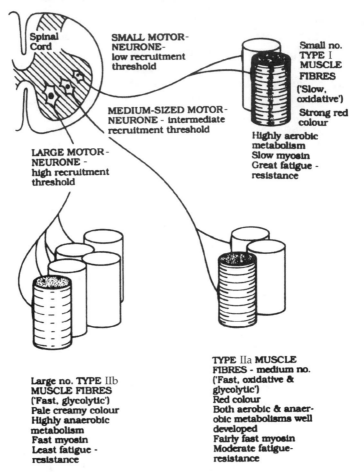

Figure 1.4. The three main types of motor unit found in mature, stable human limb muscles. (From Spurway, N.C. (1992). *British Medical Bulletin*, **48**, 569–591 reproduced by permission of the British Council)

(In some very recent literature, for example Ennion *et al.*, 1995, the IIb fibre type is referred to as IIx, because its myosin is shown to be more closely homologous to one with that label, coming between IIa and IIb in laboratory animals, than to the true IIb myosin of such species. However, until evidence is presented that, somewhere in human musculature, there is a true IIb myosin homologue, different from the IIx, one suspects that this distinction will be disregarded by the majority of writers.)

Unlike the myosins, actin molecules of fast and slow skeletal muscles are indistinguishable. Several other proteins involved in contraction differ between fast and slow fibres, though not between all three stable types. In hybrid and transitional fibres, however, some proteins may be of the faster and others of the slower types; this probably occurs because different proteins adapt to changes of use at different rates, so the textbook combinations will only be dominant when the muscle as a whole is in a stable state.

Similar considerations apply to the metabolic furniture of the different fibres. Furthermore, the separate systems are all independently flexible, responding to the particular needs of their particular motor unit. The fact that there is not a rigid relationship between metabolic systems is underlined by the situation in amphibia and fish, where fibres which are the most aerobic also have the highest anaerobic capacities (Spurway and Rowlerson, 1989). Perhaps this is because O_2 supply in these species can fall short through environmental hypoxia whereas, where mammals evolved (near sea level), shortfall only occurs when a large number of muscles are simultaneously working hard. The example warns us that general tendencies to align properties into groups must be ascribed to commonly associated influences, not to inescapable genetic couplings between myosin type, aerobic capacity and anaerobic capacity.

Influences on fibre characteristics

Within any one motor unit, all muscle fibres have similar characteristics. This correctly suggests that the nerve determines much about the kind of fibres it innervates – it 'tells the fibre not only what to do but what to be'. In classical experiments, Buller et al. (1960) showed that cross-suturing a nerve which had originally supplied a slow muscle so that it now supplied a fast one, caused that fast muscle to become slow – and conversely, when a nerve which formerly supplied a fast muscle was given control over a muscle which was formerly slow, the muscle became fast. Subsequent experiments by Vrbova and later by Salmons showed that the nerve operates, not by releasing trophic substances from its terminals on the muscle fibre membranes, as initially suspected, but by virtue of its **firing pattern**. Frequent firing, such as inevitably occurs in endurance training, slows muscle fibres and increases their aerobic capacity (making them redder). Conversely, muscle which is entirely unstimulated regresses to the extreme fast, white (IIb) form, which must therefore be considered basal. The effect of electrical stimulation has been reviewed by Salmons (1994).

Mechanical factors are another stimulus to muscle adaptation. Many forms of mechanical stress promote collagen formation. It is harder to assess whether the muscle fibres themselves in an intact human subject respond directly to mechanical influences, because increased load and stretch will both excite the stretch reflex and thereby increase motor nerve activity. Nevertheless, mechanical effects are reported even in muscle cultures devoid of innervation (Goldspink et al., 1991) so direct influences almost certainly do operate in vivo. The overall result of long repetition of high loads is that fibres increase their cross-sections until, in extreme cases (possibly only pathological ones), they may ultimately split into two i.e. 'hypertrophy' may be followed in the limit by 'hyperplasia'. One or both mechanisms underlie the muscular enlargement produced by prolonged strength training.

It is well worth noting, however, that the first 10–12 weeks of strength training elicit marked strength gains with little or no hypertrophy of the muscle. What is universally considered to be happening during this **neural phase** of strength gain is that the nervous system is 'learning' how to recruit all fibres maximally (Sale, 1988; Spurway *et al.*, 1998). The speculation has to be that, during this time, tendons, ligaments and other load-bearing structures are becoming stronger and so better able to cope with the forces produced when all motor units are fully active together in isometric or eccentric actions.

Repeated **stretch** (as in ballet training or a sustained stretch and flex programme) in turn causes muscle fibres to add sarcomeres, principally at their distal ends, and hence grow longer (Goldspink *et al.*, 1991).

How the mechanical influences operate to bring about training adaptations is not yet clear. Differences of firing frequency could produce different mean levels of ATP or Ca^{2+} in the cytoplasm, and so affect such processes as mitochondrial replication (Essig, 1996). By contrast, it is hard to see how physical forces could directly influence gene expression, for the language of the genes is chemistry. One probable contribution is that **growth factors** and other modifying chemicals are released from connective or other tissues within the loaded area, and these chemical signals elicit a muscle response. Several systemic **hormones** also circulate in increased concentration during and after exercise, and many of these also have trophic effects. Testosterone and growth hormone promote muscle growth, and these hormones are particularly elevated after resistance (strength) training. Growth hormone also enhances oxidative metabolism, as does thyroxine (perhaps more powerfully). Thyroxine in addition tends to increase contraction speeds. Prolonged regimes of endurance training somewhat raise thyroxine and growth hormone, but lower testosterone. By contrast with all the other hormones named, cortisol, the 'stress hormone', has **catabolic** (tissue-eroding) actions. Fortunately, it is never released alone due to exercise, but only in conjunction with **anabolic** (growth-inducing) agents: nevertheless, its concentration is raised by endurance training, which tends to reduce overall muscle bulk, yet its resting levels are lowered during strength training regimes, in which bulk increases. For more on hormones, see Kraemer (1992). For more on training regimes, see Chapters 4 and 11.

Fibre types in different athletes

On average, the main limb muscles of untrained people have roughly half their fibres slow and half fast, and many of these fast fibres are of the less-enduring, IIb type. However, the range of fast/slow ratios, either side of this mean, is very wide in the general population.

By contrast, if we look at top-class sprinters and top-class marathoners, we find marked differences between the two group of athletes and limited variation within each. The sprinters have more fast fibres – at least 60 per cent, and sometimes as many as 80 per cent. Generally field event athletes also have more fast than slow, though the ratio is less extreme (Figure 1.6). At the other end of the scale, top endurance performers hardly ever have fewer than 60 per cent slow fibres, and figures greater than 90 per cent have been reported. (As to the subtypes of fast fibre, in all vigorously active people IIa heavily predominates over IIb.) The advantages of the contrasting fast/slow percentages, for performance in the various events, are for the most part obvious. However, it may be surprising at first sight that weight lifters tend to have more fast than slow fibres, like field athletes. Part of the explanation is perhaps that the skills for lifting max-imal weights involve accelerating the load sharply, to carry it past unfa-vourable limb angles. Probably more importantly, however, type II fibres, when trained to the limit, reach greater diameters than type 1, and so can produce more force.

That account brings us to an interesting point, which many textbooks get wrong. They commonly say that type I fibres are of small diameter and type II (or at least IIb) are large. This is true in all small mammals and several large ones, but not in some other mammals at the larger end of the size-range, including ourselves. In untrained human muscles, fibres of all types are of similar diameters until late in life, when type II atrophy faster. In trained adults of employment age the fibres which regularly do the most work are largest. Thus an endurance athlete's type I fibres are likely to be of greater diameter than the majority or all of his/her type II fibres (cf. Figure 1.5), while in a performer trained for strength, as we saw in the last paragraph, type II will be the bigger.

The key question which is raised by the data of Figure 1.6, however, is that of 'nature versus nurture': how far did the great athlete inherit his/her muscle bulk or fibre-type proportions, and how far are they products of training? The broad spread of the type proportions in the untrained population suggests a strong influence of inheritance, with elite marath-oners being drawn from that fraction of the population who had more than 70 per cent slow fibres already ... and so on, for other groups. Research of the 1970s, on small samples of twins, pointed further in this direction; but the pendulum in the 1990s has swung rather the other way. Nevertheless, it is only when people have trained intensively for many years that their full genetic potential will be realized, and responsiveness to training is itself one of the properties in which the largest influence of genetic background can be demonstrated. Thus to expect a simple answer to the old conundrum is unrealistic. But if one thinks of nature and nur-ture as having broadly commensurate influences, one will probably not be

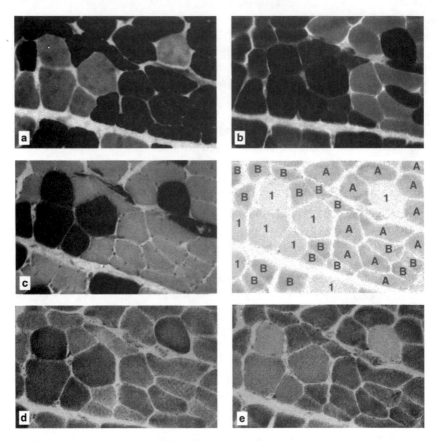

Figure 1.5. Histochemical preparation from an autopsy of human vastus later-alis after traumatic death. Serial cryostat sections reacted for: (a) myosin ATPase (the enzyme of contractile activity) after alkaline preincubation, show-ing type IIb fibres darkest and type I fibres lightest; (b) myosin ATPase after mild acid preincubation, showing type I fibres darkest and IIa lightest; (c) myosin ATPase after stronger acid preincubation, showing type I fibres still dark but type IIb as well as IIa now unreactive; (d) succinate dehydrogenase, indicating aerobic capacity, so that the fibres stained darkest in the section would have been likely to have the reddest pigmentation in the unstained specimen; (e) α-glycerophosphate dehydrogenase, indicating anaerobic capa-city. The centre right frame gives a key to fibre types: 1 = type I, A = type IIa, B = type IIb. Characteristically, the aerobic capacities of many IIa fibres overlap those of type I and, in turn, even some IIb fibres fall just within the IIa range. All type II fibres have substantial glycolytic capacity, and even the type I fibres are not devoid of it. Note that this man, who was in his 60s, is understood to have engaged in endurance activities at vigorous recreational intensity all his adult life; the fact that the type I fibres were largest and the IIbs smallest may reasonably be attributed to this. (Type-selective atrophy can also result from chronic knee pathology, but there was no report of such a condition in this instance.) (Preparation: I. Montgomery)

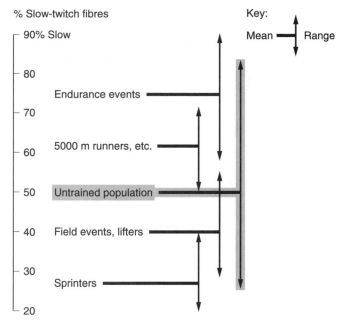

Figure 1.6. Relative percentages of slow fibres in different athletes. (Summary of data from many sources, including Gollnick, P.D. *et al.* (1972). *Journal of Applied Physiology*, **33**, 312–319 and Tesch, P. *et al.* (1984). *Journal of Applied Physiology*, **56**, 35–38)

seriously wrong. (For more on this subject compare Bouchard *et al.*, 1992 with Klissouras, 1997.)

The muscle spindle

Before going on, we should acknowledge that all discussion so far has been of the working or **extrafusal** muscle fibre. However, **muscle spindles** – groups of narrow, short, **intrafusal** muscle fibres, with afferent nerves leading from them (Figure 1.7) – are found in all muscles. They are so mounted on intramuscular connective tissue that they are passively subject to all the length changes of the muscle. However when the nerve endings in their centres are stretched they send signals to the ventral horn – a function which the extrafusal fibres have no means of achieving. These signals most directly subserve the **stretch reflex**, whereby the muscle pulls back against imposed extension. Further consideration, however, reveals that they can, in fact, be the basis of many of the control processes governing skeletal muscle action. This is because the ends of each intrafusal fibre receive motor innervation of their own, by nerve fibres rather narrower and thus slower than those to the extrafusal fibres;

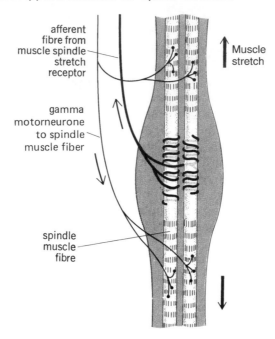

afferent
fibre from
muscle spindle
stretch
receptor

Muscle
stretch

gamma
motorneurone
to spindle
muscle fiber

spindle
muscle
fibre

Figure 1.7. The muscle spindle (highly simplified). (From Vander, A. *et al.* (1994). *Human Physiology*, 6th Edn. reproduced by permission of The McGraw-Hill Companies)

their cell bodies are classified as γ-**motoneurones**. Activation of these small-diameter, **fusimotor nerves** causes the contractile ends of the spindle fibres to shorten and stretch the centres of their fibres, just as if the whole muscle were being stretched. The potential versatility of this system is considerable, since in principle either the γ- or the α-motoneurones can be activated first. In cats, which have been extensively studied in this field of physiology, a variety of such motor patterns has been demonstrated. In humans, however, as far as the limitations of experimentation allow us to investigate, the two systems appear to be activated together (α-γ **coactivation**). This gives the contractile ends of the spindle fibres the relatively simple task of taking up the slack which extrafusal shortening would otherwise produce, thus ensuring that the stretch reflex continues to function with roughly similar sensitivity throughout the range of voluntary movement (Murphy and Martin, 1993).

This has been an exceedingly simplified account of muscle spindles, which in fact have three types of intrafusal fibre, two kinds of sensory ending with different classes of nerve fibre leading from them, and even two subclasses of motor innervation. For further detail, a good start would be Boyd and Smith (1984).

Muscle excitation

In maturity only one motor nerve makes contact with any one extrafusal muscle fibre, though before birth and in infancy two or more nerves may contribute to a single motor endplate until one of them gains ascendancy.

At all these contact points, or **neuromuscular junctions**, the transmitter substance **acetylcholine** (ACh) is released each time a nerve impulse or **action potential** (AP) invades the nerve terminal (Figure 1.8). This process involves entry of calcium ions (Ca^{2+}) from the extracellular space into the nerve terminal. After release, ACh depolarizes the subsynaptic membrane of the muscle fibre; the many folds into which this **motor endplate** is contorted have several functions, but one is to increase its area and hence its ability to carry the depolarizing current. Rapidly thereafter the ACh is hydrolysed by **acetylcholinesterase** molecules present at high concentration on the same membrane: hence not a single impulse but a train of impulses must be sent down the motor nerve if the muscle fibres are to give a sustained, **tetanic** contraction (Figure 1.9). Almost all normal movements involve fused or unfused tetani, even though the bursts concerned may be of only three to five impulses (as in the load-bearing phase of a sprinter's stride).

Endplate depolarization initiates a new AP in the adjacent regions of 'ordinary' muscle membrane exposed to the extracellular space rich in

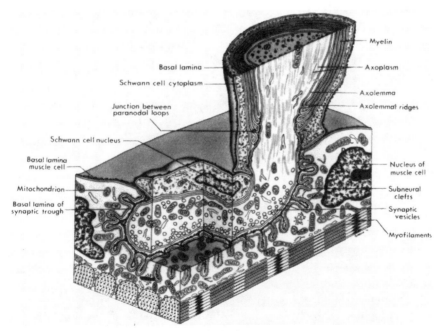

Figure 1.8. Diagram of neuromuscular junction. (Drawing by D.K. Morest from Fawcett, D.W. and Raviola, E. (1994). *Bloom and Fawcett: A Textbook of Histology*, 12th Edn. reproduced by permission of Arnold Publishers)

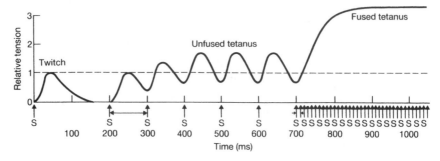

Figure 1.9. Isometric contractions produced by trains of stimuli, first at 10 Hz, then at 100 Hz, compared with a single, initial twitch. Not only does the smoothness of the contraction increase with stimulation frequency, the peak force achieved does too. The 'twitch/tetanus (peak force) ratio' is typically 3–4. (From Vander, A. *et al.* (1994). *Human Physiology*, 6th Edn. reproduced by permission of The McGraw-Hill Companies)

sodium ions (Na⁺). Despite the complex series of events involved, the **junctional delay**, between the nerve AP reaching the neuromuscular junction and the muscle AP starting to propagate away, is only 0.1–0.2 msec. The skeletal muscle AP is caused by Na⁺ inflow, followed by potassium ion (K⁺) outflow, almost exactly as in nerve: unlike the APs of cardiac and smooth muscles, it does not involve significant Ca²⁺ entry.

As the muscle AP now spreads across the fibre surface it encounters invaginations of the cell membrane which are the openings of a complex meshwork of additional membranes running transversely across the fibre – the T tubules or **T system** (Figure 1.10). Each time the muscle AP passes the mouth of one of these systems it will spread down towards the core of the fibre; the T system membranes are not identical to the surface membrane but they share the ability to propagate APs. Nevertheless the presence of these transverse membrane systems at frequent intervals along the surface has a retarding effect on progress of the AP along the fibre. Furthermore muscle fibres, unlike motor nerve fibres, are not myelinated. For these two reasons the lengthwise velocity of the muscle AP is about 4–5 m sec⁻¹ – say one-twentieth that of the preceding nerve AP.

Distributed extensively and regularly along the T system walls are closely adjoining membrane segments of the **sarcoplasmic reticulum** (SR). To be exact, these particular membranes bound the **lateral sacs** of the SR, within which Ca²⁺ ions are loosely adsorbed onto negatively charged granules of **calsequestrin**. Communication between T system and SR occurs at the interfaces between these two membrane systems, which are unmistakably structured in electron micrographs with bridging structures called 'junctional feet' at frequent and regular intervals. Different species of macromolecule, embedded within the T system and SR membranes, respectively, make up these junctional feet; they are named from pharmaceutical agents that selectively bind to, and interfere with the function of, the one macromolecule or the other (Figure 1.11). One of these agents is

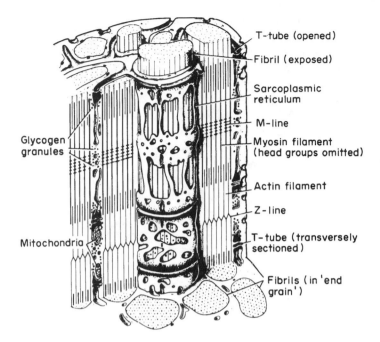

Figure 1.10. Exploded diagram of muscle fibre ultrastructure, showing T system and sarcoplasmic reticulum enveloping fibrils.(From Spurway, N.C. (1985). *Physics in Medicine and Biology Encyclopedia* (T.F. McAinsh, ed.). Pergamon)

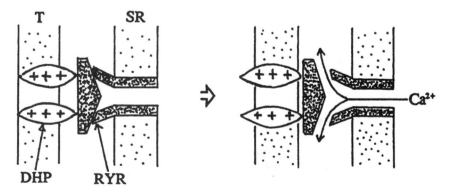

Figure 1.11. Interaction between voltage-sensitive DHP receptor in T system membrane and Ca^{2+}-carrying RyR receptor in SR membrane, as proposed by Rios *et al.* (1991). (Reprinted by permission from McComas (1996). *Skeletal Muscle, Form and Function*. Champaign, IL: Human Kinetics, 117)

dihydropyridine (DHP), the other ryanodine (RyR). The DHP **receptor** is in the T system membrane; it is positively charged, and is apparently moved transiently towards the lumen of the tubule during each AP. The resting membrane has about a 90 mV electrical gradient across it, with the cytoplasm negative relative to all parts of the extracellular space, including T tubule lumens; during an AP this polarization is reduced, and at the peak it is reversed. Thus the movement of the DHP receptor seems to be a simple electrostatic effect. The **RyR receptor** is in the SR membrane: it is a huge molecule, down the centre of which runs a Ca^{2+} channel that is, according to a tempting recent picture (Rios *et al.*, 1991), simply unplugged when the DHP receptor moves. Even if this is not the detailed mechanism, the RyR channel is evidently the route by which Ca^{2+} floods out into the cytoplasm. This chain of processes is repeated at every AP.

Calcium and the SR

In a fully relaxed skeletal muscle fibre, almost all the Ca^{2+} is in the SR, where its average concentration is in the mM (10^{-3} M) range; free in the cytoplasm of a completely resting fibre, the ion's concentration is probably less than 10^{-8} M. The flood of Ca^{2+} release following an AP raises this 1000-fold, to about 5×10^{-6} M (Gordon and Yates, 1992). After a single AP that level is maintained for only 20–30 msec before re-uptake begins to take effect. Tetanic stimulation, however, causes repeated waves of release, and maintains cytoplasmic Ca^{2+} near 10^{-5} M until the impulse volley ceases.

The effect of these relatively elevated Ca^{2+} levels – low though they still are by extracellular standards – is to promote tension generation, by mechanisms to be discussed in the following sections. The result of the concentration being lowered again is to reverse the processes, and lead to relaxation. Ca^{2+} ions are resorbed from the cytoplasm by ATP-fuelled ionic pumps in the longitudinal membranes of the SR, between the adjacent pairs of terminal cisterns. Once trapped again within the membrane-bounded space of the SR, Ca^{2+} ions probably diffuse randomly: the majority would then be quickly resorbed by the calsequestrin in the terminal cisterns, ready for the next release. Figure 1.12 summarizes the control and action of Ca^{2+} within the muscle fibre.

The contractile mechanism

The basic structure of the protein system, revealed by electron microscopy (EM) and reflected in the light-microscope (LM) striations, is summarized in Figures 1.2 and 1.13.

Note that the **thick, myosin-containing** filaments occupy the whole 1.6 mm width of the dark LM bands. The **thin, actin-containing** filaments fill the main volume of the light bands but also extend into the dark ones. Arguably the most important observation ever made with the EM (H.E.

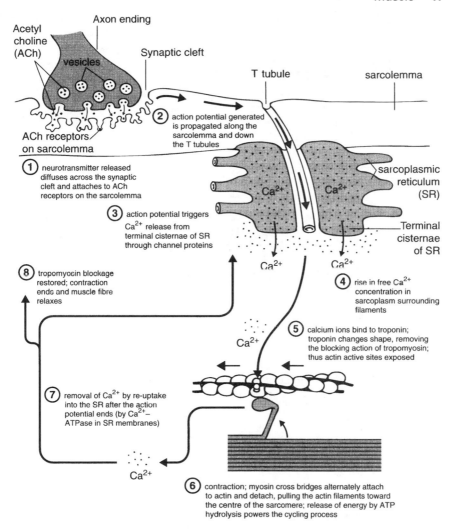

Figure 1.12. Overall sequence of events in excitation–contraction coupling (1–6) and subsequent relaxation (7–8). (From Maughan, R. *et al.* (1997). *Biochemistry of Exercise and Training.* Oxford by permission of Oxford University Press)

Huxley and Hanson, mid-1950s; see Huxley, 1969), crucially supported by LM of living muscle in the laboratory of A.F. Huxley, was that, when muscle changes length, this thin/thick overlap alters (Figure 1.13a). Whether the movements are active or passive the thick and thin filaments both stay virtually the same length, but they slide between each other as the muscle shortens and apart again as it lengthens – the **sliding filament** mechanism. Before that observation, theories of contraction assumed that the individual filaments within each muscle fibre changed length, in concertina fashion, echoing the length changes of the whole fibre.

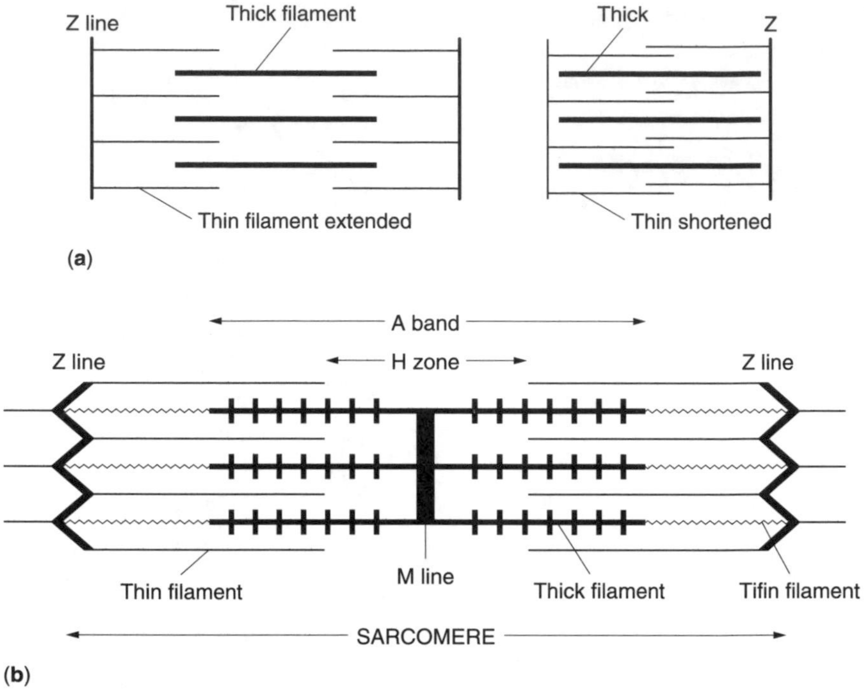

(a)

(b)

Figure 1.13. Proteins of the contractile system. (a) Key proteins of the sarcomere (left) in extended and (right) in shortened muscles. (b) More detailed diagram of an extended sarcomere, showing the elastic protein titin. XBs are shown in the relaxed position

All muscle lengthening is passive, the muscle being pulled by forces acting from outside it: muscles cannot push! Most shortening, however (except in such circumstances as the physiotherapist's couch), is due to active force generation within the muscle substance. Therefore, once the sliding filament mechanism was established, the next question was how force is generated between overlapping but separate filaments. Higher resolution EM work showed regularly spaced side-knobs on the thick filaments of relaxed muscles, and arrays of **cross-bridges** (XBs) between thick and thin filaments, unmistakably formed by these side-knobs, when the muscles had been fixed in a contracted condition. X-ray diffraction studies, first on relaxed and rigor muscle, then also on living muscle generating force, built up the picture that the XBs swung out from myosin to actin when the muscle was activated, moved longitudinally while attached to the actin, then swung back to repeat the cycle.

In parallel with this structural approach, biochemical methods showed that complete myosin molecules were rather like elongated tadpoles, 160 nm (one-tenth of an A-band) in length (Figure 1.2, bottom left). The long tails had mutual affinity and readily associated side-by-side into filaments. The other ends, the broader **head groups**, possessed powerful affinity not for one another but for actin. They also had the ability to hydrolyse ATP, releasing its energy – indeed, their only greater affinity than that for actin was for ATP. So ATP could detach myosin head groups from actin in isolated biochemical systems and restore plasticity to intact filaments which had previously been in a rigor state.

These data were synthesized in the picture of the **cross-bridge cycle** (H.E. Huxley, 1969; Taylor, 1979), most aspects of which remain the prevalent pattern of thinking to this day (Figure 1.14). An analogy with rowing may be helpful: the myosin filament is a boat with many oars (head groups) which can row it through the actin sea. Fundamental to this picture is the concept that each head group works as an 'independent force generator' (A.F. Huxley, 1974), contributing its own molecular effort (in the piconewton range) to the overall muscle output. The forces and movements of individual myosin molecules attached to single actin filaments have actually now been measured (Finer, Simmons and Spudich,

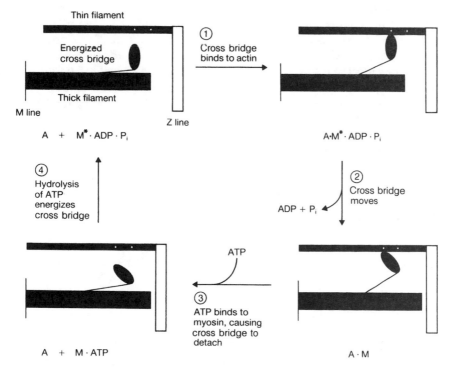

Figure 1.14. Classical representation of mechanical and chemical changes during the cross-bridge (XB) cycle. A, M, M*, P_i = actin, stable myosin, energized myosin and phosphate ion, respectively. Biochemical information deduced from rapid kinetic studies of isolated actin molecules and myosin headgroups (S1 subunits), reacting with ATP in solution. (From Vander, A. *et al.* (1994) *Human Physiology*, 6th Edn. reproduced by permission of The McGraw-Hill Companies)

1994). Between these dates, it had become generally accepted that the attachment of myosin to actin takes place in two stages: an initial, weak attachment, which holds the head group against the actin but cannot sustain any longitudinal force, and a subsequent, strong attachment which can (Geeves, 1991).

Exactly where in the myosin molecule the movement takes place has, however, long been uncertain. Recent work by Rayment and colleagues suggests that it is the head group itself which changes shape after attaching firmly to actin (Figure 1.15); the filamentous parts of each myosin molecule then have to function merely as flexible but minimally extensible strings (Rayment *et al.*, 1993). If this is correct, the oars not the arms are actually what bend in the middle!

Finally, note the account of ATP's involvement given in Figure 1.14 (and not altered in principle by Figure 1.15). After detaching the myosin head group from actin the ATP is pictured as hydrolysing (breaking the bond to its terminal phosphate group) when alone on the myosin head, and thereby energizing the recovery of the shape from which a new pull stroke can begin – the oarsman coming forward on his seat. Only after strong reattachment, however (dipping the oar in the water again), are the products of hydrolysis released into the aqueous medium. These products are an inorganic phosphate ion (P_i), an H^+ ion and an adenosine diphosphate molecule (ADP), and they are released in that order. The largest single energy pulse in the cycle is that provided by solvation of P_i – the settling of water molecules into ordered conformation around the phosphate ion when it is newly released from its macromolecular environment. It is this step which promotes strong attachment and then provides the main power for the pull stroke, whether this takes the form depicted in Figure 1.14 or that of Figure 1.15.

Control proteins

The account just given indicates no means of stopping force generation except withdrawal of ATP, which would leave the system not relaxed but locked in rigor. At the same time it fails to explain the role of Ca^{2+}. The system omitted till now is one which prevents the access of myosin head groups to their binding sites on the actin molecules – the **control proteins** – which lie alongside twin helices of actin to complete the make-up of the thin filament. These control proteins are **troponin** and **tropomyosin** (Figure 1.16a).

Troponin is a molecule with three subunits: the I (inhibitory) subunit binds to actin, the T subunit binds to tropomyosin, and the C subunit, which is in the middle, has a high affinity for Ca^{2+} ions. When Ca^{2+} concentration exceeds about 10^{-6} M the shape of the complex changes (Figure 1.16b). The usual textbook picture of what follows is that the tropomyosin rod (which is long, so that it covers seven repeating actin

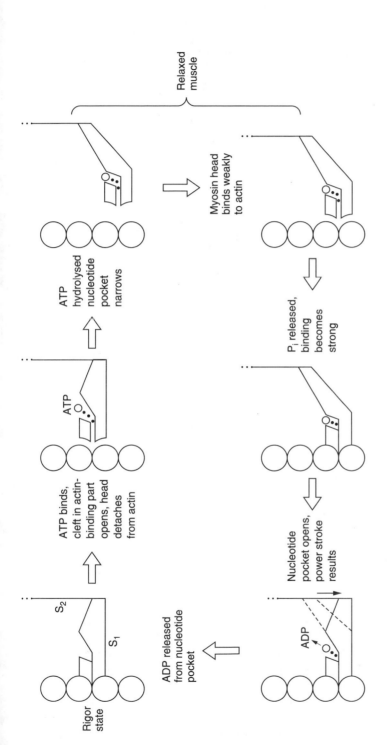

Figure 1.15. Modern concept of 'conformation' (shape) changes in myosin head group during XB cycle. Nucleotide molecules symbolized by a small open circle = adenosine; black dots = phosphate groups (3 in ATP, 2 in ADP). (Loosely derived from Rayment *et al.* (1993). *Science,* **261**, 58–65 and Reedy (1993). *Structure,* **1**, 1–15 reproduced by permission of American Association for the Advancement of Science)

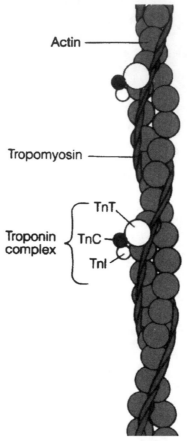

Figure 1.16a. Control proteins of thin filament. (a) Portion of filament in long-itudinal view. (Reprinted with permission from Dow, J., Lindsay, G. and Morrison, J. 1996, *Biochemistry*, Addison-Wesley)

units) is moved out of the way, allowing myosin head groups access to the actin sites. Only when head groups are bound to actin can force be generated. When Ca^{2+} concentration is lowered again by the SR, tropomyosin moves back into its blocking position as soon as the ongoing XB cycle is complete. No further force generation can now occur: the actin sea has frozen over, and the oars can no longer grip.

Without destroying the essentials, we can refine this account. Firstly, it is only the strong binding of myosin to actin which is controlled; the initial, weak binding can take place whether or not Ca^{2+} concentration is raised. When Ca^{2+} is released into the cytoplasm, and binds to troponin, strong myosin attachments can occur: and of course only strongly bound head groups can perform a pull stroke. Secondly, Ca^{2+} binding to troponin not only changes the shape of that molecule but reduces its affinity for actin. Recall that the subunit of troponin which actually binds to actin is troponin I, the 'inhibitory subunit', so called because it on its own reduces

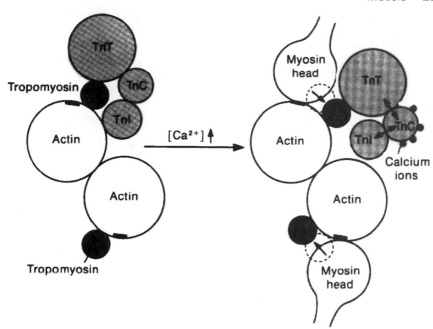

Figure 1.16b. 'Classical' interpretation of interactions of Ca²⁺ and myosin head group (S1 subunit) with actin, seen in transverse section through thin filament at troponin-binding site. Troponin has three subunits: TnT binds tropomyosin, TnC binds Ca²⁺ and changes conformation in doing so, and TnI attaches the whole complex to actin imparting its inhibitory action on that protein's interaction with myosin. *Animal Physiology* by Eckert and Randal © 1997, 1988, 1983, 1978 by W. H. Freeman and Company. Used with permission.

the affinity of myosin for the actin. It is partly a weakened association between this subunit and actin, resulting from the adsorption of Ca²⁺ to troponin C, which makes strong myosin binding possible; the effect is **reinforced**, rather than solely caused, by the tropomyosin movement of Figure 1.16b (Gordon and Yates, 1992).

Length–tension characteristics

If force is produced by XBs, each acting as an independent force generator, its magnitude must be proportional to the number of XBs pulling. It follows that, when a fully activated fibre is stretched, so that fewer myosin head groups can engage with actin partners to form XBs, less force can be produced. Over a substantial range of lengths, static (**isometric**) force should thus be proportional to overlap. This was found to be true, in a crucial experiment by Gordon *et al.* (1966) (region AB in Figure 1.17). The

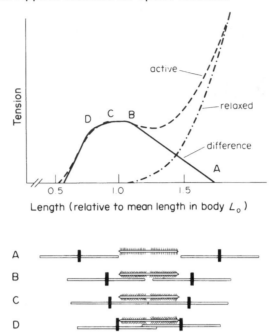

Figure 1.17. Length–tension relationships for active myofibrils (solid line) and whole muscle (broken lines). For both muscle and fibre, subtraction of the relaxed specimen's force at a given length from that of the active preparation gives the force contributed by XB activity in the fibrils. (From Spurway, N.C (1985). *Physics in Medicine and Biology Encyclopedia* (T.F. McAinsh, ed.). Pergamon)

plateau portion of this plot arises because of the 'bare zone', in the middle of each myosin filament; this exists because the orientation of individual myosin molecules has to reverse at this location, so that the actin filaments from opposite ends of the A-band are both pulled in towards the centre of the band. Parts of actin filaments which lie in this bare zone can make no contribution, positive or negative, to the force. At shorter lengths than this, the ends of actin filaments begin to interact with head groups oriented the wrong way. They probably do not get pushed back instead of pulled – and if they did, the actin filament is almost certainly not rigid enough to convey the force down its length. However, merely by blocking the access of head groups to the actin filaments upon which they could pull positively, these overshooting filaments reduce the total shortening force. Finally, at even shorter **sarcomere** lengths, the tapered ends of the myosin filaments begin to impale themselves against the transverse **Z lines**, and the force falls rapidly towards zero.

What we have just described is the **length–tension characteristic** of the force-generating system itself. In a whole fibre, however, and even more so a whole muscle, there are other elements resisting extension beyond about the plateau length just discussed – which is, for most muscles, approximately the middle of the length range in the body (symbolized by L_0). Intracellular **titin** filaments (Figure 1.13b) run through much of the length of each half of a myosin filament, extend from the ends to the adjacent Z lines, and evidently have elastic functions (Trinick, 1991). The existence of these filaments was first suggested a generation ago but has only recently received general acceptance because they are not easily identified electron microscopically; in biochemical terms this is intriguing, because titin constitutes 10 per cent of fibre protein, with only myosin and actin, at a little over 40 per cent and 20 per cent, respectively, contributing more to the cell mass. In parallel with the titin, extra-cellular fibres, principally of collagen, resist extension increasingly steeply as a muscle is drawn out beyond its biological length-range. Thus even relaxed muscle has a length–tension relationship (Figure 1.17). When stimulation occurs, the force actively generated by the XBs adds to that of the titin and collagen, to give the relationship for whole active muscle. The implications of this whole-muscle relationship for anatomical movement are exemplified by the fact that it is much easier to pull oneself about three-quarters of the way up to a bar than actually to chin it. In pulling up to the bar, one's biceps are moving from a little right of B (Figure 1.17) to a little left of C; chinning the bar requires the muscles to shorten through and perhaps even to the left of D. For fuller discussion, see Chapter 5.

Concentric force–velocity relationships

The previous section referred to fully activated muscles generating force at a series of different, set lengths. Equally important characteristics can be defined in terms of the velocity at which the fully activated muscles move under a series of different loads; in the light of the above discussion it is clearly best to take the velocity as the muscles pass through the length–tension relation's plateau. We will first consider muscles carrying loads they can actively move, so that they are therefore performing shortening (**concentric**) contractions.

As matters of everyday observation, muscles can shorten fastest under the lightest load, while above a certain maximum load they cannot shorten at all. When quantitative experiments of this kind were done on isolated muscles, Hill (1938) pointed out that the resulting **force–velocity relationship** closely approximated a segment of a hyperbola drawn on axes, respectively, to the left of and below the real ones (Figure 1.18a). Isometric force per unit cross-section (F_0) is probably higher in fast than slow muscles but the majority of evidence is that the difference is not great. By contrast, velocity under zero load (V_0) would be three to four times greater in an entirely fast muscle than in an entirely slow one (cf. 'Types of motor unit' above). In fact no human muscle consists only of fast

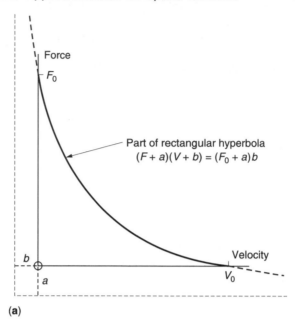

(a)

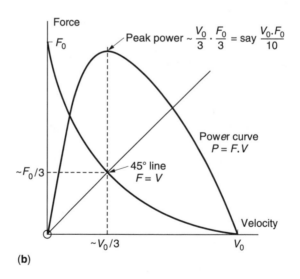

(b)

Figure 1.18. Force–velocity (F–V) curves and their consequences. Curves (a)–(c) studied in fully activated, isolated muscles. (a) F–V curve for concentric contraction, as described by A.V. Hill. (b) Power curve deduced from Hill F–V curve: with scales so chosen that F_0 and V_0 are equidistant from the origin, peak power is achieved at the point on the characteristc curve where a 45° construction line intersects it. (c) F–V curve including region of eccentric activity. (d) Torque–angular velocity curve for human knee extensors in both concentric and eccentric actions, obtained by isokinetic dynamometry

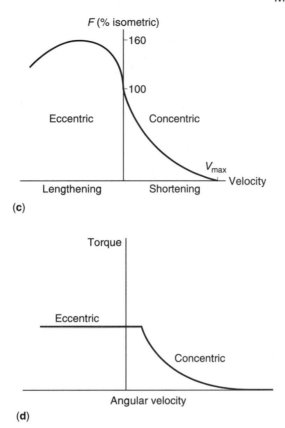

(c)

(d)

Figure 1.18. (Continued)

or only of slow fibres, but the fastest of our muscles may well be two to
two and a half times faster than the slow, 'postural' ones.

Precision experiments on single fibres indicate that the hyperbolic relation is not exact – there are deviations from the Hill curve at both ends
(Julian *et al.*, 1986; Edman *et al.*, 1997) – yet it is sufficient for almost all
sports-related purposes. In particular it enables us readily to calculate the
power (*P*) produced by a muscle at any given speed, because power, the
rate of doing work, is given simply by the product of force × velocity. For
every point on a defined force–velocity (*F–V*) curve, the power can thus be
simply calculated and a power–velocity curve deduced (Figure 1.18b). For
a typical human muscle of average fibre composition (the summed effect
of which is expressed in the values of *a* and *b* for that muscle) it emerges
that maximum power is produced at $V \cong V_0/3$, $F \cong F_0/3$, and its value is
very roughly $P = F_0V_0/10$. However, if instead of a typical mixed muscle
we consider the extreme fibre types, we find that peak *P* from a slow fibre
not only occurs at about one-quarter the speed but is typically only one-
fifth to one-eighth that of a fast one of the same cross-section (Bottinelli *et*

al., 1996). The power difference is greater than that of V_0 values, principally because the slow-muscle $F–V$ curve is also more concave than the fast one. So, even though no human muscles comprise one fibre type only, nevertheless the elite endurance athlete, with 80 per cent slow fibres, can produce only a fraction of the single-movement power available to the elite sprinter. Before leaving these curves, however, let us also note that power can be increased by raising either factor – velocity or force. It is because training can make much more difference to the latter that sprinters work so hard on strength.

Finally, we must discuss a deviation from the hyperbolic relationship which is more important for whole human work than the imprecisions shown by the best experiments on single fibres. It is that the low-speed force production of muscles under voluntary activation by the nervous system falls markedly short of the organ-bath hyperbola. Strictly speaking, one cannot measure the linear shortening velocity or the direct force of a muscle in an intact subject – that would require surgical intervention at the tendon. Instead, using an **isokinetic dynamometer**, one measures the angular (not linear) velocity of the distal limb moved by a more proximal muscle and, with most machines, the torque (not linear force) produced at different angular velocities. However, the chief mismatch between organ bath and voluntary activation has little to do with these measurement differences – it is a marked flattening of the curve at the low-speed end, such that isometric torque and force are little if at all greater than torque and force at $30–60° \, s^{-1}$ (Figure 1.18d). At the end of the next section we shall be better placed to consider what the main cause of the low-speed flattening is.

Eccentric force–velocity relationships

If the load imposed on an activated muscle is greater than the maximum it can hold stationary, i.e. greater than the **maximum isometric force** it can produce, the muscle will lengthen. As we noted early in the chapter, this lengthening under load is termed **eccentric action**.

A fully activated muscle in an organ bath typically produces 40–60 per cent greater force than the isometric level when lengthening at a velocity numerically not exceeding half of the maximum velocity at which it can shorten, V_0 (Figure 1.18c). At even higher velocities of lengthening, most experimenters have found the force to be less than this peak, but still very high over a wide range. A most important point is that ATP consumption during production of peak eccentric force is exceptionally low. In fact, it is not detectably higher than the amount which would be needed merely to fuel the surface and SR membrane pumps, suggesting that the XBs are using no ATP at all in this very high force production (Curtin and Davies, 1975). How this can come about will be discussed below. Meanwhile, we can illustrate this same phenomenon in intact humans by a vivid experiment, reported almost two generations ago. Two cycle ergometers were coupled back to back, so that subjects on them were competing as to which could pedal forward. A light, untrained female was asked to oppose a large, male athlete. Her legs were cycled backwards by his but, when he became exhausted, she was undistressed (Abbott *et al.*, 1952).

However, if we focus on force itself rather than metabolic economy, voluntarily activated human muscles, when studied in a laboratory set-up such as an isokinetic dynamometer, often show eccentric forces much less elevated over the isometric ones than those seen in isolated muscles; indeed, in quadriceps, isometric and eccentric forces are usually found to be similar, and the latter to be velocity-independent (Figure 1.18d). However, transcutaneous electrical stimulation, particularly if used as a supplement to voluntary effort, goes a considerable way to reinstating the organ bath kind of curve (Westing *et al.*, 1990).

Since direct electrical stimulation elicits more force, it must be that voluntary activation, maximal though it seems in the consciousness of the subject, fails to recruit all motor units fully in eccentric and very low-speed concentric muscle actions. At higher concentric speeds, when less force is involved, there is little or no evidence of such a shortfall in recruitment. The explanation proposed is that, to protect tendons and other vulnerable structures from damage, neural inhibitory mechanisms normally prevent recruitment of the strongest units in the very high force situations. The fact that the knee is a particularly complex and vulnerable joint tallies nicely with the effect being so marked in quadriceps. It is also compatible with the fact that the early phase of strength training, which is considered to consist largely of the overcoming of inhibition, also increases quadriceps eccentric force markedly more than the concentric or isometric force of the same muscle (Spurway *et al.*, 1998).

Finally, however, we must consider the relation between experiments in laboratories and life in the rest of the world. It seems possible that apprehensive anticipation, and perhaps other aspects of the laboratory situation, heighten the inhibitory effects in isokinetic experiments. Watching a number of high-speed sports, such as downhill skiing and hill running, it is hard to credit that eccentric forces closer to the organ bath pattern are not being generated there. One suspects that the last on this subject has not yet been heard.

Cross-bridge mechanisms in moving muscles

The general shapes of the force–velocity curves obtained in organ baths can be satisfactorily accounted for in XB terms (A.F. Huxley, 1974). Firstly, during slow movements, all head groups have time to form XBs with the nearest reactive sites on actin filaments; at high speeds, an increasing number will miss. This contributes to the fall-off of force in both concentric and eccentric high-speed contractions (the left and right ends of the plot in Figure 1.18c). Secondly, in concentric activity, as the energy of each pull stroke is given over increasingly to kinetic energy in the filaments, less is left to reveal itself as force. In eccentric actions, however, XBs which attach are bent backwards and it would be an odd machine which did not resist this with even greater force than when it was holding static.

Equally important for sport science is the question of ATP turnover and therefore of energy demand. One ATP molecule is used for every complete XB cycle (Figure 1.14). As concentric actions increase in speed, at first more cycles occur; then the effect of the 'misses' begins to predominate. Sure enough, ATP consumption, though always higher in shortening muscle than when the same muscle is producing isometric tension, goes through a maximum at something like 60 per cent of V_0, and then declines again. By contrast, XBs forced the other way never reach the point in their cycles where ADP would dissociate from the head group and allow another ATP to attach (Figure 1.19). In the extreme, therefore, the impression noted earlier is almost certainly correct: ATP is used only on the membrane pumps of the muscle, not the XBs, so that very high force is produced with very little ATP breakdown (Curtin and Davies, 1975).

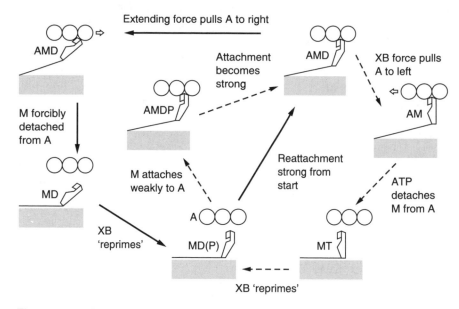

Figure 1.19. Possible mechanism for production of extreme force yet consumption of minimal ATP in eccentric contraction (left-hand cycle, solid arrows) compared with ATP-consuming concentric contraction (right-hand cycle, broken arrows). M = myosin, A = actin, T = ATP, D = ADP, P = P_i. The P is shown bracketed bottom centre because, in this hypothesis, it is present only in the concentric cycle. In its absence, reattachment in the eccentric cycle skips the weak phase. As D remains bound throughout, no new T is required however many cycles are repeated

Thus eccentric action is remarkably economical. Compare walking up and down the same hill. At a steady rate on a smooth surface, neither action involves significant acceleration or deceleration of the body mass, so effort is principally needed to hold that mass against the downward force of gravity – the same load, whether ascending or descending. But descent needs far fewer motor units because those which are active can produce so much more force in the eccentric than the concentric mode. Fewer units, each using less ATP, imply great economy. That is why, even on legs (which, one must realize, work quite unlike wheels), going downhill is so very much easier than going up at the same speed.

Although it is only during downhill movement that eccentric action dominates the stride, the runner on flat ground makes some use of it. As the foot strikes the ground, muscles are stretched and thus required to act eccentrically. Later they bounce back, and concentric work is done, for which starting from the stretched position can be shown to be an advantage. The overall effect of such a **stretch–shortening cycle** (Komi, 1988) is energy conservation. (A chapter on muscle should not, however, be blinkered: the extra energy return from tendon elasticity is also significant in such actions. See Alexander, 1988.)

Two matters arise from this account of eccentric exercise – the damage caused by high forces, and the metabolic supply of ATP. These are tackled in the following sections.

Muscle damage

Of the three modes of muscle action, eccentric causes most damage, because the forces on units which are active are greatest.

The commonest indication of this, and the least serious, is **delayed onset muscle soreness** (DOMS). Consider again the hill walkers of the last section. If one party climbed the hill, and was collected from the top by helicopter, while the other group was flown in and walked down, those who ascended would be more tired that night – but, paradoxically, those who descended would be more sore 2 days after. (This experiment has been done.) The explanation generally accepted is that micro-tears, caused by the large forces imposed on the active motor units, rupture the surface membranes of some of the fibres which have been active. Such damage is particularly common near the distal myotendinous junction. An alternative suggestion is that sarcomeres which have stretched further than others are to the right of the peak of the length–tension curve (Figure 1.17) and thus yield further and further till they disengage their actin from their myosin filaments; when the tension is released, re-engagement is sometimes imperfect, and disruption occurs (Jones *et al.*, 1997). Either origin – sarcolemmal tears or sarcomere disruption – results in intracellular damage and release of chemotactic signals into the extracellular space. These elicit invasions by successive waves of white blood cells, together with oedema – a classical inflammatory response (Smith, 1991). Swelling and discomfort are worst 2–3 days later. A secondary effect of the white cell actions is further breakdown of muscle fibre membranes and release of cytoplasmic proteins into the general circulation. Among these proteins are enzymes such as lactate dehydrogenase and creatine kinase, which can readily be detected in the plasma. Typically, the concentration of these enzymes is found to peak some 5 days after the eccentric exercise responsible. Readers will recognize the possibility of confusion with the almost identical signs of myocardial breakdown after infarction.

When damage is overt from the outset, we are faced with a lesser or greater degree of muscle tear. Detailed discussion of these injuries must be found elsewhere (e.g. Renstrom, 1988; Salmons, 1997) but some comments on the biology of the tissue response are appropriate. Two points are key:

● That repair is a balance between connective tissue invasion and muscle regeneration, the purpose of most physiotherapy being to tilt the balance more in favour of the muscle fibres.
● That all such regeneration is achieved by nuclei which had not been part of the torn fibres themselves. The latter are the nuclei of **satellite cells** (Figure 1.20). These are really quiescent myoblasts with minimal cytoplasm, yet they lie beneath the sarcolemma of each adult muscle fibre, and can be distinguished from fibre nuclei only by the EM. Doubtless the fact that satellite cells are mononucleate underlies their ability to replicate in response to an injury, while the multiple nuclei of the fibre cannot do so – probably because mitotic spindles do not form.

Regrowth of muscle following a severe tear follows what was in fact the original growth history of the tissue: mononucleate **myoblasts** invade the damaged area, fuse endways into **myotubes** (still with central nuclei), and gradually mature into fibres with peripheral nuclei, deep to which is the contractile cytoplasm. If reinnervation is required, the history of the initial innervation may also be repeated, with a period of multiple innervation preceding the dominance of one nerve branch and elimination of competitors. However, success in this contest usually goes to the nerve with its main branch closest to hand, so the original mosaic distribution of motor units is lost and fibres in the once-damaged area tend to clump into the separate domains of different nerves.

Perhaps the ultimate illustration of the power of satellite cells is that, if a muscle is ablated from an experimental animal, minced (but coarsely, so that many of the mononucleate cells remain undamaged) and injected back whence it came, something close to the original muscle in bulk and properties will ultimately regrow – provided only that the original nerve can also rebuild its access.

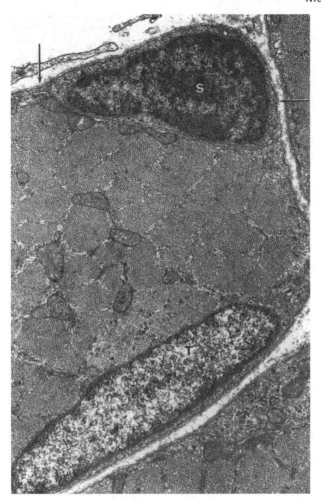

Figure 1.20. Electron micrograph of muscle fibres in transverse section, with parts of two satellite cells. A true muscle fibre nucleus (T) is surrounded by muscle cytoplasm. However, two narrowly-separated membranes (the plasma membranes of the muscle fibre and the satellite cell) separate this cytoplasm from the narrow ring of different cytoplasm surrounding a satellite cell nucleus (S). A slightly greater quantity of cytoplasm (SC), part of another satellite cell, is seen right. The muscle nucleus, T, is in its characteristic quiescent state, whereas the satellite nucleus, S, has clumped chromatin – a characteristic but not universal feature from Moss, F.P. and Leblond, C.P. (1961). *Anatomical Record*, **170**, 421–435 reprinted by permission of Wiley-Liss, Inc. a subsidiary of John Wiley & Sons, Inc.)

Muscle metabolism: basics

Muscles are 'chemical machines' – they perform mechanical work only on the basis of chemical energy supply. The immediate currency, both for the ionic pumps underlying the excitation mechanisms (SR Ca^{2+} uptake, plasmalemma Na^+/K^+ exchange) and the XB cycle generating force is, of course, ATP. Metabolism is required to regenerate the ATP.

The efficiency of the whole system is about 25 per cent in cycling and less than 20 per cent in walking, running or arm cranking. The 75 per cent or more of the total energy input which does not appear as mechanical energy output is degraded into heat – which is helpful in cold weather but a challenge to our mechanisms of thermoregulation when it is warm. Inefficiency, however, does not arise significantly in the XBs, which (at the optimum speed of shortening) convert the energy released by ATP hydrolysis almost totally into work. Part of our cellular inefficiency lies in the ionic pumps, which use ATP to power the muscular control system instead of the production of mechanical work. At the other extreme of the scale are the inefficiencies of our biomechanics and in particular those due to repeated acceleration and decelerations of limbs and those due to the maintenance of posture (which in itself involves no external work, yet is the essential basis against which the working muscles must produce their force). It is chiefly because the whole body beneath the shoulders must be braced for arm cranking that this exercise is less efficient than leg cycling. Another gross loss is the heating of the ground by every impact of a foot: this is the main reason why running is less efficient than cycling.

However, up to 50 per cent of our total inefficiency arises not from any of the above causes but during the biochemical processes of ATP regeneration, to which we must now turn. (More detail about many aspects of these processes will be found later in Chapter 3.) The regeneration route is termed **aerobic** when it is in balance with O_2 intake and **anaerobic** when it is not. But each of these categories has two subdivisions. Which of the four systems predominates at a given moment is determined partly by the intensity of the work and partly by how long it has gone on.

Anaerobic pathways

For the first few seconds of any new effort or a marked increase of effort, muscles draw on their internal supplies of high-energy phosphates: ATP and the **creatine phosphate** (CP) store. If the effort is maximal, this store will be depleted with a half-time of 3–5 s, but the ATP and CP entirely suffice for any single throw or jump, for overhead smashes, diving saves and kicks for touch. When first recognized, this was termed the 'alactic' phase of energy supply (Margaria *et al.*, 1964).

However, a track race, even of 100 let alone 400 m, cannot be fuelled principally this way. Still less can the 'sprints' in other sports, like cycling and swimming, where times are of the same order as those of 400 m on the track. Within 5 sec of the start the athlete is having to make new high-energy phosphate as fast as it is used. The first pathway to become available for this (and the one able to supply energy at the highest rate in the type 2 muscle fibres which dominate in such events) is that of **anaerobic**

glycolysis. This is the route which begins with dissociation of individual hexose phosphate units from glycogen stores within the fibre (glycogen-olysis), splits each of them into two 3-carbon units with regeneration of three molecules of ATP, and ends in the reduction of pyruvate to lactic acid. However, work cannot be continued for more than 30–60 s at the kind of rate we are discussing, before being inhibited by the accumulation of its own products. Lactic acid in particular builds up, probably contributing substantially to the inhibition (see sections on Muscle fatigue below) and appearing more slowly in the circulation; peak blood concentration is reached 3–6 min after an event of this kind has stopped.

Before moving on, it is appropriate to note that recovery from strenuous anaerobic exercise is less well understood than used to be thought. Stores of ATP and CP are replenished with time constants of $\sim$ 2–6 min. Most of the excess lactate is removed only a little slower, though the last few per cent may take the following hour or so. The O_2 necessary for these two processes (termed the 'oxygen debt' by Hill *et al.*, 1924) has turned out, however, to be considerably less than the total of the **excess post-exercise O_2 consumption** (EPOC) actually observed. The extra elevation of metabolism during recovery is largely attributable to hormonal effects and raised body temperature, but additional mechanisms cannot be excluded.

Aerobic pathways

Returning to the exercise period itself, suppose the runner did not set off at 400 m pace, but at that of the marathon. Then the initial lactate would accumulate much more slowly, and long before contraction became inhibited another metabolic pathway would take over the main burden of ATP resynthesis. This is the aerobic pathway, operating in mitochondria. Pyruvate molecules and hydrogen atoms, instead of producing further lactic acid, are taken up by these organelles. There they are oxidized via the tricarboxylic acid (TCA) cycle and the electron transport chain, producing a total of 36 ATP molecules per original hexose unit ('oxidative phosphorylation').

If exercise continues long enough to make substantial inroads into the glycogen stores, fatty acids can increasingly fuel this same mechanism, especially in the trained endurance performer, thus 'sparing' glycogen. The overall process is termed **aerobic glycolysis** or **aerobic lipolysis** according to the substrate. Figure 1.21 represents the balances between the four systems we have described, as they change with time at a steady work-rate. Note, however, that the maximum rates at which they can supply energy vary in the same sequence. In round figures, taking aerobic lipolysis as our unit, aerobic glycolysis can operate at least twice as fast in an average individual, anaerobic glycolysis five times and CP breakdown ten times as fast (cf. Chapter 3, Table 3.1). Exact figures, however, will

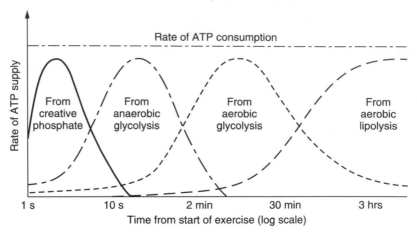

Figure 1.21. Sketch-diagram of phases of metabolism in an endurance-trained subject performing steadily at about 70 per cent of $\dot{V}O_2$ max. Note logarithmic time-scale

vary with fibre type distributions, states of training, nutrition and the type of exercise used in the comparison.

A further point can be made by reference to Figure 1.21: it suggests why exercise undertaken for weight reduction is likely to be actually more effective (quite apart from being cardiovascularly safer) if it is long and slow.

By contrast, in competitive sport, it is only in a relatively small number of race events that a performer even approximates to an even pace, such as considered in this figure. A 'multiple sprint sport', such as soccer or hockey, requires bursts of intense anaerobic activity, some of them in the first instance largely alactic, alternating with aerobic repositioning runs and jogging or walking recovery periods. Tactical imperatives are, however, bringing an incidental benefit here: even after a track race, **active recovery** (typically by jogging) is recommended, as it accelerates the clearance of lactate from the blood. Jogging back to position can achieve this *en passant*.

Adjustments between the systems

Type IIb fibres have so few mitochondria that their metabolism during exercise is almost entirely anaerobic. When they are recruited, it is unavoidable that the activity will have a large anaerobic component for as long as the work rate can be maintained. However, type IIa fibres and, in humans though not many animals, type I also, have significant anaerobic capacity alongside their generous supply of mitochondria. This anaerobic capacity probably contributes substantially to ATP supply during the first 2–3 min of any exercise, even one that is being performed at a rate which will settle down to be maintained aerobically later (see Chapter 3). The mechanisms which effect these adjustments are partly cardiovascular, partly intracellular. It appears that the latter are normally rate-limiting. They are outlined in the next two paragraphs.

Ca^{2+} ions, released by the activation mechanism, activate phosphorylase to initiate glycogenolysis and feed glucose-6-phosphate into the glycolytic chain. If adrenaline is flowing in anticipation of the event, it will act synergistically at this step. The next rate-limiting enzyme, phosphofructokinase, is stimulated by the products of ATP breakdown (for details see Chapter 3). By these mechanisms, the glycolytic rate is quickly stepped up and has been calculated to reach 2000-fold above its resting rate by the time CP stores are beginning to run down. Initially only lactate can be produced as the glycolytic end-point; however, pyruvate and reducing equivalents begin crossing the mitochondrial outer wall to initiate increased activity in the TCA cycle. When, after a few seconds, ADP and P_i also enter, oxidative phosphorylation can begin. The resulting ATP has to diffuse out again into the cytoplasm before it can begin inhibiting the cytoplasmic enzymes – a property it possesses in counterbalance to the stimulatory effects of the lower adenosine phosphates. (If two molecules are sufficiently alike to have affinity for the same enzymic site, and one is stimulatory, the other, by competitively displacing it, can be expected to be inhibitory.) When the steady state is finally attained, some 3–5 min into the race, glycolysis need proceed only at one-twelfth the initial rate to maintain the same flow of ATP. Lactate production will have fallen even further, because of the flow of pyruvate and reducing equivalents into the mitochondria.

Thus the adjustment from anaerobic to aerobic glycolysis is entirely performed within the muscle fibre, though it would of course not succeed if there were not a sufficiently increased supply of O_2 from the blood. By contrast, the gradual modulation towards lipolysis, in the period from 30 to 90 min into the exercise, is initiated by the actions of several hormones. Predictably, one effect (mediated by a **hormone-sensitive lipase**) is to mobilize the fat stores visible as microscopical droplets within the muscle fibres themselves. The principal action, however, takes place not within the muscle fibres but on fat cells anywhere in the body. In particular, noradrenaline and growth hormone, aided by a lowering of insulin level, promote breakdown of **adipose tissue triglycerides** and the release of **fatty acids** into the blood stream, from whence they are taken up by the active muscles. Some direct uptake of lipids from the circulation also occurs, catalysed by lipases in the muscle capillary endothelium. All three mechanisms raise the concentration of fatty acids within the red (types I and IIa) muscle fibres; there, simply by their physical presence ('**mass action**' is the chemical term) they increasingly contribute to the mitochondrial metabolism and reduce the demand on the remaining glycogen.

Significance of lactate

Aerobic athletes working for periods of at least several minutes at rates more than about two-thirds of their maximum aerobic capacity (and untrained people working above about half this capacity) produce lactate at elevated rates. The IIb fibres, which cannot supply themselves with adequate ATP by the aerobic pathway, are unlikely to be recruited at such relatively modest work-rates in any healthy person, and certainly not in the trained athlete. Until the 1980s it was universally accepted that lactate production in these circumstances indicated a shortfall in O_2 supply to working muscles, which forced them, despite an ample furniture of mitochondria, to draw significant proportions of their ATP direct from the anaerobic pathway. The account of the last two sections is entirely compatible with this, but not committed to it, and experiments seeking to assess whether O_2 supply is in fact deficient in lactate-producing muscles have rarely found it so. One alternative explanation, in terms of pyruvate decarboxylase, is offered by Greenhaff and Hultman (see Chapter 3). Another, placing its emphasis after rather than before the TCA cycle, notes that the metabolic intermediary, NADH, has to reach a substantial concentration within the mitochondrion in order to drive the electron transport chain at a high rate by mass action (Connett *et al.*, 1990; for review, see Spurway, 1992). Because of this increased drive, the overwhelming percentage of ATP resynthesis remains aerobic. However, exchange of reducing equivalents across the mitochondrial wall causes cytoplasmic NADH concentration to rise in concert, and this leads to an increased conversion of pyruvate to lactate. This is the lactate which appears in the blood. The crucial difference from the oxygen-shortfall assumption is that the extra energy derived from the anaerobic pathway is, on Connett's model, less than 1 per cent.

Among the facts of human performance with which accounts of this kind are more compatible than the older view are:

- that when an athlete, by training, lowers his/her lactate production, O_2 consumption at the work rates concerned has never been shown to increase; and
- that muscles, relaxed or working, can take up lactate when the blood concentration is high, convert it to pyruvate, and utilize this in aerobic metabolism (Bradley *et al.*, 1994).

Thus lactate production in itself does not indicate a 'last recourse' commitment to anaerobic metabolism. Only when the individual can take in no more O_2 (i.e. is working above maximum aerobic capacity, VO_2max) does a demand for yet-faster ATP provision have to be met by glycolysis which is really anaerobic. Exercise at such intensities can at most be maintained for a matter of minutes – say, up to the duration of a 3000 m track race in the most highly trained.

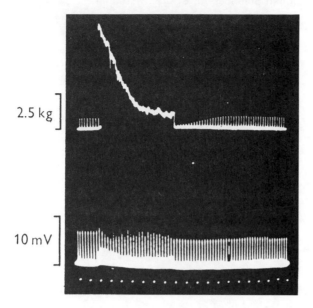

Figure 1.22a. EMG studies of human muscle fatigue. (a) During MVC of thumb adductor, force declines massively but externally-stimulated synchronous APs in ulnar nerve (large deflections, lower trace) do not consistently diminish (from Merton, P. A. (1965) Voluntary strength and fatigue, *Journal of Physiology*, **123**, pp. 553–564 reproduced by permission of Cambridge University Press)

Muscle fatigue: principles

Overall bodily and mental fatigue involves countless factors. Even within the muscles, many processes are involved, and they vary with the nature and duration of the exercise. In very intensive efforts there may be some failure of neuromuscular transmission. Logic suggests that this is particularly likely during sustained isometric efforts, since these occlude their own blood supply to the most active muscles, and release of chemical transmitter substances is especially vulnerable to hypoxia. However, transmission failure is probably not a major contributory factor in most circumstances (see, for example, Figure 1.22). Metabolic factors within the muscle fibres must therefore be the main focus of attention in the space available here. Before leaving Figure 1.22b, however, note that the greatest percentage torque loss experienced by this subject was at the highest angular velocity. This is typical. Expressing the same feature in other terms, we may say that muscle fatigue consists of loss of speed as well as force. And if we lose both force and speed their product, power, is sacrificed worst of all.

The most important single realization about fatigue is that it does not involve a metabolically significant reduction of ATP concentration. ATP is in fact protected at the cost of all other substrates (Figure 1.23). In any case, if ATP does fall to submillimolar levels, in an experimental system or death, the result is not force loss but the opposite – rigor.

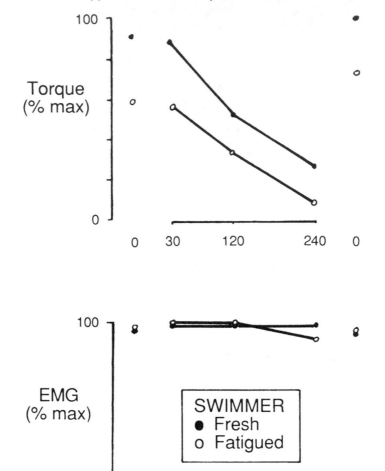

Figure 1.22b. (b) Isokinetic knee-extension torques at three angular velocities, showing massive fall-off at higher speeds after an 80 min exhausting swim; yet EMG from quadriceps is negligibly reduced. (Part (a) from Merton, P.A. (1954). *Journal of Physiology*, **123**, 553–564; (b) from Robertson, E. and Spurway, N.C., figure unpublished but cf. *Journal of Physiology*, **409**, 19 reproduced by permission of Cambridge University Press)

Analysis of traces such as those shown in Figure 1.23, or of biopsy samples from intensively exercising muscles, shows that CP concentration falls greatly and H^+ and P_i rise as fatigue develops. CP is not considered to play a direct part in force production, but the two small ions are both

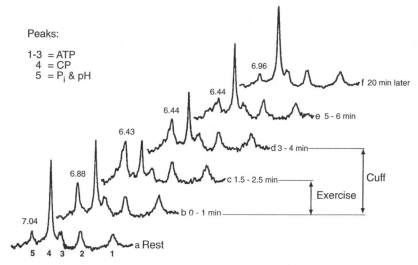

Peaks:

1-3 = ATP
4 = CP
5 = P$_i$ & pH

Figure 1.23. Phosphorus nuclear magnetic resonance (NMR) study of short-term fatigue (handgrip exercise under arterial occlusion) in human forearm muscles. Chemical significance of each peak is stated on trace; height of each peak indicates concentration of that substance, while pH is deduced from position (not height) of P$_i$ peak. When exercise reached its limit (start of trace c, P$_i$ has risen markedly at the expense of CP and pH has fallen ~ 0.6 units from its resting-muscle value; ATP, however, has been maintained without detectable change. (From Ross *et al.* (1981). *New England Journal of Medicine*, **304**, 1338–1342 reproduced by permission of the Massachusetts Medical Society)

released into the cytoplasm during the reaction which drives contraction, namely the hydrolysis of ATP:

$$ATP <=> ADP + P_i + H^+ + energy$$

Like all other chemical reactions, this one is in principle liable to proceed to the right, i.e. in the direction of hydrolysis less vigorously when substances on the right-hand side accumulate. The generic term for this category of influence is **'product inhibition'**. Thus inhibitory effects of both H$^+$ and P$_i$ on force generation would be predicted on first principles, and have been repeatedly confirmed in experiments at laboratory temperatures (Cooke and Pate, 1990).

Sprint fatigue

At the end of brief bursts of intense activity, such as a 400 m track race, muscle pH may be as low as 6.4 – due essentially to accumulation of pyruvic and lactic acids in the cytoplasm. It has thus long been assumed that H$^+$ accumulation was the major agent of the short-term fatigue which operates at the end of such an event. However, at least three arguments point against this. Firstly, force production recovers to a near-original level several minutes quicker than pH. Secondly, several laboratories have recently shown that force impairment by H^+, though marked at room temperature, is not substantial near $37°C$ (Westerblad *et al.*, 1997). Finally, sufferers from McArdle's syndrome, who lack phosphorylase and so cannot perform glycolysis and do not 'go acid', nevertheless fatigue severely. The possibility that accumulation of H^+ and P_i together can account for short-term fatigue in the normal subject should perhaps not be dismissed, but one is bound to conclude that the mechanism of this form of fatigue is less clear at the time of writing than it had seemed for many years.

Middle-distance fatigue

For fatigue in events lasting 5–10 min, a considerably larger number of fatigue mechanisms can be proposed. Of the earlier mechanisms, P_i accumulation remains a valid candidate, but pH fall is less marked than in briefer, more intensive bursts of activity. However, laboratory simulations show that less Ca^{2+} is released by each muscle AP when repeated short tetani are continued for some minutes (Allen *et al.*, 1995). One among a range of mechanisms which might bring this about is accumulation of K^+ ions in the lumens of the T system. K^+ outflow occurs in the falling phase of each AP, and it cannot all be instantly pumped back into the fibres from which it came; mixed venous blood often contains 6–7 mmol l^{-1} K^+ after 10 min of vigorous exercise. In that circumstance it can be calculated that the restricted diffusion zone deep in the T tubes must contain K^+ at 15–20 mmol l^{-1}, and this concentration would suffice to block further AP propagation there. So the centres of the fibres will cease to be excited until activity stops; then the K^+ rapidly clears again.

Endurance fatigue

The classic observation here (Bergstrom and Hultman, 1967) is that fatigue sets in when glycogen concentration in the working muscles has fallen to one-fifth to one-tenth of its normal rested-muscle value. Since any IIb motor units contributing to the biopsied sample are unlikely to have been active at all, this overall figure suggests that glycogen concentration in the low-threshold motor units required for endurance activities must be very low indeed. The practice of **carbohydrate loading** to defer fatigue in sports activities lasting about 90 min or more has arisen from this. Even in such a well established situation, however, we should not assume that everything is clear. If no more metabolism at all were possible in a fibre, it would go into rigor. Presumably, when glycogen is as depleted as it ever is physiologically, metabolism slows down but does not stop. Several factors probably contribute to the indications of fatigue: P_i accumulation remains relevant, it most likely being this which directly inhibits XB action (Chin and Allen, 1997). Membrane pumps, being also ATP driven, may be inhibited similarly. Other metabolite changes, however, appear to directly inhibit E–C coupling. An interesting hypothesis in this connection notes that glycogen is particularly depleted in immediate juxtaposition to the structures linking T tubes to SR (Figure 1.11), and proposes that ATP concentration falls particularly severely in that region; if the function of either of the proteins of Figure 1.11 depends on its being phosphorylated, Ca^{2+} release would be markedly impaired in that circumstance (Chin and Allen, 1997).

Almost certainly, at least as many mechanisms as we have listed contribute to endurance fatigue – and microscopic damage impairs performance too (Hikida *et al.*, 1983). Nothing is simple in this field!

Low-frequency fatigue

In the days following a strenuous activity of medium or long term, even though the immediate insurmountable fatigue is over, it is common to find that more effort is needed to summon up maximum force – though by now it *can* again be done. Edwards *et al.* showed (1977) that this was a matter of stimulation rate; the aftermath of intense, sustained effort is that electrical stimulation at higher frequencies than usual (the equivalent of a more determined willed effort) is required to persuade the muscle into full action. Because it shows at low but not high stimulation frequencies, this is classified as **low-frequency fatigue**. Submicroscopic damage, somewhere in the excitation/contraction coupling pathway, seemed as likely a cause as could be proposed in 1977. Now, however, we may wonder if the glycogen concentration nearest to the E–C coupling structures takes longer than 1 day to recover.

Isometric fatigue

Sustained isometric effort is relatively unusual in sport, and consequently has been less studied than the fatigue due to various intensities of dynamic (and therefore cyclic) exercise. The key difference is that, in a large muscle like quadriceps, the attempt to sustain forces above about 30 per cent of maximum voluntary contraction (MVC) cuts off the muscle's own blood supply, because intramuscular pressure occludes the inflow vessels. In smaller muscles, such as biceps, rather higher percentages of MVC may be necessary to do this, but anything approaching 100 per cent MVC will always have such a consequence (Asmussen, 1981).

Isometric fatigue, or at least **quasi-isometric** fatigue (the present author's term for fatigue attributable to the muscle's sustained occlusion of its own blood flow, even where some movement may occur) is encountered in dinghy and board sailing, in rock climbing, and in riding both horses and motor cycles. Extracellular accumulation of metabolites is likely to be a major influence in all these situations: K^+ (compare

'Middle-distance fatigue' above) is almost certainly one important agent, adenosine (a powerful pain inducer) may well be another. What does *not*, even here, appear to be a substantial contributor is failure of junctional transmission (Merton, 1954; Figure 1.22a above). However, it is the case that firing rates of the motoneurones decline in these circumstances. After a period of controversy, the explanation which has emerged is intriguing. Because the relaxation time of a single twitch is markedly slowed early in the onset of fatigue, tetanic fusion will occur after a minute or two at frequencies ~ 50 per cent of the firing rate required by fresh muscle. Slowed firing from the spinal cord has been shown to be a reflex adjustment to this changed situation (Bigland-Ritchie *et al.*, 1986). The adjustment keeps the firing rate just a little above fusion frequency, with the result that only a small reduction of firing rate would be needed to elicit less tension. This, being advantageous for continued fine control, has been termed **'muscular wisdom'** by Merton and colleagues.

Complexity

Far from fatigue being the single condition which the use of a single word implies, we have concluded that each of the various situations discussed involves a substantially different group of mechanisms. Nor have we been confident that any of the situations was actually as simple as our account, even where that account was itself quite complex. Yet should we expect them to be simple? Intensive exercise, in its varied forms, must have carried with it critical survival value during evolution. If one mechanism were consistently the weak point, or even very much the weakest point in a single category of fatigue, natural selection would surely have eliminated the problem by now. To be left with a variety of mechanisms, all contributing on terms not too far from equal, is surely just what one should expect.

References

Abbott, B.C., Bigland, B. and Ritchie, J.M. (1952). The physiological cost of negative work. *J. Physiol.*, **117**, 380–390.

Alexander, R. McN. (1988). *Elastic Mechanisms in Animal Movement*. Cambridge University Press.

Allen, D.G., Lannergren., J. and Westerblad, H. (1995). Muscle cell function during prolonged activity: cellular mechanisms of fatigue. *Exp. Physiol.*, **80**, 497–527.

Asmussen, E. (1981). Similarities and dissimilarities between static and dynamic exercise. *Circulation Res.*, **48** (Supplement 1), 3–10.

Bergstrom, J. and Hultman, E. (1967). A study of the glycogen metabolism during exercise in man. *Scand. J. Clin. Lab. Invest.*, **19**, 218–228.

Bigland-Ritchie, B., Dawson, N.J., Johansson, R.S. and Lippold, O.C.J. (1986). Reflex origin for the slowing of motoneurone firing rates in fatigue of human voluntary contractions. *J. Physiol.*, **379**, 451–459.

Billeter, R., Weber, H.L., Lutz, H. *et al*. (1980). Myosin types in human skeletal muscle fibres. *Histochemistry*, **65**, 249–279.

Bottinelli, R., Canepari, M., Pellegrino, M.A. and Reggiani, C. (1996). Force–velocity properties of human skeletal muscle fibres: myosin heavy chain isoform and temperature dependence. *J. Physiol.*, **495**, 573–586.

Bouchard, C., Dionne, F.T., Simoneau, J.A. and Boulay, M.R. (1992). Genetics of aerobic and anaerobic performances. *Exerc. Sport Sci. Rev.*, **20**, 27–58.

Boyd, I.A. and Smith, R.S. (1984). The muscle spindle. In *Peripheral Neuropathy* (P. Jones Dyck, P.K. Thomas, E.H. Lombert and R. Bunge, eds), pp. 171–202. Saunders.

Bradley, J.L., Spurway, N.C. and Hood, S. (1994). Preliminary investigation into the effects of exercising small and large muscle groups on the blood flow and extracellular lactate concentrations of the forearm. *J. Sports Sci.*, **12**, 129–130.

Brooke, M.H. and Kaiser, K.K. (1970). Muscle fibre types: how many and what kind? *Arch. Neurol.*, **23**, 369–379.

Buller, A.J., Eccles, J.C. and Eccles, R.M. (1960). Interactions between motoneurones and muscles in respect of the characteristic speeds of their responses. *J. Physiol.*, **150**, 417–439

Burke, R.E., Levine, D.N., Zajac, F.E. *et al*. (1971). Mammalian motor units: physiological–histochemical correlation in three types in cat gastrocnemius. *Science*, **174**, 709–712.

Chin, E.R. and Allen, D.G. (1997). Effects of reduced muscle glycogen concentration on force, Ca^{2+} release and contractile protein function in intact mouse skeletal muscle. *J. Physiol.*, **498**, 17–29.

Connett, R.J., Honig, C.R., Gayeski, T.E.J. and Brooks, G.A. (1990). Defining hypoxia: a systems view of VO_2, glycolysis, energetics and intracellular PO_2. *J. Appl. Physiol.*, **68**, 833–842.

Cooke, R. and Pate, E. (1990). The inhibition of muscle contraction by the products of ATP hydrolysis. In *Biochemistry of Exercise*, Vol.VII (A.W. Taylor, P.D. Gollnick, H.J. Green *et al*., eds), pp. 59–72. Human Kinetics.

Curtin, N.A. and Davies, R.E. (1975). Very high tension with very little ATP breakdown by active skeletal muscle. *J. Mechanochem. Cell Motility*, **3**, 147–154.

Dawson, M.J., Gadian, D.G. and Wilkie, D.R. (1978). Muscular fatigue investigated by phosphorus nuclear magnetic resonance. *Nature*, **274**, 861–866.

Edman, K.A.P., Mansson, A. and Caputo, C. (1997). The biphasic force–velocity relationship in frog muscle fibres and its evaluation in terms of cross-bridge function. *J. Physiol.*, **503**, 141–156.

Edwards, R.H.T, Hill, D.K., Jones, D.A. and Merton, P.A. (1977). Fatigue of long duration in human muscle after exercise. *J. Physiol.*, **272**, 769–778.

Ennion, S., Sant-Ana Pereira, J., Sargeant, A.J. *et al*. (1995). Characterization of human skeletal muscle fibres according to the myosin heavy chains they express. *J. Muscle Res. Cell Motility*, **16**, 35–43.

Enoka, R.M. (1996). Eccentric contractions require unique activation strategies by the nervous system. *J. Appl. Physiol.*, **81**, 2339–2346.

Essig, D.A. (1996). Contractile activity-induced mitochondrial biogenesis in skeletal muscle. *Exerc. Sports Sci. Rev.*, **24**, 289–319.

Finer, J.T., Simmons, R.M. and Spudich, J.A. (1994). Single myosin molecule mechanics: piconewton forces and nanometre steps. *Nature*, **368**, 113–119.

Geeves, M.A. (1991). The dynamics of actin and myosin association and the crossbridge model of muscle contraction. *Biochem. J.*, **274**, 1–14.

Goldspink, G., Scutt, A., Martindale, J. *et al*. (1991). Stretch and force generation induce rapid hypertrophy and isoform gene switching in adult skeletal muscle. *Biochem. Soc. Trans.*, **19**, 369–373.

Gordon, A.M., Huxley, A.F. and Julian, F.J. (1966). The variation in isometric tension with sarcomere length in vertebrate skeletal muscle fibres. *J. Physiol.*, **184**, 170–192.

Gordon, A.M. and Yates, L.D. (1992). Regulatory mechanisms of contraction in skeletal muscle. In *Muscle Contraction and Cell Motility: Molecular and Cellular Aspects* (H. Sugi, ed.). Springer.

Henneman. E., Somjen, G. and Carpenter, D.O. (1965). Functional significance of cell size in spinal motoneurones. *J. Neurophysiol.*, **28**, 560–580.

Hikida, R.S., Staron, R.S., Hagerman, F.C. *et al.* (1983). Muscle fibre necrosis associated with human marathon runners. *J. Neurological Sci.*, **59**, 185–203.

Hill, A.V., Long, C.N.H. and Lupton, H. (1924). Muscular exercise, lactic acid and the supply and utilization of oxygen: VI. The oxygen debt at the end of exercise. *Proc. Royal Soc., B*, **97**, 122–138.

Hill, A.V. (1938). The heat of shortening and the dynamic constants of muscle. *Proc. Royal Soc., B*, **126**, 136–195.

Huxley, A.F. (1974). Muscular contraction. *J. Physiol.*, **243**, 1–43.

Huxley, H.E. (1969). The mechanism of muscular contraction. *Science*, **164**, 1356–1366.

Jones, C., Allen, T., Morgan, D.L. and Proske, U. (1997). Changes in the mechanical properties of human and amphibian muscle after eccentric exercice. *Eur. J. Appl. Physiol. Occupational Physiol.*, **76**, 21–31.

Julian, F.J., Rome, L.C., Stephenson, D.G. and Stritz, S. (1986). The maximum speed of shortening in living and skinned frog muscle fibres. *J. Physiol.*, **370**, 181–199.

Klissouras, V. (1997). Heritability of adaptive variation revisited. *J. Sports Med. Physical Fitness*, **37**, 1–6.

Komi, P.V. (1988). The musculoskeletal system. In *The Olympic Book of Sports Medicine* (A. Dirix, H.G. Knuttgen and K. Kittel, eds), pp. 23–39. Blackwell.

Kraemer, W.J. (1992). Hormonal mechanisms related to the expression of muscular strength and power. In *Strength and Power in Sport* (P.V. Komi, ed.), pp. 64–76. Blackwell.

Margaria, R., Ceretelli, P. and Mangili, E. (1964). Balance and kinetics of anaerobic energy release during strenuous exercise in man. *J. Appl. Physiol.*, **26**, 623–628.

Merton, P.A. (1954). Voluntary strength and fatigue. *J. Physiol.*, **123**, 553–564.

Murphy, P.R. and Martin, H.A. (1993). Fusimotor discharge patterns during rhythmic movements. *Trends Neurosci.*, **16**, 273–278.

Rayment, I., Holden, H.M., Whittaker, M. *et al.* (1993). Structure of the actin–myosin complex and its implications for muscle contraction. *Science*, **261**, 58–65.

Renstrom, P. (1988). Muscle injuries. In *The Olympic Book of Sports Medicine* (A. Dirix, H.G. Knuttgen and K. Tittel, eds), pp. 413–427. Blackwell.

Rios, E., Ma, J.J. and Gonzalez, A. (1991). The mechanical hypothesis of excitation–contraction (EC) coupling in skeletal muscle. *J. Muscle Res. Cell Motility*, **12**, 127–135.

Sale, D.G. (1988). Neural adaptation to resistance training. *Med. Sci. Sports Exerc.*, **20**, S135–145.

Salmons, S. (1994). Exercise, stimulation and type transformation of skeletal muscle. *Int. J. Sports Med.*, **15**, 136–141.

Salmons, S. (1997). *Muscle Damage*. Oxford.

Sherrington, C.S. (1904). The correlation of reflexes and the principle of the final common path. *British Assoc. Reports*, **74**, 728–741.

Smith, L.L. (1991). Acute inflammation: the underlying mechanism in DOMS? *Med. Sci. Sports Exerc.*, **23**, 542–551.

Spurway, N.C. (1992). Aerobic exercise, anaerobic exercise and the lactate threshold. *Brit. Med. Bull.*, **48**, 569–591.

Spurway, N.C., Watson, H., McMillan, K. and Connelly, G. (1998). The effect of strength training on the apparent inhibition of eccentric force production in voluntarily activated human quadriceps. *Eur. J. App. Physiol. Occupational Physiol.* (submitted).

Spurway, N.C. and Rowlerson, A.M. (1989). Quantitative analysis of histochemical and immunohistochemical reactions in skeletal muscle fibres of *Rana* and *Xenopus*. *Histochem. J.*, **21**, 461–474.

Taylor, E.W. (1979). Mechanism of actomyosin ATPase and the problem of muscle contraction. *CRC Critical Revs Biochem.*, **6**, 103–164.

Trinick, J. (1991). Elastin filaments and giant proteins in muscle. *Current Opin. Cell Biol.*, **3**, 112–119.

Westerblad, H., Bruton, J.D. and Lannergren, J. (1997). The effect of intracellular pH on contractile function of intact, single fibres of mouse muscle declines with increasing temperature. *J. Physiol.*, **500**, 193–204.

Westing, S.H., Seger, J.M. and Thorstensson, A. (1990). Effects of electrical stimulation on eccentric and concentric torque–velocity relationships during knee-extension in man. *Acta Physiol. Scand.*, **140**, 17–22.

Further reading

General textbooks

Vander, A.J., Sherman, J.H. and Luciano, D.S. (1994). *Human Physiology: The Mechanisms of Body Function*, VIth Edn, Chap. 11, pp. 303–337. McGraw-Hill.

Greger, R. and Windhorst, U. (1996). *Comprehensive Human Physiology: From Cellular Mechanisms to Integration*, Chaps 45–48, pp. 911–985. Springer.

Monographs

Bagshaw, C.R. (1993). *Muscle Contraction*, 2nd Edn. Chapman and Hall.

Jones, D.A. and Round, J.M. (1990). *Skeletal Muscle in Health and Disease*. Manchester University Press.

Komi, P.V. (1992). *Strength and Power in Sport*. Blackwell. (See especially: Noth, J., Motor units, Chap. 2B, pp. 21–28; Billeter, R. and Hoppeler, H., Muscular basis of strength, Chap. 3, pp. 39–63; Edman, K.A.P., Contractile performance of skeletal muscle fibres, Chap. 6A, pp. 96–114.)

McComas, A.J. (1996). *Skeletal Muscle Form and Function*. Human Kinetics.

2

Cardiorespiratory responses to exercise

Adrianne E. Hardman

During dynamic exercise skeletal muscle metabolism dominates whole-body metabolism. There are two reasons for this: first, its large mass – in a young man typically 30 kg or 40 per cent of body mass; and second, its unique capability to increase its metabolic rate – as much as 50-fold. Even light exercise therefore results in marked increases in whole-body oxygen uptake. The oxygen store in muscle is very limited and sustained muscular activity necessitates an increased delivery of oxygen which is co-ordinated with tissue requirements. This taxes the functional capacity of the cardiovascular and respiratory systems more than any other stressor. Consequently, exercise with the body's large muscles provides an appropriate model for study of the operation and regulation of these systems. This chapter describes the main features of the cardiorespiratory adjustments to exercise. In addition, the evidence which sheds light on the relative importance of different aspects of oxygen transport and utilization will be considered. Finally, brief reference will be made to changes with training and increasing age.

Whole-body oxygen uptake response

The rate of uptake of oxygen, the ultimate hydrogen ion acceptor, by the body provides a measure of metabolic rate. As would be expected, this is closely coupled to exercise intensity as measured by work-rate on a cycle ergometer or speed of walking or running on a treadmill. Oxygen uptake rises rapidly during the first minutes of exercise to a steady-state value which matches the demands of the tissues. Differences in mechanical efficiency are small and so the oxygen uptake shows rather small variation between individuals at a standard work-rate during weight-supported exercise, for example on a cycle or rowing ergometer (Figure 2.1a). In contrast, for tasks where the body weight is not supported, oxygen uptake can differ markedly between people; most of this variation is attributable to differences in body mass, however, and the rate of uptake *per kg* is rather similar (Figure 2.1b). Average values for women tend to be somewhat lower than for men in both types of exercise, probably because

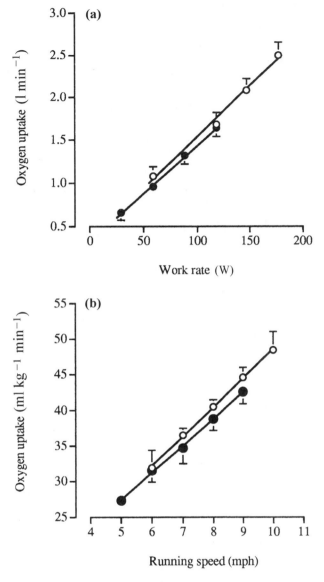

Figure 2.1. Linear relationship between oxygen uptake and exercise intensity for cycle ergometry (a) and treadmill running (b). Unpublished observations and (b) adapted from Bransford and Howley (1977)

their lower body mass and muscle mass confer a lower resting metabolic rate. Longitudinal study of young athletes shows that the oxygen uptake at a standard running speed is higher than in adults, decreasing through adolescence (Sjödin and Svedenhag, 1992), possibly as a consequence of maturational changes in biomechanical factors.

For each individual, there is a ceiling to oxygen uptake known as the maximum oxygen uptake ($\dot{V}O_{2max}$). This was first described by Hill and Lupton in 1923 when they showed that oxygen uptake reaches a plateau at intolerable levels of exertion. Although individuals can exercise for brief periods at levels beyond that which elicited $\dot{V}O_{2max}$, oxygen uptake had reached its upper limit. Hill and Lupton (1923) argued that this is because of limitations imposed by the cardiovascular and respiratory systems and much evidence supports this view.

Maximum oxygen uptake is a fundamental characteristic of the individual which shows day-to-day variability of only 2–4 per cent, despite the fact that not all individuals demonstrate the 'classic' plateau. This measure is an essential reference point in understanding human physiological responses to exercise and in explaining interindividual differences in the capability for endurance exercise. The factors contributing to $\dot{V}O_{2max}$ can best be considered through reference to the Fick principle, i.e.

$$\dot{V}O_{2\,max} = HR_{max} \times SV_{max} \times (a-v)O_2 \ diff_{max}$$

where HR_{max} is the maximum heart rate, SV_{max} is the maximum stroke volume and $(a-v)\ O_2\ diff_{max}$ is the maximum difference between the oxygen content of arterial and mixed venous blood.

Clearly, both the capacity of the cardiovascular system to deliver oxygen and the capacity of tissues to extract oxygen are potentially important determinants of $\dot{V}O_{2max}$. Values for men of contrasting physical activity status, i.e. patients whose cardiac performance is compromised by mitral stenosis, sedentary men who are 'normally' active and endurance athletes (Table 2.1) show that the difference in $\dot{V}O_{2max}$ between these groups is attributable mostly to differences in maximum stroke volume (Rowell, 1993). Stroke volume and the arterial–mixed venous difference for oxygen are not easily measured, however, so the usual approach is to determine the oxygen content of a sample of expired air obtained over a known time period at maximum exertion and obtain the oxygen taken up by subtraction of this value from the calculated intake. At $\dot{V}O_{2max}$, cardiac output (the product of maximum heart rate and maximum stroke volume) typi-

Table 2.1   Range of maximal values for different groups (after Rowell, 1993)

Training status	$\dot{V}O_{2max} =$ $(1 \cdot min^{-1})$	$HR_{max} \times$ $(beat \cdot min^{-1})$	$SV_{max} \times$ (ml)	$(a-v)O_2 difference_{max}$ $(ml \cdot 100ml$ $blood^{-1}$
Low (M.S.)	1.40	190	43	17
Average (Sedentary)	3.50	195	112	16
High (Endurance athletes)	6.25	190	205	16

cally may be four- to seven-fold above resting values and oxygen extraction increased more than three-fold, i.e. from 4.5 ml per 100 ml of blood at rest to 16 ml per 100 ml.

There is little interindividual variation in the oxygen 'cost' of running at a given speed, so it follows that the $\dot{V}O_{2max}$ is the single most important determinant of endurance performance. When individuals with a wide range of values are studied, the relationship with performance time is strong and correlation coefficients of the order of -0.9 are commonly reported (Costill *et al.*, 1973; Williams, 1981). Figure 2.2 shows the relationship, for 16 distance runners with varied abilities, between performance in a 10 mile time-trial and $\dot{V}O_{2max}$ measured during uphill treadmill running (Costill *et al.*, 1973). However, when a relatively homogeneous sample is studied, there is no relationship between performance and $\dot{V}O_{2max}$. In the latter circumstances running economy, i.e. the oxygen uptake at a standard running speed, accounts for a large proportion of the interindividual variation in running performance (Conley and Krahenbuhl, 1980).

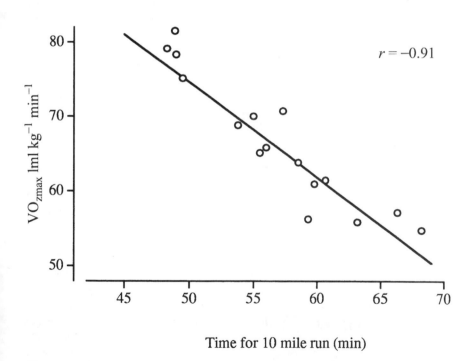

Figure 2.2. Relationship between maximal oxygen uptake and performance in a 10-mile road race in male distance runners. (Adapted from Costill *et al.*, 1973)

Cardiovascular adjustments to exercise

During exercise, the need is for marked increases in muscle blood flow. This provides for removal of waste products and controls local temperature, as well as ensuring delivery of oxygen and metabolic substrates. Tissue blood flow can increase 20- to 40-fold at maximum exertion, and the vasodilation needed to effect such flows represents a profound challenge to maintenance of arterial blood pressure. This challenge is met remarkably effectively, through synchronized and complementary adjustments of central and peripheral cardiovascular functions.

Central adjustments

The principal feature of the cardiovascular response is a tight coupling between cardiac output and systemic metabolic demand. For each increase in oxygen uptake of $1 \, \mathrm{l \, min^{-1}}$, cardiac output increases by about $5 \, \mathrm{l \, min^{-1}}$. Increases in heart rate and stroke volume both contribute. The rapid increase in heart rate to about 100 beats per minute (bpm) is attributed to withdrawal of the vagal tone which, at rest, exerts a restraining effect. Above this level, usually representing about 40 per cent of $\dot{V}O_{2max}$, sympathetic activity is the mechanism involved. This can be seen because at this intensity noradrenaline from sympathetic nerve endings begins to appear in plasma (Savard et al., 1989).

The main effect of upright exercise on stroke volume is to allow it to regain values evident during rest in the supine position. The increase is achieved through both better filling (greater end diastolic volume) and more complete emptying (lower end systolic volume), but the former is the more important influence. The weight of evidence is that stroke volume is maintained even during exercise approaching $\dot{V}O_{2max}$, but there are reports of a decrease above 70 per cent of $\dot{V}O_{2max}$. Given the decrease in filling time associated with increased heart rate (from 0.55 sec at 70 bpm to 0.12 sec at 195 bpm), it is surprising that stroke volume is not diminished. Major simultaneous adjustments in ventricular filling pressure are needed in order to compensate, despite the increases in the contractile state of the myocardium attributable to increased adrenaline and to enhanced sympathetic activity.

The necessary increase in filling pressure is achieved through the so-called 'muscle pump', which provides the energy to drive blood back to the heart against gravity. Its importance in allowing cardiac output to increase cannot be over-stressed and its capacity has been described as similar to that of the left ventricle (Rowell, 1993). It raises central venous volume and pressure but also increases muscle perfusion. Immediately after each contraction, the local veins are empty and venous valves prevent backflow; thus net perfusion pressure is increased. The importance of the muscle pump in maintaining stroke volume is demonstrated by its relation with the mass of active muscle; when this is small, venous return is lower, so that stroke volume is lower for a given oxygen uptake, with a compensatory increase in heart rate. The respiratory pump exerts a smaller additional effect on ventricular filling. During inspiration, intrathoracic pressure is reduced and intra-abdominal pressure increased. These pressure differences are transmitted through the rather thin walls of the great veins, so enhancing venous return.

Peripheral circulation

Muscle blood flow at rest is $0.75–1.0\,l\,min^{-1}$ or 15–20 per cent of cardiac output, but in maximum exercise can increase to about $20\,l\,min^{-1}$, 80–85 per cent of output. Thus muscle flow increases by more than 20-fold, more than can be accounted for by the increased cardiac output. The additional increase is achieved through locally stimulated vasodilation in contracting muscle.

In muscle, as in other tissues, vascular smooth muscle is innervated by sympathetic fibres. This outflow is increased during exercise but opposed by locally induced vasodilation which relaxes precapillary sphincters, so opening up more capillaries. The mechanisms involved are not well defined, but increases in potassium concentration and osmolarity, as well as local decreases in the partial pressure of oxygen, may play a part in the rapid increase in flow at the start of exercise. The maintenance of enhanced flow as exercise continues is less easy to explain. The possibility has been explored that endothelium-derived relaxing factors (maybe nitric oxide) may contribute, but the magnitude and time-course of exercise-induced hyperaemia cannot be mimicked by infusing combinations of known vasodilator metabolites, and so some other factor is involved. The muscle pump may itself increase local flow through sudden release of a high compressive force. Elastic recoil would serve to pull open empty veins and increase the pressure gradient across muscle, and flow would be enhanced through the rhythmic cycle of contraction and relaxation. Whatever mechanism is involved, the relation between exercise intensity and local autoregulatory vasodilation in active muscle is linked most elegantly (directly or indirectly) to the tissue metabolic rate.

Vasodilation of arterioles and precapillary sphincters has a profound effect on muscle's potential for oxygen uptake. At rest, only a small fraction of capillaries are perfused in resting muscle. The enormous increase in the numbers of capillaries which are patent in active muscle greatly reduces diffusion distances. Capillary blood volume is increased, opposing a decrease in mean capillary transit time as flow rates increase. This protects diffusion capability and blood leaving active muscle may contain as little as 2 ml of oxygen per 100 ml, compared with about 14 ml at rest. Off-loading during exercise is assisted by a rightward shift of the oxyhaemoglobin dissociation curve caused by the associated fall in muscle pH and rise in temperature.

Regional blood flows

Without compensatory systemic vasoconstriction in non-active tissues, vasodilation in a large active muscle mass would threaten the body's ability to maintain adequate arterial blood pressure. The necessary increased in peripheral resistance is achieved through widespread vaso-constriction via adrenergic activity. In particular, marked decreases in flow are evident in splanchnic and hepatic circulations. At rest, these tissues have high flow rates but extract only a small fraction of available oxygen, i.e. they are overperfused for their metabolic need. For example, splanchic flow in a resting human is about 1500 ml min^{-1}, 25 per cent of cardiac output, but only 15–20 per cent of arterial oxygen is extracted and so large reductions in splanchnic flow can occur without compromising oxygen provision. In fact, nearly 250 ml of oxygen per minute can be redistributed by these means to active muscle at VO_{2max} (Rowell, 1993).

Coronary blood flow must, of course, increase as the metabolic cost of increasing output rises during exercise. Estimates suggest that this may be from 5 per cent of an output of some 5 l min^{-1} at rest, rising linearly with heart rate to about 1.0 l min^{-1} at 195 bpm. Cutaneous blood flow changes during exercise are complex and difficult to measure. The veins here are very compliant and can accommodate very high flows, being described sometimes as a 'blood sink'. Although increased vasoconstrictor activity probably causes skin blood flow to fall during the early minutes of exercise, subsequent increases to above pre-exercise levels as body temperature rises represent both withdrawal of vasoconstrictor outflow and increase of active vasodilation (vasodilatory nerve fibres or neurohumoral effects linked to sympathetic cholinergic activation of sweat glands).

Because the cutaneous beds are so capacious, increases in their perfusion greatly affect the central circulation. As skin per fusion rises during exercise, the peripheral displacement of central blood volume can cause venous return to fall, so that a compensatory and progressive rise in heart rate is necessary to maintain cardiac output. This phenomenon is known as cardiovascular drift and is particularly marked during exercise in a hot, humid environment when the body's capability for heat loss is challenged. Cutaneous vasodilation is not inexorably linked to deep body temperature, however. When this reaches about 38°C, skin blood flow reaches an upper limit (Brengelmann et al., 1977). The mechanisms responsible are not clear, but the effect is to prevent decline in blood pressure. Total blood flow to the brain is maintained relatively constant during exercise.

Integration of cardiovascular adjustments

Maintenance of stroke volume and cardiac output during exercise requires a balance between the mechanical effects of muscle contraction and the unselective, passive effects of sympathetic vasoconstrictor outflow. When the exercising muscle groups are large, as in cycling or running for example, the large increases in conductance in active tissues oppose a rise in blood pressure. In contrast, during exercise with small muscles there is little increase in conductance and blood pressure rises. This is most marked when the exercise is essentially isometric because increases in intramuscular pressure may hinder or stop flow of blood out of veins.

At $\dot{V}O_{2max}$, whole-body oxygen extraction is commonly 80–85 per cent and the oxygen content of mixed venous blood falls as low as 2–3 ml per 100 ml of blood. This reflects compensatory increases in extraction by non-active tissues in response to decreased flow as well as increased oxygen extraction by active muscle.

The tight coupling between muscle metabolism and muscle blood flow was mentioned above. This relationship is a key feature of the integration of cardiovascular adjustments to exercise. Thus:

- muscle metabolism dictates muscle blood flow;
- muscle blood flow dictates venous return;
- venous return dictates cardiac output; *and so*
- muscle metabolism dictates cardiac output.

Ventilation during exercise

The healthy human lung has vast reserves of ventilatory capacity and successfully defends arterial oxygen saturation in the face of four- to six-fold increases in cardiac output.

Resting ventilatory values of 6–7 l min^{-1} increase during dynamic exercise to 100 or 150 l min^{-1} and even, in extreme cases, to 200 l min^{-1} (Åstrand and Rodahl, 1986). Ventilation increases linearly with oxygen uptake during light and moderate exercise, but the increases become curvilinear as $\dot{V}O_{2max}$ is approached. At maximum effort, however, ventilation is still somewhat less than that which can be achieved by voluntary effort, i.e. maximum voluntary ventilation. The work done by respiratory muscles rises markedly; the oxygen cost increases from a resting value of between 0.5 and 1.0 ml per litre of ventilation and may reach up to 10 per cent of total oxygen uptake. This leads to a progressive ventilatory inefficiency which is reflected in changes in the ventilatory equivalent for oxygen, i.e. the ventilation necessary to achieve an increase of 1 l min^{-1} in oxygen uptake; this is typically 20–25 during moderate exercise but can rise to 30–35 l min^{-1} during maximum exercise. Values may be even higher in children.

Increases in both frequency and depth of breathing contribute to the increased ventilation of exercise. In light exercise, increases in the tidal volume are the more important – although rarely is more than 60 per cent of vital capacity deployed. The relative contribution of these two to increased ventilation is often dependent on the exercise rhythm, for example pedal rate frequency or stride cadence, which tends to dictate the breathing frequency.

At rest in the standing position, perfusion of the lower areas of the lungs is increased, at the expense of upper areas, leading to inequalities of the ratio of alveolar ventilation to perfusion. These effects of gravity are offset during exercise and there is improved matching of ventilation to perfusion. In the healthy lung this is not a major factor for increasing gas transport, however. On the other hand, the three-fold expansion of pulmonary capillary blood volume is important because it maintains mean transit time and hence gas equilibration. Overall, the diffusion capacity rises three-fold.

Ventilation is more closely coupled to carbon dioxide production than to oxygen uptake and marked interindividual differences are apparent at a standard oxygen uptake. At rest, pulmonary ventilation is chiefly regulated by the chemical state of the blood. The partial pressure of carbon dioxide in plasma (and hence in cerebrospinal fluid) – a value highly related to the hydrogen ion concentration – appears to have the major role. There is little consensus, however, concerning the nature of the factors responsible for increased ventilation during exercise. Chemical changes in the arterial blood are small even during intense exercise and cannot explain the ventilation rates achieved. Neurogenic stimuli, perhaps from active muscles and joints, may play a part but the consensus is that they are probably more important in activation of the ventilatory drive rather than in regulation of a sustained high ventilatory rate.

In sharp contrast to the close coupling between muscle metabolism and cardiovascular function, there appears to be no such association between metabolic rate and ventilatory changes. The concept of an 'anaerobic threshold' was developed in an attempt to define the exercise intensity where glycolysis becomes an increasingly important means of ATP resynthesis. Proponents take the view that this can be identified either as a marked increase in the concentration of lactate in blood (or attainment of a reference value for this, often $4 \text{ mmol } l^{-1}$) or as the point at which a non-linear increase in ventilation or carbon dioxide production occurs. The theoretical basis for this is that lactate accumulation reduces blood pH and hence the central chemoreceptor drive to ventilation. One fundamental problem with this approach is that patients with McArdle's syndrome, who lack myophosphorylase and so cannot produce lactate, show a perfectly normal ventilatory response (Hagberg *et al.*, 1982). A detailed discussion of the evidence for and against the existence of a well-defined 'point' which can be measured reproducibly is beyond the scope of this chapter and the interested reader is referred to specific reviews (see, for example, Brooks, 1985). What is certain, however, is that training does increase the oxygen uptake which an individual can sustain in a 'metabolic steady state', i.e. where muscle metabolism is predominantly oxidative, with little lactate accumulation.

Relative exercise intensity

It was mentioned above that $\dot{V}O_{2max}$ is a key determinant of endurance performance. The reason for this is that this quantity plays such an important role in dictating human responses to the challenge of exercise. This can be illustrated by reference to cardiovascular, thermoregulatory, metabolic and humoral responses.

Early studies in Sweden first examined the reasons behind the wide variation in heart rate at a standard oxygen uptake (Åstrand, 1960). Most of this was attributable to the proportion of $\dot{V}O_{2max}$ which this oxygen uptake represented for an individual. Thus, at 50 per cent of $\dot{V}O_{2max}$ the average heart rate of a young man is 128 bpm, whereas at 70 per cent of $\dot{V}O_{2max}$ it is 154 bpm. Corresponding values are slightly higher for women, i.e. 138 bpm and 168 bpm respectively (the standard deviation for all these values is 9–10 bpm). Maximum heart rate decreases with age, however, so it is important to note that the relationship between relative exercise intensity (per cent $\dot{V}O_{2max}$) and heart rate is quantitatively different in older people; e.g. for a 65-year-old man the heart rate at 50 per cent $\dot{V}O_{2max}$ would be about 110 bpm.

The relative exercise intensity also determines circulatory changes in non-active peripheral tissues during exercise. In a series of studies in the late 1960s, hepatic-splanchnic blood flow was compared in three groups of subjects with widely differing $\dot{V}O_{2max}$ values, i.e. normally active controls, endurance athletes and patients with mitral stenosis (data summarized in Rowell, 1993). At a given submaximum level of oxygen uptake, the decrements in hepatic-splanchnic flow varied markedly among subjects. In contrast, when oxygen uptake was expressed relative to individual $\dot{V}O_{2max}$ the differences between individuals virtually disappeared. In other words, the decrease in hepatic-splanchnic flow from rest is related to the proportion of $\dot{V}O_{2max}$ which a particular exercise represents for the individual.

Thermoregulatory responses are also governed by the intensity of exercise relative to $\dot{V}O_{2max}$. Variation in deep body tempterature is considerable at a given absolute oxygen uptake but, in contrast, small at a given relative oxygen uptake. For example, at an oxygen uptake of $1.5 \, l \, min^{-1}$ oesophageal temperature was $38.2°C$ in one subject with a $\dot{V}O_{2max}$ of $2.61 \, l \, min^{-1}$ but only $37.1°C$ in a subject with a $\dot{V}O_{2max}$ of $5.35 \, l \, min^{-1}$ (Saltin and Hermansen, 1966). During exercise at 50 per cent $\dot{V}O_{2max}$, however, these subjects had identical temperatures, despite the fact that the subject with the higher $\dot{V}O_{2max}$ was producing more than twice as much heat as the subject with the lower $\dot{V}O_{2max}$. Typically the steady-state deep body temperature at 50 per cent of $\dot{V}O_{2max}$ is $38°C$, i.e. about $1°C$ above the resting level.

Muscle metabolism also appears to be linked to the relative intensity of exercise, although this can be modified with training. For example, both the rate of glycogen breakdown (Saltin and Karlsson, 1971) and the change in blood lactate concentration are largely dependent on the percentage of $\dot{V}O_{2max}$ the individual is utilizing. Figure 2.3 shows blood lactate concentrations for three subjects during treadmill running. When concentrations are expressed relative to speed of running (approximating to oxygen uptake) the responses of these subjects are very different (Figure 2.3a). When expressed relative to individual values for $\dot{V}O_{2max}$ they are remarkably similar (Figure 2.3b).

The level of all these responses contributes to a subject's performance potential and to their perception of the intensity of effort during exercise. The relative intensity typically adopted across a range of competitive distances decreases with distance (Figure 2.4). For example, recreational runners at the half marathon distance (21 km) typically select a running pace representing about 80 per cent of $\dot{V}O_{2max}$ (Williams and Nute, 1983). Again, there are changes here with more prolonged and intensive training so that elite endurance runners can sustain this relative intensity over the full marathon distance (Costill, 1984).

Limitations to maximum oxygen uptake ($\dot{V}O_{2max}$)

Theoretically, any one (or more) of the different steps in the transport of oxygen from the air to the site of utilization in the mitochondria of skeletal muscle could be rate-limiting. Many of these possibilities have been examined experimentally and there is now much evidence to help answer the question 'what limits oxygen transport during exercise?'.

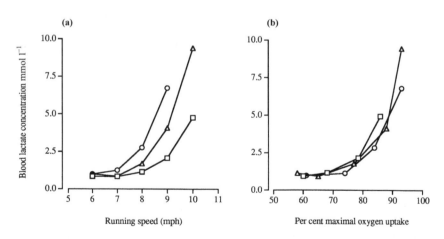

Figure 2.3. Blood lactate concentrations in three individuals during treadmill running at common speeds (a). (b) Shows concentrations plotted against the oxygen uptake of the runners expressed as a proportion of each individual's $\dot{V}O_{2max}$, i.e. as relative exercise intensity. Data courtesy of Professor Clyde Williams

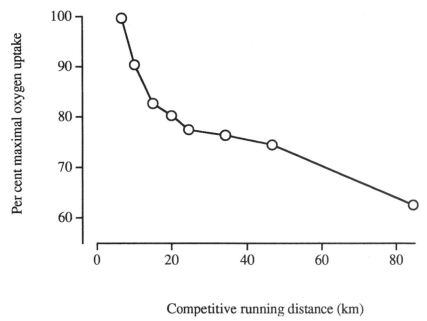

Per cent maximal oxygen uptake

Competitive running distance (km)

Figure 2.4. Typical relative exercise intensity of maximal efforts over a range of competitive running distances. (Adapted from Costill, D.L. (1979). A scientific approach to distance running, *Track and Field News*)

The main candidates are: (1) the pulmonary diffusion capacity; (2) the maximum cardiac output; (3) the capacity of circulation in skeletal muscle; and (4) the metabolic capacity of skeletal muscle. When $\dot{V}O_{2max}$ is measured at sea-level, the diffusion capacity of the lung can probably be excluded, based on observations that there is little evidence of arterial oxygen desaturation during intense exercise. An exception may be endurance-trained athletes with extremely high $\dot{V}O_{2max}$ values. In such individuals a degree of desaturation may occur, indicating that the lungs' ability to transfer oxygen from air to blood may not be able to match central cardiovascular capacity. If these subjects breathe oxygen-rich air (26 per cent oxygen) their haemoglobin saturation and their $\dot{V}O_{2max}$ values increase, proving a pulmonary diffusion limitation when breathing atmospheric air (Powers *et al.*, 1989).

The view of most physiologists is that $\dot{V}O_{2max}$, with this exception, is limited mainly by central cardiovascular capacity when exercise is performed with large muscle groups. However, the quantity of muscle recruited influences $\dot{V}O_{2max}$; values determined during cycling are somewhat lower than during running, with skiing eliciting the highest values.

Observational studies point to a cardiovascular rather than a metabolic limitation. For example, Table 2.1 shows that the characteristic explaining the higher $\dot{V}O_{2max}$ values in athletes is the maximum stroke volume and not the maximum arterio-venous difference for oxygen. Similarly, training studies show that most of the increase in $\dot{V}O_{2max}$ with training is attributable to increased maximum stroke volume. Both lines of evidence tie in persuasively with the dissociation between the time-scale of changes in $\dot{V}O_{2max}$ and indices of muscle oxidative metabolism during changes in training status. Figure 2.5 shows parallel changes in these variables in subjects studied during 8–10 weeks of training, followed by 6 weeks of detraining (Henriksson and Reitman, 1977). Although rates of change (expressed relative to baseline values) were initially similar for $\dot{V}O_{2max}$ and for muscle indices of oxidative capacity, these quickly diverged. During the first week of detraining differences were particularly clear; $\dot{V}O_{2max}$ remained rather stable in the face of enormous, rapid decreases in muscle oxidative enzyme activities.

The results of experimental manipulation of the oxygen supply to muscle have strengthened the view that the metabolic capacity of muscle does not limit $\dot{V}O_{2max}$. The rationale here is that if $\dot{V}O_{2max}$ is not enhanced when oxygen availability increases, then the capacity of the muscle to take up and utilize oxygen is not limiting. Arterial oxygen content has been enhanced by asking subjects to breathe a hyperoxic gas mixture (usually 50 per cent oxygen) and, in separate experiments, by reinfusion of red blood cells to temporarily increase blood haemoglobin content. The two interventions make additional oxygen available by different means, of course; the first 'loads up the plasma' with more oxygen, the second increases the oxygen carried by haemoglobin. Both interventions result in a statistically significant increase in $\dot{V}O_{2max}$, showing that the limitation to oxygen uptake is in the cardiovascular delivery system (Ekblöm *et al.*, 1975, 1976).

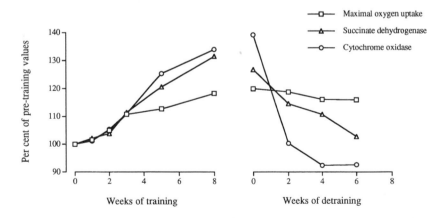

Figure 2.5. Percentage changes in maximal oxygen uptake and in activities of skeletal muscle succinate dehydrogenase and cytochrome oxidase measured in vastus lateralis during 8–10 weeks of training, followed by 6 weeks of detraining. (Adapted from Henriksson and Reitman, 1977)

Elegant one-leg studies (Andersen and Saltin, 1985) have demonstrated conclusively that neither the microcirculation in skeletal muscle nor its oxidative capacity limits $\dot{V}O_{2max}$. These workers developed a knee-extension model which allowed them to measure the blood flow to, and the oxygen uptake by, a carefully defined muscle mass (the quadriceps). Through measurements made when flow into and out of the lower leg was prevented by a tourniquet below the knee, it was shown that muscle blood flow can increase to 2.5 l kg^{-1} muscle min^{-1} and take up oxygen at a rate of about 0.35 l kg^{-1} muscle min^{-1}. If these values are extrapolated to exercise with most of the body's skeletal muscle mass (say, 30 kg), then maximum cardiac output would be more than 70 l min^{-1} and $\dot{V}O_{2max}$ nearly 10 l min^{-1}. Such values are clearly not attained, even by elite athletes, and these data show that the capacity of a small muscle mass to dilate and accept flow far exceeds that which can be accommodated by the cardiac output during exercise with the large muscle groups. Similar maximum values for blood flow and oxygen uptake are attained by older men (aged 44–69 years) performing the same exercise (Magnusson *et al.*, 1994).

These studies, besides helping address the limitation to $\dot{V}O_{2max}$, allow some further appreciation of the mechanisms of cardiovascular regulation during extreme challenge. The interpretation is that when the muscle mass engaged exceeds some threshold, there exists the possibility for a mismatch between cardiac output and vascular conductance. Put another way, the maximum output cannot maintain blood pressure in the face of this degree of vascular conductance in active muscle. In these circumstances it is likely that sympathetically induced vasoconstriction reduces flow in active muscle, preventing a fall in pressure. This suggestion is consistent with increased noradrenaline 'spill-over' when additional muscle mass is activated (Savard *et al.*, 1989). The proportion of muscle mass that needs to be engaged before this mechanism is evident is not known but is probably somewhat less than that involved during dynamic exercise with two legs (Savard *et al.*, 1987). This speculation fits with observations by Davies and Sargeant who used a one-leg training model to provide indirect evidence on this (Davies and Sargeant, 1975). Their subjects trained each leg separately on three occasions over a 5–6 week period, i.e. each leg was trained during every training session but always whilst the contralateral leg remained inactive. Before and after the training period $\dot{V}O_{2max}$ was determined during exercise with each leg separately and also during two-leg cycling. The main finding was that the increment in oxygen uptake during two-leg cycling (0.14 l min^{-1} or 4.7 per cent) did not approach that observed during one-leg cycling (on average 0.34 l min^{-1} or 14 per cent). The enhanced capability of each well-trained leg for oxygen uptake could not be met by the cardiac output in circumstances where the muscle groups of both legs were active at the same time.

This speculation is supported by direct observations of cardiac output, leg blood flow and oxygen uptake when an already large active muscle mass is increased further (Secher *et al.*, 1977). Measurements were made first when subjects were exercising on a cycle ergometer at nearly 70 per cent $\dot{V}O_{2max}$ and repeated after the addition of arm cranking, whilst maintaining the same power output with the legs. The addition of arm exercise caused a reduction in leg blood flow and leg oxygen uptake, with no change in mean arterial pressure. These findings demonstrate again that vasoconstriction of active muscle is needed during intense exercise with a large muscle mass in order for cardiac output to be maintained at a level sufficient to maintain arterial blood pressure.

In summary, the limitation to $\dot{V}O_{2max}$ for most ordinarily active individuals is the central cardiovascular capacity, or maximum cardiac output. For a few elite endurance athletes who can generate a remarkably high output, the pulmonary diffusion capacity may be exceeded and impose a limit to uptake. Different factors are also limiting in some patients where specific pathology impairs one aspect of oxygen transport. For example, in patients with chronic obstructive lung disease inadequate diffusion capacity will restrict oxygen uptake and oxygen desaturation on effort is a common feature of the disease. Peak values in this group range from 9 ml kg^{-1} min^{-1} in those with end-stage lung disease (Cahalin *et al.*, 1995) to, more typically, 14–22 ml kg^{-1} min^{-1} (Punzal *et al.*, 1991), and exercise capacity is low accordingly. (The term 'peak' is to be preferred when the maximum value for oxygen uptake is not dictated by central cardiovascular capacity.) Patients with myocardial infarction also possess low values but these can be increased through exercise rehabilitation, reflecting both recovery of pathology and improved fitness (Hardman, 1998). In peripheral vascular disease the local blood flow is inadequate, but here again regular exercise can contribute to disease management through increasing the oxidative capacity of the leg muscles, delaying the onset of fatigue and increasing walking tolerance (Mannarino *et al.*, 1989).

Changes in cardiorespiratory responses with training

This is an area that has been the subject of considerable research which can only be referred to briefly here. The increase in $\dot{V}O_{2max}$ with training was first 'mapped out' in the late 1960s. In healthy but initially inactive young men this is commonly of the order of 16 per cent, changing from, say, 44 to 53 ml kg^{-1} min^{-1} (see Saltin and Rowell, 1980). The magnitude of the increase is dependent, however, on the initial level of $\dot{V}O_{2max}$, persons with lower values showing the greater increase with training. Deconditioning results in a reduction in $\dot{V}O_{2max}$; for example, a decrease of 26 per cent was observed over 21 days of complete bed-rest, all of this accounted for by a decrease in stroke volume at $\dot{V}O_{2max}$ (Saltin *et al.*, 1968).

The close coupling between arterially delivered oxygen and $\dot{V}O_{2max}$ over a wide range of situations points to the heart's capability for oxygen delivery as being crucial to the training response (Figure 2.6). In line with cross-sectional studies (Table 2.1), most of the increase is due to increased maximum cardiac output and specifically to maximum stroke volume as maximum heart rate shows little change. Explanations for the training-induced improvements in stroke volume vary but commonly involve increased filling pressure (sometimes referred to as preload) which, by the Frank–Starling mechanism, will increase stroke volume. Certainly end diastolic volume is reported to be higher in well-trained people and there is evidence of an increase with training. However, the size of the left ventricular cavity (measured using echocardiography) also increases with endurance training and might contribute. Significant relationships have been found between heart size, $\dot{V}O_{2max}$, cardiac output and stroke volume, and cardiac dimensions increase with training. Changes in the myocardial state are unlikely to contribute as the ventricle empties well

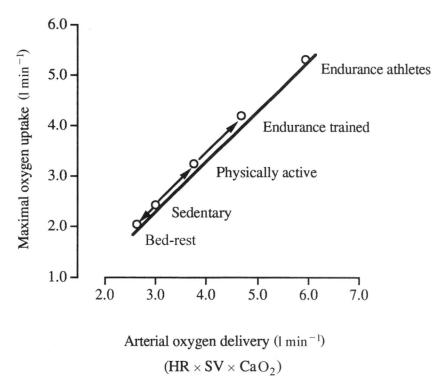

Figure 2.6. Schematic illustration of the close relationship between arterially delivered oxygen during exhausting exercise and maximal oxygen uptake. (After Saltin, 1990)

even in untrained individuals, the left ventricular ejection fraction being about 85 per cent.

Increased maximum cardiac output means a higher rate of blood flow through skeletal muscle in the trained state but capillary transit time is protected through improvements in the microcirculation which maintain capillary blood volume. Increases in this factor of about 20 per cent are reported after short periods of training, and of up to 60 per cent after many years of training (Saltin and Rowell, 1980).

There are profound changes in the responses to submaximum exercise at a standard level. The total metabolic demand, measured by the oxygen uptake, remains largely unaltered, as does the cardiac output to which this is tightly coupled. Heart rate is lowered – the classic bradycardia of training – so output is maintained through enhancement of stroke volume. Diffusion is improved in muscle as a result of better capillarization, particularly around the fibres which exhibit the highest oxidative capacity (type I). This, together with the considerable metabolic changes within muscle, improves oxygen extraction across muscle so that the unchanged metabolic demand can be met through lower muscle blood flow. Consequently, the restriction of blood flow in peripheral circulation is less pronounced with training, i.e. flow to hepatic and splanchnic beds is compromised less.

Metabolic adaptations in skeletal muscle influence oxygen kinetics at the start of exercise or when adjusting to a new, higher level so that a steady state is more rapidly achieved after endurance training (Hagberg *et al.*, 1980). This reflects better metabolic regulation probably arising from more rapid response to imbalance between concentrations of ADP and ATP.

In contrast to its profound effects on cardiovascular functioning, there is little effect of training on pulmonary function – as might be expected if the limitation to oxygen transport lies elsewhere. Vital capacity remains unchanged but the ventilation during standard, submaximum exercise is reduced, particularly at high intensities. This probably arises from a reduction in ventilatory drive following the fall in pH associated with a high glycolytic rate in skeletal muscle. Reduced ventilation is thus a consequence of metabolic adaptations in skeletal muscle. During maximum exercise ventilation is higher in the trained state, probably through increased carbon dioxide production associated with the increased $\dot{V}O_{2max}$.

Changes in $\dot{V}O_{2max}$ with aging

Evidence from cross-sectional and longitudinal studies shows that, as sedentary men age, their $\dot{V}O_{2max}$ decreases at a rate of approximately 0.45 ml kg^{-1} min^{-1} per year (Hagberg, 1987). For the average 25 year old this is equivalent to some 10 per cent per decade after the age of 25. Not all the decline is attributable directly to the aging process *per se*, as people generally become less physically active as they age and, in Western societies at least, tend to become fatter. In addition, the incidence of relevant pathologies increases. Physiological determinants of the age-related decline include a decrease in the maximum heart rate that can be achieved and a decrease in muscle mass.

The extent to which continued training over years alters the age-related decline is uncertain. The prevailing view used to be that the rate of decline is smaller in endurance-trained individuals than in sedentary men (Hagberg, 1987). Doubt exists now, however, as other evidence suggests that the decline in endurance athletes is as least as great as in sedentary men (Saltin, 1990). Less information is available for women but meta-analysis of such data (total of 4884 subjects) found a slower rate of decline in $\dot{V}O_{2max}$ in sedentary women (3.5 ml kg^{-1} min^{-1} per decade) than in endurance-trained women (6.2 ml kg^{-1} min^{-1} per decade) (Fitzgerald *et al.*, 1997). These findings may be explained on the basis of 'baseline' effects; initially high levels of both $\dot{V}O_{2max}$ and the overall exercise stimulus, i.e. physical activity level, may change proportionately more over the years than low levels. This fits with the fact that percentage decline in $\dot{V}O_{2max}$ from levels at about 25 years was similar. However, the declines in maximum heart rate did not differ according to activity level (7.0–7.9 bpm per decade), suggesting that other factors were responsible for the different rates of decline in $\dot{V}O_{2max}$.

Even if the age-related decline in $\dot{V}O_{2max}$ is greater in trained individuals, it should be emphasized that these men and women retain higher values than their sedentary peers, with an associated advantage in the ability to perform physical tasks. Differences in endurance capacity, a parameter which depends on the oxidative capacity of muscle rather than on $\dot{V}O_{2max}$, are especially clear between sedentary and endurance-trained men. An example is given by Grimby (Grimby, 1986) who reports data for middle-aged orienteers who were studied for 18 years. Despite a 30 per cent decrease in $\dot{V}O_{2max}$ (52 to 38 ml kg^{-1} min^{-1}) the muscles of these men retained a high oxidative capacity – much higher than in young men with comparable $\dot{V}O_{2max}$ values.

During the late 1980s and the 1990s much new information has emerged to describe the responses to increased physical activity levels in older people. The consensus is that the cardiorespiratory adaptations are qualitatively similar to those recorded for young people (Haskell and Phillips, 1995). Training causes a marked bradycardia during submaximum exercise which, together with a decrease in mean arterial blood pressure, must decrease cardiac work. Improvements in $\dot{V}O_{2max}$ between 22 and 30 per cent have been reported and, perhaps because of the low initial fitness levels, increases are found even after rather low-intensity training.

Summary

Cardiorespiratory responses to dynamic exercise serve to maintain delivery of oxygen and removal of carbon dioxide at rates which match the metabolic demand of active skeletal muscle. Thus the muscle metabolic rate and the mass of muscle engaged are major determinants of the magnitude of these responses. Cardiac output is closely coupled to muscle metabolic rate through haemodynamic and local metabolic mechanisms. Whilst this relationship is fixed, and has to be to fulfil the laws of bioenergetics, other responses (heart rate, peripheral distribution of cardiac output, rise in deep body temperature) are determined instead by the proportion of the individual's $\dot{V}O_{2max}$ that a particular exercise elicits. In turn, these factors dictate the individual's perception of the intensity of effort and the potential of that effort to stimulate a training response.

References

Andersen, P. and Saltin, B. (1985). Maximum perfusion of skeletal muscle in man. *J. Physiol.,* **366**, 233–249.

Åstrand, I. (1960). Aerobic work capacity in men and women with special reference to age. *Acta Physiol. Scand.,* **49** (Suppl.), 169.

Åstrand, P.-O. and Rodahl, K. (1986). *Textbook of Work Physiology. Physiological Bases of Exercise.* McGraw-Hill.

Brengelmann, G.L., Johnson, J.M., Hermansen, L. and Rowell, L.B. (1977). Altered control of skin blood flow during exercise at high internal temperature. *J. Appl. Physiol.,* **43**, 790–794.

Brooks, G. A. (1985). Anaerobic threshold: review of the concept and directions for future research. *Med. Sci. Sports Exerc.,* **17**, 22–31.

Cahalin, L. P., Pappagianopoulos, P., Prevost, S. *et al.* (1995). The relationship of the 6-minute walk test to maximum oxygen consumption in transplant candidates with end-stage lung disease. *Chest,* **108**, 452–459.

Conley, D. L. and Krahenbuhl, G. (1980). Running economy and distance running performance of highly trained athletes. *Med. Sci. Sports,* **12**, 357–360.

Costill, D. L. (1984). Energy supply during endurance activities. *Int.J. Sports Med.,* **5**, 19–21.

Costill, D. L., Thomason, H. and Roberts, E. (1973). Fractional utilization of the aerobic capacity during distance running. *Med. Sci. Sports,* **5**, 248–252.

Davies, C. T. M. and Sargeant, A. J. (1975). Effects of training on the physiological responses to one- and two-leg work. *J. Appl. Physiol.,* **38**, 377–381.

Ekblöm, B., Huot, R., Stein, E.M. and Thorstensson, A.T. (1975). Effect of changes in arterial oxygen content on circulation and physical performance. *J. Appl. Physiol.,* **39**, 71–75.

Ekblöm, B., Wilson, G. and Åstrand, P.-O. (1976). Central circulation during exercise after venesection and reinfusion of red blood cells. *J. Appl. Physiol.,* **40**, 379–383.

Fitzgerald, M. D., Tanaka, H., Tran, Z. V. and Seals, D. R. (1997). Age-related declines in maximum aerobic capacity in regularly exercising vs. sedentary women: a meta-analysis. *J. Appl. Physiol.,* **83**, 160–165.

Grimby, G. (1986). Physical activity and muscle training in the elderly. In *Physical Activity in Health and Disease* (P.-O. Åstrand and G.Grimby, eds), pp. 233–237. Almqvist and Wiskell.

Hagberg, J. M. (1987). Effect of training on the decline of $\dot{V}O_{2max}$ with aging. *Fed. Proc.,* **46**, 1830–1833.

Hagberg, J. M., Coyle, E.F., Carroll, J. E., Miller, J. M., Martin, W. H. and Brooke, M. H. (1982). Exercise hyperventilation in patients with McArdle's disease. *J. Appl. Physiol.*, **52**, 991–994.

Hagberg, J. M., Hickson, R. C., Ehsani, A. A. and Holloszy, J. O. (1980). Faster adjustment to and recovery from submaximum exercise in the trained state. *J. Appl. Physiol.*, **48**, 218–224.

Hardman, A. E. (1998). The exercise component. In: *Cardiac Rehabilitation: Guidelines and Audit Standards* (D. R. Thompson, G. S. Bowman, D. de Bono and A. Hopkins, eds), pp. 61–77. Royal College of Physicians.

Haskell, W. L. and Phillips, W. T. (1995). Exercise training, fitness, health, and longevity. In *Perspectives in Exercise Sciences and Sports Medicine. Volume 8: Exercise in Older Adults* (D.R. Lamb, C.V. Gisolfi and E. Nadel, eds), pp. 11– 52. Cooper, Carmel.

Henriksson, J. and Reitman, J. S. (1977). Time course of changes in human skeletal muscle succinate dehydrogenase and cytochrome oxidase activities and maximum oxygen uptake with physical activity and inactivity. *Acta Physiol. Scand.*, **99**, 91–97.

Hill, A. V. and Lupton, H. (1923). Muscular exercise, lactic acid, and the supply and utilization of oxygen. *Quart. J. Med.*, **16**, 135–171.

Magnusson, G., Kaijser, L., Isberg, B. and Saltin, B. (1994). Cardiovascular responses during one- and two-legged exercise in middle-aged men. *Acta Physiol. Scand.*, **150**, 353–362.

Mannarino, E., Pasqualini, L., Menna, M., Maragoni, G. and Orlandi, V. (1989). Effects of physical training on peripheral vascular disease: a controlled study. *Angiology*, **40**, 6–10.

Powers, S.K., Lawler, J., Dempsey, J.A., Dodd, S. and Landry, G. (1989). Effects of incomplete pulmonary gas exchange of VO_{2max}. *J. Appl. Physiol.*, **66**, 2491–2495.

Punzal, P.A., Ries, A.L., Kaplan, R.M. and Prewitt, L.M. (1991). Maximum intensity exercise training in patients with chronic obstructive pulmonary disease. *Chest*, **100**, 618–623.

Rowell, L.B. (1993). *Human Cardiovascular Control*. Oxford University Press.

Saltin, B. (1990). Cardiovascular and pulmonary adaptation to physical activity. In *Exercise, Fitness, and Health: A Consensus of Current Knowledge* (C. Bouchard, R.J. Shephard, T. Stephens, J.R. Sutton and B.D. McPherson, eds), pp. 187–203. Human Kinetics.

Saltin, B., Blomqvist, G., Mitchell, J.H., Johnson, R.L., Wildenthal, K. and Chapmann, C.B. (1968). Response to exercise after bed rest and after training. *Circulation*, **38**, VII-1–VII-78.

Saltin, B. and Hermansen, L. (1966). Esophageal, rectal, and muscle temperature during exercise. *J. Appl. Physiol.*, **21**, 1757–1762.

Saltin, B. and Karlsson, J. (1971). Muscle glycogen utilization during work of different intensities. In *Muscle Metabolism During Exercise* (B. Pernow and B. Saltin, eds), pp. 289–299. Plenum.

Saltin, B. and Rowell, L.B. (1980). Functional adaptations to physical activity and inactivity. *Fed. Proc.*, **39**, 1506–1513.

Savard, G., Kiens, B. and Saltin, B. (1987). Central cardiovascular factors as limits to endurance; with a note on the distinction between maximum oxygen uptake and endurance fitness. In *Exercise: Benefits, Limits and Adaptations* (D. Macleod, R. Maughan, M. Nimmo, T. Reilly and C. Williams, eds), pp. 162–180. Spon.

Savard, G.K., Richter, E.A., Strange, S., Kiens, B., Christensen, N.-J. and Saltin, B. (1989). Norepinephrine spillover from skeletal muscle during exercise in humans: role of muscle mass. *Am. J. Physiol.*, **257**, H1812–H1818.

Secher, N.H., Clausen, J.P. and Klausen, K. (1977). Central and regional circulatory effects of adding arm exercise to leg exercise. *Acta Physiol. Scand.*, **100**, 288–297.

Sjödin, B. and Svedenhag, J. (1992). Oxygen uptake during running as related to body mass in circumpubertal boys: a longitudinal study. *Eur. J. Appl. Physiol.*, **65**, 150–157.

Williams, C. (1981). The biological basis of aptitude; the endurance runner. *J. Biosocial Sci.*, **13**, Suppl. 710, 103–112.

Williams, C. and Nute, M.L.G. (1983). Some physiological demands of a half-marathon race on recreational runners. *Br. J. Sports Med.* **17**, 152–161.

Further reading

Babcock, M.A. and Dempsey, J.A. (1994). Pulmonary system adaptations: limitations to exercise. In *Physical Activity, Fitness and Health* (C. Bouchard, R.J. Shephard and T. Stephens, eds), pp. 320–330. Human Kinetics.

Howley, E.T, Bassett, D.R. and Welch, H.G. (1995). Criteria for maximal oxygen uptake: review and commentary. *Med. Sci. Sports Exerc.*, **27**, 1292–1301.

Mitchell, J.H. and Raven, P.B. (1994). Cardiovascular adaptation to physical activity. In *Physical Activity, Fitness and Health* (C. Bouchard, R.J. Shephard and T. Stephens, eds), pp. 286–301. Human Kinetics.

Saltin, B. (1990). Cardiovascular and pulmonary adaptation to physical activity. In *Exercise, Fitness and Health. A Consensus of Current Knowledge* (C. Bouchard, R.J. Shephard, T. Stephens, J.R. Sutton and B.D. McPherson, eds), pp. 187–215. Human Kinetics.

Saltin, B. and Rowell, L.B. (1980). Functional adaptations to physical activity and inactivity. *Fed. Proc.*, **39**, 1506–1513.

3

The biochemical basis of exercise

Paul L. Greenhaff and Eric Hultman

During exercise the energy demands of muscle contraction will fluctuate enormously. For muscle contraction to occur, chemical energy stored in the form of ATP must be converted into mechanical energy at rates appropriate to the needs of the muscle. However, the muscle store of ATP is relatively small (24 mmol kg^{-1} dry muscle (dm)), and for exercise to continue beyond a few seconds ATP must be resynthesized using free energy liberated by phosphocreatine (PCr), carbohydrate and fat degradation. Compared with other tissues, skeletal muscle contains a large reservoir of PCr, amounting to 70–80 mmol kg^{-1} dm at rest. PCr utilization occurs at the immediate onset of contraction to buffer the rapid accumulation of ADP resulting from ATP hydrolysis in the multitude of energy-requiring processes of muscle contraction and relaxation. Indeed, the momentary rise in ADP concentration is the primary stimulus to PCr hydrolysis via the creatine kinase reaction. For each mole of PCr degraded one mole of ATP is resynthesized via creatine kinase.

It is generally accepted that carbohydrate is the major substrate for ATP resynthesis during intense exercise. The carbohydrate stores of the body are principally located in skeletal muscle and liver, with small amounts also being found in the form of circulating glucose. The amount of energy stored as glycogen amounts to $\sim$ 6000 kJ and 1500 kJ in muscle and liver, respectively, which is very small compared with the body store of triacylglycerol (340 000 kJ), the alternative fuel for ATP resynthesis. Triacylglycerol is the preferred substrate for energy production in resting muscle and can cover the energy demands of exercise up to $\sim$ 50% of maximal oxygen consumption. At higher exercise intensities the relative contribution of fat to total energy production falls and carbohydrate oxidation increases, such that carbohydrate is the sole fuel oxidized at the highest exercise intensities. This is due to the increased recruitment of glycolytic type II muscle fibres and the activation of glycolytic enzymes when ATP turnover is increased. Further, the maximal rate of ATP production from lipid is lower than that of carbohydrate, as is the ATP yield per mole of oxygen utilized. In contrast with lipid, carbohydrate can be metabolized anaerobically via glycolysis. The resynthesis of ATP and lactate accumulation that occurs almost instantaneously at the onset of contraction demonstrates that the activation of this pathway is extremely rapid. It should be noted that the anaerobic utilization of carbohydrate will be indispensable during the transition from rest to steady-state exercise and during maximal exercise. Furthermore, the relatively small store of body carbohydrate will limit exercise performance during prolonged intense exercise due to the depletion of muscle and liver glycogen stores.

The body store and maximal rates of ATP resynthesis from phosphocreatine, carbohydrate and lipid are shown in Table 3.1.

ATP: the energy currency of the cell

As depicted in Figure 3.1, the free energy released during the degradation of PCr, carbohydrates and fat is stored in the compound ATP; hence the terms 'high-energy phosphate' or 'phosphagen', which are commonly used to describe this compound. ATP is the only form of chemical energy that can be converted into other forms of energy used by living cells. For example, the hydrolysis of ATP to ADP and P_i by skeletal muscle liberates free energy enabling contraction to occur. Furthermore, the cellular concentrations of ATP, ADP and P_i are such that the ΔG of the adenylate kinase reactions (also known as the myokinase reactions) depicted below are large and negative, thereby enabling enough chemical energy to be converted into mechanical work to produce movement.

$$ATP \rightarrow ADP + P_i \text{ and } ATP \rightarrow AMP + 2P_i$$

It has been shown that muscles can perform up to 24 kJ of work for each mole of ATP degraded. It follows, therefore, that the ΔG for ATP hydrolysis must be greater than 24 kJ mol^{-1}. It is also worth noting that the component parts of the adenylate kinase reaction are interconvertible without any net change in ΔG:

Table 3.1. The amounts of substrate available and the maximal rates of energy production from phosphocreatine, carbohydrate and lipid in a 70 kg man (of estimated muscle mass 28 kg)

	Amount available (mol)	Production rate (mol)(mol min^{-1})
ATP, PCr → ADP, Cr	0.67	4.40
Muscle glycogen → lactate	6.70*	2.35
Muscle glycogen → CO$_2$	84	0.85–1.14
Liver glycogen → CO$_2$	19	0.37
Fatty acids → CO$_2$	4000*	0.40

* These pathways of substrate utilization will not be fully utilized during exercise.

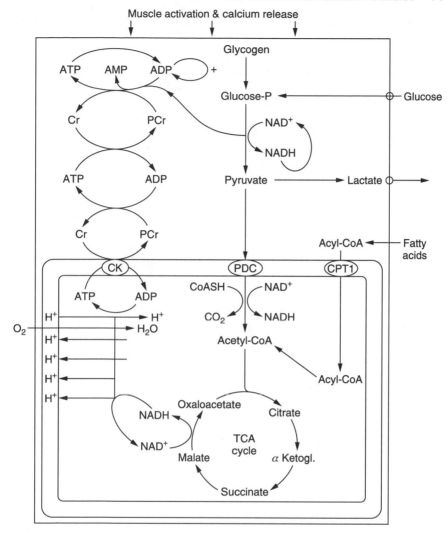

Figure 3.1. Schematic illustration of skeletal muscle energy turnover

$$ATP + AMP \leftrightarrow ADP + ADP$$

Adenosine triphosphate is an adenine nucleotide consisting of a purine base adenine, a five-carbon sugar ribose and a triphosphate unit. Generally, the most metabolically active form of ATP is the magnesium salt and the most interesting part of the compound in terms of exercise metabolism is the triphosphate unit. The sequential hydrolysis of the two terminal phosphate bonds in the adenylate kinase reactions releases a substantial amount of free energy that is used to drive a myriad of energy requiring reactions and processes, including muscle contraction, the pumping of ions across membranes and all reactions involved in the synthesis of complex compounds:

$$ATP + H_2O \rightarrow ADP + P_i + H^+ \Delta G = -31 \text{ kJ mol}^{-1}$$

$$ATP + H_2O \rightarrow AMP + P_i + H^+ \Delta G = -31 \text{ kJ mol}^{-1}$$

It should be noted that there is nothing particularly special about the phosphate bonds in the above reactions. Their importance lies in that they release free energy when hydrolysed.

Due to its unique role in energy production, ATP has been termed the energy currency of the cell. However, unlike currency, ATP cannot be accumulated in large amounts and the intramuscular ATP store is limited to 24 mmol kg^{-1} dry material. Indeed, as will be discussed later, given that changes in the cellular concentrations of ATP, ADP and AMP are involved in the regulation of many metabolic processes, it would be unwise to simply increase the cellular store of ATP.

Phosphocreatine: the spatial and temporal energy buffer

Phosphocreatine is restricted to the cytoplasm of the muscle cell where it is present at a concentration of about 75 mmol kg^{-1} dm. The rapid degradation of PCr at the onset of submaximal exercise and during high intensity exercise occurs because it has a higher phosphate group transfer potential than ATP. This means that the free energy of PCr hydrolysis (-43 kJ mol^{-1}) is greater than that of ATP (-31 kJ mol^{-1}), resulting in a greater likelihood for free energy transfer to occur from PCr to ADP to re-form ATP:

$$ADP + PCr + H^+ \rightarrow ATP + Cr$$

The above reaction is catalysed by creatine kinase and functions to maintain ATP homeostasis during contraction. Indeed, the rate at which this reaction can occur is far in excess of any of the ATP utilizing reactions occurring in the cell, and it is not unusual for the muscle PCr store to be completely degraded during maximal exercise.

It is now clear that creatine kinase has a number of isoenzymes (variations of the enzyme, having a slightly different structure but the same substrate specificity), which are located at different intracellular locations. At least three are known to be present in skeletal muscle. For example, MM-CK is located near the sites of muscle cross-bridge formation (i.e. near a site of ATP utilization) and Mi-CK is located at the mitochondrial membrane (i.e. near the site of ATP production). The discovery of the existence of isoenzymes of creatine kinase with discrete cellular locations has led to the hypothesis that PCr may have a number of different functions within skeletal muscle. The first, and possibly the most important, relates to its function described above, i.e. acting as a temporal buffer to maintain the cellular ATP concentration and ATP:ADP ratio. A second function, which is currently the subject of much debate, is that PCr may act as a spatial energy buffer, i.e. an energy transport system between the site of ATP production (the mitochondria) and the sites of ATP utilization (e.g. the myofibrils). This suggested function has resulted in the use of the phrase 'the PCr shuttle'. Those researchers in favour of its existence have gone on to suggest that the primary role for PCr in type I muscle fibres may be to operate as a spatial buffer, which contrasts with its suggested principal role in type II fibres as a temporal energy buffer. The 10–20 mmol kg^{-1} dm higher concentration of PCr found in type II fibres supports this suggestion. A third suggested function for PCr is its functional coupling with several other cellular reactions, which facilitates the integration of energy metabolism during muscle contraction. For example, it is clear from the reactions described above that the adenylate kinase reaction will result in the generation of H$^+$ and the creatine kinase reaction will result in the sequestering of H$^+$; it is the functional coupling of these two reactions that prevents the rapid acidification of the cell at the onset of contraction. Similarly, the rapid liberation of Pi by PCr hydrolysis during contraction plays an integral part in the activation of glycogen phosphorylase at the onset of exercise, thereby ensuring that energy production is maintained.

During the early 1960s, it was thought that the initial 10–15 sec of maximal exercise was fuelled almost solely by PCr degradation. This belief arose as a consequence of PCr being stored in the cytosol in close proximity to the sites of energy utilization and because PCr hydrolysis does not depend on oxygen availability or necessitate the completion of several metabolic reactions before energy is liberated to fuel ATP resynthesis. Whilst it is now accepted that anaerobic metabolism of glycogen also makes a significant contribution to ATP resynthesis during the initial seconds of high intensity exercise, the importance of PCr hydrolysis lies in the extremely rapid rates at which it can resynthesis ATP (Table 3.1). As will be discussed later, this is especially important during maximal short-duration exercise.

Muscle carbohydrate utilization: the principal mainstay of ATP resynthesis

Glycogenolysis is the hydrolysis of muscle glycogen to glucose-1-phosphate, which is transformed to glucose-6-phosphate via a phosphoglucomutase reaction. The glucose-6-phosphate formed, together with that derived from the phosphorylation of blood glucose by hexokinase at the muscle cell membrane, enters the glycolytic pathway which is a series of reactions involved in the degradation of glucose-6-phosphate to pyruvate (Figure 3.1).

Glycogenolysis

The integrative nature of energy metabolism ensures that the activation of muscle contraction by Ca^{2+} and the accumulation of the products of ATP and PCr hydrolysis (ADP, AMP, IMP, NH_3 and P_i) act as stimulators of glycogenolysis, and in this way guarantee that ATP production is maintained. The control of glycogenolysis during muscle contraction is a highly complex mechanism which can no longer be considered to centre only around the degree of Ca^{2+}-induced transformation of less active glycogen phosphorylase b to the more active a form, as is suggested in many textbooks. For some time it has been known that glycogenolysis can proceed at a negligible rate, despite almost total transformation of phosphorylase to the a form, for example following adrenaline infusion (Chasiotis et al., 1983). Conversely, an increase in glycogenolytic rate has been observed during circulatory occlusion, despite a relatively low mole fraction of the phosphorylase a form (Chasiotis, 1983). From this and other related work, it was concluded that P_i accumulation arising from ATP and PCr hydrolysis played a key role in the regulation of the glycogenolytic activity of phosphorylase a, and by doing so served as a link between the energy demand of the contraction and the rate of carbohydrate utilization (Chasiotis, 1983). However, the findings that glycogenolysis can occur within 2 sec of the onset of muscle contraction in conjunction with only a small increase in P_i, and more recently, that glycogenolysis can proceed at a low rate despite a high phosphorylase a form and P_i concentration, suggests that factors other than the degree of Ca^{2+}-induced phosphorylase transformation and P_i availability are involved in the regulation of glycogenolysis (Ren and Hultman, 1989, 1990).

Classically both IMP and AMP have been associated with the regulation of glycogenolysis during exercise (Aragon et al., 1980; Lowry et al., 1964). IMP is thought to exert its effect by increasing the activity of phosphorylase b during contraction (apparent K_m of phosphorylase b for IMP ~ 1.2 mmol l^{-1} intracellular water). AMP has also been shown to increase the activity of phosphorylase b, but it is thought to require an unphysiological accumulation of free AMP to do so (apparent K_m of phosphorylase b for AMP ~ 1.0 mmol l^{-1} intracellular water). In vitro experiments have demonstrated that AMP can bring about a more marked effect on glycogenolysis by increasing the glycogenolytic activity of phosphorylase a (Lowry et al., 1964). However, because 90 per cent or more of the total cell content of AMP has been suggested to be bound to cell proteins in vivo, it has in the past been questioned whether the increase in free AMP during contraction is of a sufficient magnitude to affect the kinetics of phosphorylase a. More recent work, however, demonstrates that a small increase in AMP concentration (10 μmol l^{-1}) can markedly increase the *in vitro* activity of phosphorylase *a* (Ren and Hultman, 1990). Furthermore, *in vivo* evidence demonstrating a close relationship between muscle ATP turnover and glycogen utilization, suggests that an exercise-induced increase in free AMP and inorganic phosphate may be the key regulators of glycogen degradation during muscle contraction (Ren and Hultman, 1990).

Glycolysis

From the preceding discussions it can be seen that the rate of glycogen-olysis is determined by the activity of glycogen phosphorylase. However, it is the activity of phosphofructokinase (PFK) that dictates the overall rate of glycolytic flux (Tornheim and Lowenstein, 1976). Phosphofructokinase acts as a gate to the flow of hexose units through glycolysis and there is no other enzyme subsequent to PFK that is capable of matching flux rate with the physiological demand for ATP. Stimulation of glycogen phosphory-lase by adrenaline and/or exercise results in the accumulation of glucose-6-phosphate, demonstrating that PFK is the rate-limiting step in the degradation of hexose units to pyruvate (Richter *et al.*, 1986).

ATP is known to be the most potent allosteric inhibitor of PFK. The most important activators or deinhibitors of PFK are ADP, AMP, P_i, fructose-6-phosphate, glucose-1,6-bisphosphate, fructose-1,6- and -2,6-bisphosphates and, under extreme conditions, ammonia. Removal of the ATP-mediated inhibition of PFK during contraction, together with the accumulation of the positive modulators of PFK, is responsible for the increase in flux through the enzyme during exercise and thereby is responsible for matching glycolytic flux with the energy demand of contraction.

Hydrogen ion and citrate accumulation during contraction have been suggested to be capable of decreasing the activity of PFK, and thereby, the rate of glycolysis during intense exercise. However, it is now generally accepted that the extent of this inhibition of glycolysis during exercise is overcome in the *in vivo* situation by the accumulation of PFK activators (Spriet *et al.*, 1987).

Pyruvate oxidation

It has been accepted for some time that the rate-limiting step in carbohydrate oxidation is the decarboxylation of pyruvate to acetyl-CoA, which is controlled by the pyruvate dehydrogenase complex (PDC), and is essentially an irreversible reaction committing pyruvate to entry into the TCA cycle and oxidation (Wieland, 1983; Figure 3.1). The PDC is a conglomerate of three enzymes located within the inner mitochondrial membrane. Adding to its complexity, PDC also has two regulatory enzymes, a phosphatase and a kinase which regulate an activation/inactivation cycle. Increased ratios of ATP/ADP, acetyl-CoA/CoA and NADH/NAD$^+$ activate the kinase, resulting in the inactivation of the enzyme. Conversely, decreases in the above ratios and the presence of pyruvate will inactivate the kinase, whilst increases in calcium will activate the phosphatase, together resulting in the activation of PDC. Thus, it can be seen that the increases in calcium and pyruvate availability at the onset of contraction will result in the rapid activation of PDC. These factors, together with the subsequent decrease in the ATP/ADP ratio as contraction continues, will result in continued flux through the reaction (Constantin-Teodosiu *et al.*, 1991).

Following decarboxylation of pyruvate by the PDC reaction, acetyl CoA enters the TCA cycle resulting in the formation of citrate, which is catalysed by citrate synthase (Figure 3.1). The rate of flux through the TCA cycle is thought to be regulated by citrate synthase, isocitrate dehydrogenase and α-ketoglutarate dehydrogenase. The activity of these enzymes is controlled by the mitochondrial ratios of ATP:ADP and NADH:NAD$^+$. Good agreement has been found between the maximal activity of α-ketoglutarate dehydrogenase and flux through PDC and the TCA cycle.

The last stage in pyruvate oxidation involves NADH and FADH generated in the TCA cycle entering the electron transport chain. In the electron transport chain, NADH and FADH are oxidized and the energy generated is used to rephosphorylate ADP to ATP. The rate of flux through the electron transport chain will be regulated by the availability of NADH, oxygen and ADP (Chance and Williams, 1955). Finally, the translocation of ATP and ADP across the mitochondrial membrane is thought to be dependent on creatine in the mitochondrial creatine kinase reaction (Moreadith and Jacobus, 1982), thereby linking mitochondrial ATP production to the ATPase activity in the contractile system (Figure 3.1).

Lactate production

Considerable controversy exists concerning the exact mechanism responsible for lactate accumulation during intense muscle contraction. The most widely accepted theory attributes this to a high rate of energy demand coupled with an inadequate oxygen supply. In short, when tissue oxygen supply begins to limit oxidative ATP production, resulting in the accumulation of mitochondrial and cytosolic NADH, the flux through glycolysis and a high cytosolic NAD$^+$/NADH ratio are maintained by the reduction of pyruvate to lactate (Figure 3.1). However, it has been suggested that the reduction in mitochondrial redox state during contraction is insignificant, thereby indicating that reduced oxygen availability is not the only cause of lactate accumulation during contraction (Graham and Saltin, 1989). In addition, there are data to indicate that it is the activation of the PDC and acetyl group availability, and not oxygen availability, which primarily regulate lactate production during intense muscle contraction (Timmons *et al.*, 1996). Furthermore, it has also been shown that for any given workload, lactate accumulation can be significantly altered by pre-exercise dietary manipulation (Putman *et al.*, 1993). Taken together, these findings suggest that an imbalance between pyruvate formation and decarboxylation to acetyl-CoA will dictate the extent of lactate formation during exercise as seen, for example, during the transition period from rest to steady-state exercise.

Muscle fat utilization: the inadequately understood phenomenon

On a weight to weight basis, fat is approximately five times more efficient than carbohydrate as a storage fuel and, therefore, in terms of energy supply there would be a distinct advantage if fat was the principal fuel oxidized during prolonged exercise. Furthermore, Table 3.1 clearly demonstrates that fat constitutes the largest energy reserve in man, but unfortunately it also exhibits a low maximal rate of oxidation relative to muscle glycogen oxidation. Thus, fat oxidation has the ability to provide all of the muscle energy requirements during highly prolonged low intensity exercise (50 per cent of maximal oxygen consumption). However, as exercise intensity increases, the contribution of fat to energy delivery declines. The factors responsible for limiting the rate of fat oxidation during exercise are presently unclear and are the subject of intense debate. It would seem however that the limiting step must precede acetyl-CoA formation as from this point fat and carbohydrate share the same fate (Figure 3.1).

It is important to appreciate that the simultaneous utilization of fat and carbohydrate by skeletal muscle becomes increasingly important to maintaining muscle ATP production as exercise intensity and duration increase. By way of example, it can be calculated that if the elite marathon runner depended solely on carbohydrate as an energy source he would be exhausted after $\sim$ 90 min of running. As the world record for the marathon is close to 130 min, this clearly exemplifies the importance of fuel integration during prolonged exercise. However, the mechanisms by which muscle integrates the use of fat and liver and muscle glycogen during prolonged exercise are complex and unresolved.

It is widely accepted that the accumulation of acetyl-CoA and NADH resulting from fat oxidation can reduce the amount of PDC activation and its catalytic activity, thereby resulting in an inhibition of carbohydrate oxidation (Figure 3.1). This interaction forms the basis of the 'glucose–fatty acid cycle' proposed by Randle *et al.* (1963) which has for many years been accepted to be the key regulatory cycle in the integration of carbo-hydrate and fat utilization by skeletal muscle. However, a growing body of evidence is accumulating to suggest that the glucose-fatty acid cycle does not operate in contracting human skeletal muscle (Putman *et al.*, 1993; Dyke *et al.*, 1993; Putman *et al.*, 1995). For example, when acetyl group availability was forcibly increased using both intra-lipid and acet-ate infusion, consistent with the glucose–fatty acid cycle, PDC activation was reduced at rest. However, during subsequent intense cycling exercise the decrease in PDC activation seen at rest following infusion was over-come, such that no differences in PDC activation status was observed between the control and treatment groups. Despite this lack of an effect on PDC, muscle glycogen utilization during exercise was reduced by ~ 40 per cent following intra-lipid infusion. This led to the proposal that the glucose–fatty acid cycle does not operate in human skeletal muscle during prolonged moderate-intensity exercise and that the regulation of the inte-gration of carbohydrate and fat oxidation must reside elsewhere (e.g. at the level of muscle glucose uptake or glycogen phosphorylase). It should be stressed, however, that the exercise intensities performed in most, if not all, studies relating to PDC and exercise have been sufficient to saturate PDC activation by calcium and, therefore, outweigh any effect of acetyl-CoA and NADH on PDC transformation. It is not yet known whether the glucose–fatty acid cycle operates during very prolonged low-intensity exercise when calcium activation of PDC will be at its lowest.

An alternative focal point for the integration of carbohydrate and fat oxidation resides at the level of malonyl-CoA. It has been suggested that an increase in acetyl-CoA formation via the PDC reaction during exercise could result in the rapid formation of malonyl-CoA. The accumulation of malonyl-CoA has been shown to directly inhibit the enzyme carnitine palmityle transferase I (CPT I), which catalyses the rate-limiting step in the transport of long chain fatty acyl-CoA into the mitochondria, and would therefore presumably decrease fat oxidation (Figure 3.1). Conversely, its concentration has been shown to decline rather rapidly in rat skeletal muscle during contraction, presumably thereby increasing mitochondrial fat transport. The relevance of this finding to fuel substrate utilization is difficult to interpret because of a lack of other relevant mea-surements and time-course data. Furthermore, because the sensitivity of rat muscle CPT I for malonyl-CoA is relatively high, it has been calculated that even at low malonyl-CoA concentrations, CPT I and, therefore, fat oxidation would be completely inhibited which is clearly not the case. To date, the role of malonyl-CoA in the regulation of mitochondrial fat trans-port in human skeletal muscle during contraction has received relatively little attention, but the limited amount of information available indicates that it is not of any principal importance (Odland *et al.*, 1996). Undoubtedly future research will provide us with more information on this topic.

The integration of substrate utilization with respect to exercise intensity

Maximal exercise

During submaximal (steady state) exercise, ATP resynthesis can be adequately achieved by oxidative combustion of fat and carbohydrate stores. However, during high intensity (non-steady state) exercise the relatively slow activation and rate of energy delivery of oxidative phosphorylation cannot meet the energy requirements of contraction. In this situation, anaerobic energy delivery is essential for contraction to continue. Typically, oxidative energy delivery requires several minutes to reach a steady state, due principally to the number and complexity of reactions involved. Once achieved, the maximal rate of ATP production is in the region of ~ 2.5 mmol kg^{-1} dm sec^{-1}. On the other hand, anaerobic energy delivery is restricted to the cytosol and its activation is almost instantaneous and can deliver ATP at a rate in excess of 11 mmol kg^{-1} dm sec^{-1}. The downside, however, is that this can be maintained for only a few seconds before beginning to decline. Of course, oxidative and anaerobic ATP resynthesis should not be considered to function independently of one another. It has been demonstrated that as the duration of exercise increases the contribution from anaerobic energy delivery decreases, whilst that from aerobic is seen to increase.

Figure 3.2 shows that maximal ATP resynthesis from PCr and glycogen degradation can only be maintained for short time periods during maximal contraction in man (Hultman *et al.*, 1991). The rate of PCr degradation is at its maximum immediately after the initiation of contraction and begins to decline after only 1.3 sec. Conversely, the corresponding rate of glycolysis does not peak until after ~ 5 sec of contraction and does not begin to decline until after 20 sec of contraction. This suggests that the rapid utilization of PCr may buffer the momentary lag in energy provision from glycolysis, and that the contribution of the latter to ATP resynthesis rises as exercise duration increases and PCr availability declines. This point exemplifies the critical importance of PCr at the onset of contraction. Without this large hydrolysis of PCr, it is likely that muscle force production would almost instantaneously be impaired, which is indeed the case in muscles in which the PCr store has been replaced with a Cr analogue (Meyer *et al.*, 1986). It is also important to note that ultimately there is a progressive decline in the rate of ATP resynthesis from both substrates during this type of exercise. For example, during the last 10 sec of exercise depicted in Figure 3.2, the rate of ATP production from PCr hydrolysis had declined to ~ 2 per cent of the peak rate. Similarly, the corresponding rate of ATP resynthesis from glycogen hydrolysis had fallen to ~ 40 per cent.

The above example concerns exercise of maximal intensity lasting about 30 sec. However, non-steady state exercise, albeit less intense, can

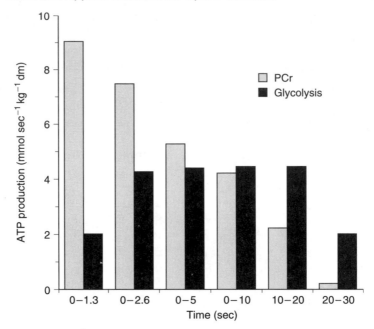

Figure 3.2. Rates of anaerobic ATP formation from phosphocreatine (PCr) and glycolysis during maximal intermittent electrically evoked isometric contraction in man (see Hultman *et al.*, 1991). Note that the reference base for the muscle date in the figures and text is dry muscle (dm). This is because the muscle samples were freeze dried prior to biochemical analysis. To convert to wet weight, values should be divided by 4.3. This assumes 1 kg of wet muscle contains 70 ml of extracellular water and 700 ml of intracellular water

be sustained for durations approaching 5 min before fatigue is evident. Under these conditions carbohydrate oxidation can make a major contribution to ATP production and therefore its importance should not be underestimated. For example, it has been demonstrated that during 3.2 min of fatiguing exercise oxidative phosphorylation can contribute as much as 55 per cent of total energy production (Bangsbo *et al.*, 1990). This indicates the importance of substrate oxidation during high intensity exercise. Under these conditions, muscle glycogen is the principal fuel utilized as muscle glucose uptake is inhibited by glucose-6-phosphate accumulation and adipose tissue lipolysis is inhibited by lactate accumulation.

Submaximal exercise

The term submaximal exercise is typically used to define exercise intensities which can be sustained for durations falling between 30–180 min. In practice, this is usually exercise intensities between 60–85 per cent of maximal oxygen consumption. Continuous exercise of any longer duration (i.e. an intensity <60 per cent of maximal oxygen consumption) is probably not limited by substrate availability and, providing adequate hydration is maintained, can probably be sustained for several hours or even days! Unlike maximal intensity exercise, the rate of muscle ATP production required during prolonged exercise is relatively low (<2.5 mmol sec^{-1} kg^{-1} dm) and, therefore, PCr, carbohydrate and fat can all contribute to ATP resynthesis. As already mentioned, it is important to note that anaerobic ATP delivery from PCr and glycogen utilization will make a significant contribution to ATP turnover at the onset of submaximal exercise, and that the magnitude of this contribution will be directly related to the intensity of the exercise performed (Hultman et al., 1967). Indeed, it has been demonstrated that there is a clear relationship between the rates of PCr hydrolysis, lactate production and exercise intensity at the onset of submaximal exercise. It is currently under debate whether these responses occur because of a lag in oxygen delivery and/ or inertia in the activation of mitochondrial ATP resynthesis (TCA cycle and oxidative phosphorylation) at the onset of contraction. Whatever the cause, this rapid hydrolysis of PCr and glycogen during the rest to exercise transition period is stimulated by the rapid rise in ADP concentration which occurs as consequence of energy delivery not matching ATP utilization. In physiological terms, this contribution from anaerobic metabolism to ATP resynthesis, whether at the onset of submaximal exercise or during high intensity exercise, appears as the oxygen deficit.

It can be calculated that the maximum rate of ATP production from carbohydrate oxidation will be $\sim$ 2.0–2.8 mmol sec^{-1} kg^{-1} dm (based upon a maximum oxygen consumption of 3–4 l min^{-1}), which corresponds to a glycogen utilization rate of $\sim$ 4 mmol min^{-1} kg^{-1} dm. Therefore, it can be seen that carbohydrate could meet the energy requirements of prolonged exercise. However, because the muscle store of glycogen is in the region of 350 mmol kg^{-1} dm, under normal conditions, it can be calculated that it could only sustain in the region of 80 min of exercise. This was first demonstrated in the 1960s by Bergstrom and Hultman (1967). The authors also demonstrated that if the glycogen store of muscle was increased by dietary means, exercise duration increased in parallel (Bergstrom et al., 1967). Of course, carbohydrate is also delivered to skeletal muscle from hepatic stores in the form of blood glucose and this can generate ATP at a maximum rate of $\sim$ 1 mmol sec^{-1} kg^{-1} dm.

The majority of hepatic glucose released during exercise (1.5–5.5 mmol min^{-1}) is utilized by skeletal muscle. Only 0.5 mmol min^{-1} is utilized by extramuscular tissue during exercise. Muscle glucose utilization is dependent on glucose supply, transport and metabolism. If blood glucose is unchanged, as in the majority of exercise conditions, glucose supply to muscle is dictated by muscle blood flow, which increases linearly with exercise intensity and can increase by 20-fold from rest to maximal exercise. The increase in muscle glucose delivery as a result of the exercise mediated increase in blood flow is probably more important for muscle glucose uptake during exercise than the insulin- and contraction-induced increase in membrane glucose transport capacity (see Richter and Hespel, 1996). As exercise continues, plasma insulin concentration declines which facilitates hepatic glucose release and reduces glucose utilization by extra-muscular tissue. However, insulin supply to muscle probably remains elevated above basal supply due to the contraction induced elevation in muscle blood flow.

Hexokinase is responsible for the phosphorylation of glucose by ATP when it enters the muscle cell (Figure 3.1). The enzyme is allosterically inhibited by glucose-6-phosphate, the product of the hexokinase reaction and an intermediate of glycolysis. Thus, during short-term, high-intensity exercise and at the onset of prolonged submaximal exercise, glucose phosphorylation by hexokinase will be inhibited by glucose-6-phosphate accumulation. This will increase the concentration of glucose in the extra- and intracellular water and will contribute to the increase in blood glucose observed during high intensity exercise. However, as submaximal exercise continues, the decline in muscle glucose-6-phosphate results in an increase in glucose phosphorylation.

In comparison with muscle glycogen metabolism relatively little is known about the interaction between exercise and hepatic glycogen metabolism in man. This is not because of a lack of interest but because of the invasive nature of the liver biopsy technique. The few studies that have been performed in healthy volunteers using this technique have demonstrated that the rate of liver glucose release in the post-absorptive state is in the region of 0.8 mmol glucose min^{-1}, which is sufficient to meet the carbohydrate demands of the brain and obligatory glucolytic tissues. Approximately 60 per cent of this release (0.5 mmol min^{-1}) is derived from liver glycogen stores and the remainder is synthesized by gluconeogenesis in the liver using lactate, pyruvate, glycerol and amino acids as substrates (Hultman and Nillson, 1971; Nilsson and Hultman, 1973).

The rate of hepatic glucose release during exercise in the post-absorptive state has been shown to be mainly a function of exercise intensity (Ahlborg et al., 1974; Ahlborg and Felig, 1982; Wahren et al., 1971; Hultman, 1967). The uptake of gluconeogenic precursors by the liver is only marginally increased during the initial 40 min of submaximal exercise but increases as exercise continues (Ahlborg et al., 1974). Most (>90 per cent) of the glucose release is derived from liver glycogenolysis resulting in a decline and ultimately depletion of liver glycogen stores. Direct measurements of liver glycogen concentration in the post-absorptive state and following 60 min of exercise at 75 per cent of maximal oxygen consumption showed a 50 per cent decrease in the liver glycogen concentration with exercise (Hultman and Nilsson, 1971). This corresponded to a glycogen degradation rate of 4.2 mmol min^{-1} (assuming 1.8 kg of liver) and suggested that the liver glycogen store would have been depleted within 120 min of exercise at this intensity.

The exact mechanisms responsible for the regulation of liver glucose release at the onset and during exercise are still unresolved. However, it is known that the decline in blood insulin concentration and increases in adrenaline and glucagon with increasing exercise duration together with afferent nervous feedback from contracting muscle will stimulate liver glucose release (for more complete information, see Kjar, 1995).

Biochemical responses across muscle fibre types

The conclusions presented so far have been based on metabolite changes measured in biopsy samples obtained from the quadriceps femoris muscle group. However, it is known that human skeletal muscle is composed of at least two functionally and metabolically different fibre types. Type I fibres are characterized as being slow contracting, fatigue resistant, having a low power output and favouring aerobic metabolism for ATP resynthesis during contraction. Conversely, in comparison, type II fibres are fast contracting, fatigue rapidly, have a high power output and favour mainly anaerobic metabolism for ATP resynthesis (Burke and Edgerton, 1975).

Maximal exercise

Evidence from animal studies performed on muscles composed of predominantly type I or type II fibres and from one study performed using bundles of similar human muscle fibre types, suggest that the rapid and marked rise and subsequent decline in maximal power output observed during intense muscle contraction in man may be closely related to activation and rapid fatigue of type II fibres during contraction (Faulkner *et al.*, 1986).

Figure 3.3 demonstrates glycogen degradation in type I and type II muscle fibres during maximal exercise under four different experimental conditions. Notice that during intense contraction the rates of glycogenolysis are higher in type II compared with type I fibres. This is true for both dynamic exercise (Greenhaff *et al.*, 1994, treadmill sprinting) and electrically induced isometric contractions (Greenhaff *et al.*, 1991, 1993). The rates of glycogenolysis observed in both fibre types during treadmill sprinting and intermittent isometric contraction with circulation occluded are in good agreement with the V_{max} of phosphorylase measured in both fibre types (Harris *et al.*, 1976), suggesting that glycogenolysis is occurring at a near maximal rate during intense exercise. Surprisingly, during intermittent isometric contraction with circulation intact, when the rest interval between contractions is of the order of 1.6 sec, the rate of glycogenolysis in type I fibres is almost negligible. The corresponding rate in type II fibres is almost maximal and similar to that seen during contraction with circulatory occlusion. This suggests that during maximal exercise glycogenoly-

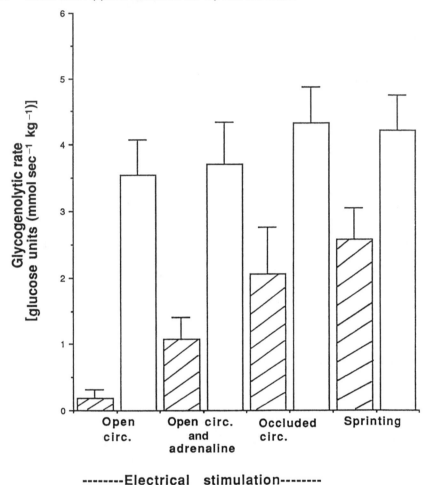

Figure 3.3. Glycogenolytic rates in type I (hatched bars) and type II (open bars) human muscle fibres during 30 s of intermittent electrically evoked maximal isometric contraction with intact circulation (circ.), intact circulation with adrenaline infusion, occluded circulation and during 30 s of maximal sprint running. (Based on Greenhaff *et al.*, 1991, Greenhaff *et al.*, 1993 and Greenhaff *et al.*, 1994)

sis in type II fibres is invariably occurring at a maximal rate, irrespective of the experimental conditions, while the rate in type I fibres is probably very much related to cellular oxygen availability.

Submaximal exercise

In contrast to maximal exercise, the rate of glycogenolysis during submaximal exercise is greatest in type I fibres, especially during the initial period of exercise (Ball-Burnett et al., 1990). This phenomenon is likely to be the result of differences in the recruitment pattern between muscle fibre types. If exercise is continued, glycogen utilization occurs in both fibre types but depletion is observed first in the type I muscle fibres. The consumption of carbohydrate during exhaustive submaximal treadmill running has been shown to offset the depletion of glycogen specifically in type I fibres (Tsintzas et al., 1996).

The biochemical basis of exercise-induced fatigue

What is clear from the literature is that glycogen availability *per se* is not usually considered to be responsible for fatigue development during maximal exercise, providing the pre-exercise glycogen store is not depleted to below 100 mmol kg^{-1} dm. It is even unlikely that glycogen availability will limit performance during repeated bouts of exercise, due to the decline in glycogenolysis and lactate production that occurs under these conditions. It is more probable that fatigue development during maximal exercise will be caused by a gradual decline in anaerobic ATP production caused by the depletion of PCr and a fall in the rate of glycogenolysis.

Lactic acid accumulation during high intensity exercise is considered to produce muscle fatigue as a result of H^+ and P_i accumulation. An increase in hydrogen ion concentration will negatively affect phosphorylase activity, thereby decreasing the rate of glycogenolysis, by delaying transformation of the *b* form to the *a* form (Danforth, 1965; Chasiotis, 1983) and by decreasing the availability of HPO_4^-, which is the substrate for phosphorylase. The inhibition of PFK discussed previously seems to be at least partly offset by an increase in the activators of PFK, especially ADP, AMP and P_i, when the rate of ATP utilization is higher than the rate of oxidative ATP resynthesis. The increase in P_i, especially the $H_2PO_4^-$ form, in acidotic muscle is known to have inhibitory effects on contractile function (Cook and Pate, 1985; Nosek et al., 1987). However, there is no evidence of a direct relationship between the decline in muscle force during contraction and H^+ accumulation. For example, studies involving human volunteers have demonstrated that muscle force generation following fatiguing exercise can recover rapidly, despite having a very low muscle pH value (Sahlin and Ren, 1989). The general consensus at the moment appears to be that the initial generation of muscle force production is dependent on the capacity to generate ATP but the maintenance of force generation is also pH dependent.

Despite the wealth of information showing that carbohydrate availability is essential to performance during submaximal exercise, the exact biochemical mechanism(s) by which fatigue is brought about in the carbohydrate-depleted state are still unclear. Recent evidence suggests that carbohydrate depletion will result in an inability to rephosphorylate ADP to ATP at the required rate, possibly because of a decrease in the rate of flux through the TCA cycle as a result of a decline in muscle TCA cycle intermediates (Sahlin *et al.*, 1990). The consequent rise in ADP concentration will bring about fatigue, perhaps as a direct inhibitory effect of ADP and/or P_i on contraction coupling.

Conclusions

It has been demonstrated that there is a direct relationship between exercise intensity and the magnitude of phosphocreatine degradation during exercise (Hultman *et al.*, 1967). Subsequently, studies indicated that the creatine kinase and adenylate kinase reactions are essentially at equilibrium under most conditions *in vivo* (Connett, 1988). This indicates there is a tight coupling between the components of the phosphate energy system (PCr, ATP, ADP, AMP and P_i), such that the decline in PCr during contraction will be matched by increases in free ADP and AMP concentrations.

Glycogen degradation is initiated by the release of Ca^{2+} from the sarcoplasmic reticulum at the immediate onset of contraction. The rate of glycogen hydrolysis and subsequent metabolism of glucose-1-phosphate is governed by the activation of glycogen phosphorylase, PFK and PDC. All three enzymes are regulated by complex control mechanisms through which metabolic signals reflecting exercise intensity and substrate availability are conveyed. In general, however, it would appear that the control of glycogenolysis, following the initial transformation of glycogen phosphorylase by Ca^{2+}, as well as the control of glycolysis by PFK, could be governed by changes in the components of the phosphate energy system. In the same way, the flux through PDC, following transformation by Ca^{2+} and pyruvate, will be dependent on the rate of pyruvate delivery from glycolysis and on the mitochondrial $NADH/NAD^+$ ratio, which will be determined by the extent of stimulation of the electron transport chain by ADP. Thus, taken together, these suggestions point to the phosphorylation state of the cell as being pivotal in the control of PCr and carbohydrate utilization during exercise.

Fat is the most abundant substrate available to man and has the ability to provide all of the muscle energy requirements during low-intensity exercise. It is known that as exercise intensity increases the contribution of fat oxidation to energy delivery declines. However, the mechanism by which this phenomenon occurs has not been resolved. This aside, it is important to appreciate that the contribution of fat oxidation to ATP resynthesis is important to the maintenance of energy delivery at most exercise intensities, and especially as exercise duration increases. However, the mechanisms by which muscle integrates the use of fat and liver and muscle glycogen during prolonged exercise are complex and uncertain.

References

Ahlborg, G., Felig, P., Hagenfeldt, L., Hendler, R. and Wahren, J. (1974). Substrate turnover during prolonged exercise in man. Splanchnic and leg metabolism of glucose, free fatty acids and amino acids. *J.. Clin. Investigation*, **53**, 1080–1090.

Ahlborg, G. and Felig, P. (1982). Lactate and glucose exchange across the forearm, legs and splanchnic bed during and after prolonged leg exercise. *J. Clin. Investigation*, **69**, 45–54.

Aragon, J.J., Tornheim, K. and Lowenstein, J.M. (1980). On a possible role of IMP in the regulation of phosphorylase activity in skeletal muscle. *FEBS Letts*, **117**, K56–K64.

Ball-Burnett, M., Green, H.J. and Houston, M.E. (1991). Energy metabolism in human slow and fast twitch fibres during prolonged cycle exercise. *J. Physiol.*, **437**, 257–267.

Bangsbo, J., Gollnick, P.D., Graham, T.E., Juel, C., Kiens, B., Mizuno, M. and Saltin, B. (1990). Anaerobic energy production and O_2 deficit–debt relationship during exhaustive exercise in humans. *J. Physiol.*, **422**, 539–559.

Bergstrom, J. and Hultman, E. (1967). A study of glycogen metabolism during exercise in man. *Scand. J. Clin. Lab. Investigation*, **19**, 218–228.

Burke, R.W. and Edgerton, V.R. (1975). Motor unit properties and selective involvement in movement. *Exerc. Sports Sci. Revs*, **3**, 31–81.

Chance, B. and Williams, G.R. (1955). Respiratory enzymes in oxidative phosphorylation. I. Kinetics of oxygen utilisation. *J. Biolog. Chem.*, **217**, 383–393.

Chasiotis, D., Sahlin, K. and Hultman, E. (1983). Regulation of glycogenolysis in human muscle in response to epinephrine infusion. *J. Appl. Physiol.*, **54**, 45–50.

Chasiotis, D. (1983). The regulation of glycogen phosphorylase and glycogen breakdown in human skeletal muscle. *Acta Physiol. Scand.*, **518** (Supplement), 1–68.

Connnett, R.J. (1988) Analysis of metabolic control: new insights using a scaled creatine kinase model. *Am. J. Physiol.*, **254**, R949–R959.

Constantin-Teodosiu, D., Carlin, J.J, Cederblad, G., Harris, R.C. and Hultman, E. (1991). Acetyl group accumulation and pyruvate dehydrogensae activity in human muscle during incremental exercise. *Acta Physiol. Scand.*, **143**, 367–372.

Cook, R. and Pate, E. (1985). The effects of ADP and phosphate on the contraction of muscle fibres. *Biophysical J.*, **48**, 789–798.

Cori, G.T. (1945). The effect of stimulation and recovery on the phosphorylase a content of muscle. *J. Biolog. Chem.*, **158**, 333–339.

Cori, G.T., Colowick, S.P. and Cori, C.F. (1938). The action of nucleotides in the disruptive phosphorylation of glycogen. *J. Biol. Chem.*, **123**, 381–389.

Cori, G.T. and Illingworth, B. (1956). The effect of epinephrine and other glycogenolytic agents on the phosphorylase a content of muscle. *Biochem. Biophys. Acta*, **21**, 105–110.

Danforth, W.H. (1965) Activation of glycolytic pathway in muscle. In *Control of Energy Metabolism* (B. Chance and R.W. Estabrook, eds), pp. 287–296. Academic Press.

Dyke, D.J., Putman, C.T., Heigenhauser, G.J.F., Hultman, E. and Spriet, L,L. (1993). Regulation of fat–carbohydrate interaction in skeletal muscle during intense aerobic cycling. *Am. J. Physiol.*, **265**, E852–E859.

Faulkner, J.A., Claflin, D.R. and McCully, K.K. (1986). Power output of fast and slow fibres from human skeletal muscles. In *Human Power Output* (N.L. Jones, N. McCartney and A.J. McComas, eds), pp. 81–89. Human Kinetics.

Graham, T.E. and Saltin, B.. (1989). Estimation of the mitochondrial redox state in human skeletal muscle during exercise. *J. Appl. Physiol.*, **66**, 561–566.

Greenhaff, P.L., Ren, J-M., Soderlund, K. and Hultman, E. (1991). Energy metabolism in single human muscle fibres during contraction without and with epinephrine infusion. *Am. J. Physiol.*, **260**, E713–E718.

Greenhaff, P. L., Soderlund, K., Ren, J.-M. and Hultman, E. (1993). Energy metabolism in single human muscle fibres during intermittent contraction with occluded circulation. *J. Physiol.*, **460**, 443–453.

Greenhaff, P.L., Nevill, M.E., Soderlund, K., Bodin, K., Boobis, L.H., Williams, C. and Hultman, E. (1994). The metabolic responses of human type I and II muscle fibres during maximal treadmill sprinting. *J. Physiol.*, **478**, 149–155.

Harris, R.C., Essen, B. and Hultman, E. (1976). Glycogen phosphorylase in biopsy samples and single muscle fibres of musculus quadriceps femoris of man at rest. *Scand. J. Clin. Lab. Investigation*, **36**, 521–526.

Hultman, E. (1967). Studies on muscle of glycogen and active phosphate in man with special reference to exercise and diet. *Scand. J. Clin. Lab. Investigation*, **19** (Suppl. 94), 1–63.

Hultman, E., Bergstrom, J. and McLennan-Anderson, N. (1967). Breakdown and resynthesis of phosphocreatine and adenosine triphosphate in connection with muscular work. *Scand. J. Clin. Lab. Investigation*, **19**, 56–66.

Hultman, E. and Nilsson, L.H. (1971). Liver glycogen in man, effects of different diets and muscular exercise. In *Muscle Metabolism during Intense Exercise* (B. Pernow and B. Saltin, eds), pp. 143–151. Plenum Press.

Hultman, E., Greenhaff, P.L., Ren, J.-M. and Soderlund, K. (1991). Energy metabolism and fatigue during intense muscle contraction. *Biochem. Soc. Trans.*, **19**, 347–353.

Kjar, M. (1995). Hepatic fuel metabolism during exercise. In *Exercise Metabolism* (M. Hargreaves, ed.), pp. 73–97. Human Kinetics.

Lowry, O.H., Schulz, D.W. and Passoneau, J.V. (1964). Effects of adenylic acid on the kinetics of muscle phosphorylase *a*. *J. Biol. Chem.*, **239**, 1947–1953.

Meyer, R.A., Brown, T.R., Krilowicz, B.L. and Kushmerick, M.J. (1986). Phosphagen and intracellular pH changes during contraction of creatine-depleted rat muscle. *Am. J. Physiol.*, **250**, C264–C274.

Moreadith, R.W. and Jacobus, W.E. (1982). Creatine kinase of heart mitochondria: functional coupling to ADP transfer to the adenine nucleotide translocase. *J. Biol. Chem.*, **257**, 899–905.

Nilsson, L.H. and Hultman, E. (1973). Liver glycogen in man – the effect of total starvation or a carbohydrate-poor diet followed by carbohydrate feedings. *Scand. J. Clin. Lab. Investigation*, **32**, 325–330.

Nosek, T.M., Fender, K.Y. and Godt, R.E. (1987). It is diprotonated inorganic phosphate that depresses force in skinned skeletal muscle fibres. *Science*, **236**, 191–193.

Odland, L.M., Heigenhauser, G.J.F., Lopaschuk, G.D. and Spriet, L.L. (1996). Human skeletal muscle malonyl-CoA at rest and during prolonged exercise. *Am. J. Physiol.*, **270**, E541–E544.

Putman, C.T.,. Spriet, L.L., Hultman, E., Lindinger, M.I., Lands, L.C., McKelvie, R.S., Cederblad, G., Jones, N.L. and Heigenhauser, G.J.F. (1993). Pyruvate dehydrogenase activity and acetyl group accumulation during exercise after different diets. *Am. J. Physiol.*, **265**, E752–E760.

Putman, C.T., Spriet, L.L., Hultman, E., Dyke, D.J. and Heigenhauser, G.J.F. (1995). Skeletal muscle pyruvate dehydrogenase activity during acetate infusion in humans. *Am. J. Physiol.*, **268**, E1007–E1017.

Randle, P.J., Garland, P.B., Hales, C.N. and Newsholme, E.A. (1963). The glucose–fatty acid cycle: its role in insulin sensitivity and the metabolic disturbances of diabetes mellitus. *Lancet*, **1**, 786–789.

Ren, J.M. and Hultman, E. (1989). Regulation of glycogenolysis in human skeletal muscle. *J. Appl. Physiol.*, **67**, 2243–2248.

Ren, J.M. and Hultman, E. (1990). Regulation of phosphorylase *a* activity in human skeletal muscle. *J. Appl. Physiol.*, **69**, 919–923.

Richter, E.R., Sonne, B., Ploug, T., Kjaer, M., Mikines, K. and Galbo, H. (1986). Regulation of carbohydrate metabolism in exercise. In *Biochemistry of Exercise IV* (B. Saltin, ed.), pp. 151–166. Human Kinetics.

Richter, E.R. and Hespel, P. (1996). Determinants of glucose uptake in contracting muscle. In *Biochemistry of Exercise IX* (R. Maughan and S. Shirreffs, eds), pp. 51–60. Human Kinetics.

Sahlin, K. and Ren, J.-M. (1989). Relationship of contraction capacity to metabolic changes during recovery from fatigueing contraction. *J. Appl. Physiol.*, **67**, 648–654.

Sahlin, K., Katz, A. and Broberg, S. (1990). Tricarboxylic cycle intermediates in human muscle during submaximal exercise. *Am. J. Physiol.,* **259**, C834–C841.

Spriet, L.L., Soderlund, K., Bergstrom, M. and Hultman, E. (1987). Skeletal muscle glycogenolysis, glycolysis and pH during electrical stimulation in man. *J. Appl. Physiol.,* **62**, 611–615.

Timmons, J.A., Poucher, S.M., Constantin-Teodosiu, D., Worrall, V., Macdonald, I.A. and Greenhaff, P.L. (1996). Increased acetyl group availability enhances contractile function of canine skeletal muscle during ischemia. *J. Clin. Investigation*, **97**, 879–883.

Tornheim, K. and Lowenstein, J.M. (1976). Control of phosphofructokinase from rat skeletal muscle. *J. Biol. Chem.,* **251**, 7322–7328.

Tsintzas, O.-K., Williams, C., Boobis, L. and Greenhaff, P.L. (1996). Carbohydrate ingestion and single muscle fibre glycogen metabolism during prolonged running in man. *J. Appl. Physiol.,* **81**, 801–809.

Wahren, J., Felig, P., Ahlborg, G. and Jorfelt, L. (1971). Glucose metabolism during leg exercise in man. *J. Clin. Investigation,* **50**, 2715–2725.

Wieland, O.H. (1983). The mammalian pyruvate dehydrogenase complex: structure and regulation. *Rev. Physiol. Biochem. Pharmacol.,* **96**, 123–170.

4

Physiological adaptations to exercise training

Karyn L. Hamilton, Jeff S. Coombes, Haydar A. Demirel and Scott K. Powers

Exercise training results in many physiological adaptations which improve the body's ability to maintain homeostasis during submaximal exercise as well as improve maximal exercise performance. Over the past 30 years, numerous studies have carefully described changes in both systemic and cellular physiology resulting from regular exercise; this chapter will discuss these changes at the cellular, tissue and systemic levels. Our focus in this chapter is on endurance exercise-induced changes in the cardiovascular, respiratory and neuromuscular systems. Further, we also provide an overview of the rapidly expanding body of knowledge regarding the interactions between exercise training, oxygen radicals and the antioxidant capacity of skeletal muscle. Finally, we provide a brief overview of skeletal muscle adaptations to resistance exercise training.

Principles of training

Principle of individuality

Genetics play a significant role in determining the growth, metabolic rate and neuroendocrine responses of an individual (Astrand and Rodahl, 1970). While physiological responses to specific stimuli are somewhat predictable, no two individuals adapt to exercise training in the same way, a concept known as the **principle of individuality**. Because of this individuality, the same exercise training programme may not lead to the same benefits for each participant. For example, it has been estimated that 25–50 per cent of the variation in maximum oxygen consumption is due to genetics (Bouchard *et al.*, 1992). Research comparing maximum oxygen consumption of identical twins, fraternal twins and non-twin siblings has revealed that identical twins have nearly identical maximum oxygen consumption, while fraternal and non-twin siblings have significantly greater variability (Klissouras, 1971). Another factor influencing an individual's response to a training regimen is the initial fitness level of that individual. When the initial fitness level is low, gains achieved from training will be of greater magnitude when compared to those of an individual who is initially fit.

Progressive overload principle

The **progressive overload principle** forms the basis for all exercise training. The overload principle states that methodically overloading a system causes it to respond and adapt. Progressive overload means that, as a system responds and adapts, a proportionately greater stressor must be applied for further adaptation. Progression may be achieved via increasing either the intensity or the duration of the activity, the end result being an increase in the total work accomplished in the exercise session. Whether the goal of training is to achieve strength gains or to improve endurance, the principle of progressive overload must be applied.

Principle of specificity

To improve performance of a specific activity, athletes must train the energy systems and muscle groups specific to their events. This notion, the **principle of specificity**, is critical for obtaining performance enhancement from a training programme. For example, an endurance runner would not improve the muscular endurance for his/her event by embarking on a training programme that emphasizes high-intensity, low-volume resistance training. This does not mean that resistance training should be completely eliminated in training for an endurance event; rather, athletes must emphasize training the muscles and bioenergetic systems used predominantly in their events.

Principle of reversibility

While the expression 'use it or lose it' is often used in jest, it is an important principle that applies to training. The **principle of reversibility** or disuse is based on findings that when a trained individual stops training, the physiological gains made from the training will decrease gradually back to pre-training levels. While the time-course for loss of training effects is variable, 'detraining' occurs relatively rapidly. Within 7 to 20 days of cessation of training, significant decreases in $\dot{V}O_{2\,max}$, cardiac output, oxygen extraction, work capacity and blood volume have been noted (Coyle *et al.*, 1984, 1985; Friman, 1979; Saltin, 1968).

Cardiovascular adaptations to endurance training

Endurance training results in profound changes in many aspects of the cardiovascular system. These changes (summarized in Table 4.1) translate to an improved capacity to deliver blood and oxygen to the working

Table 4.1. Cardiovascular adaptations following endurance training

	Rest	Submax.	Max.
Heart rate	↓	↓	no Δ
Stroke volume	↑	↑	↑
Cardiac output	no Δ or ↓	no Δ or ↑	↑
Systolic BP	no Δ or ↓	no Δ or ↓	no Δ
Diastolic BP	no Δ or ↓	no Δ or ↓	no Δ
VO₂	no Δ	no Δ	↑
a–v O₂ difference	no Δ or ↓	↑	↑
Blood volume	↑	N/A	N/A
Plasma volume	↑	N/A	N/A
Inactive muscle blood flow	no Δ	no Δ	no Δ
Active muscle blood flow	no Δ or ↓	no Δ or ↓	↑

no Δ = no change; N/A = not applicable.

muscles. The following discussion provides a summary of the specific adaptations that occur in response to endurance training.

Maximal oxygen consumption

Maximal oxygen consumption ($\dot{V}O_{2\,max}$) is increased following endurance training (Figure 4.1). The magnitude of improvement in $\dot{V}O_{2\,max}$ following endurance training depends on a number of factors including initial fitness level, age and type of training. The greatest training-induced increases in $\dot{V}O_{2\,max}$ can be achieved in individuals with initially low fitness levels. Typically, increases in $\dot{V}O_{2\,max}$ of 15–25 per cent are observed, though increases of up to 93 per cent have been reported in severely deconditioned individuals (Pollock, 1973).

Maximal oxygen consumption in the body can be calculated using the Fick equation:

$$\dot{V}O_{2max} = \text{Cardiac output}_{max} \times (a - v\ O_2\ \text{difference})_{max}$$

where cardiac output = heart rate (HR) (stroke volume (SV) × and a–v O_2 difference = arterio-venous oxygen difference.

Therefore, $\dot{V}O_{2\,max}$ can be increased by increasing either maximal cardiac output or the maximal arterio-venous oxygen difference. In the following sections, we will discuss specific adaptations which account for the increases in $\dot{V}O_{2\,max}$ observed with endurance training.

Heart rate

Resting heart rate (HR), normally 60–80 beats per minute (bpm), decreases following an endurance-training programme, frequently resulting in rates less than 60 bpm, a condition referred to as exercise-induced bradycardia

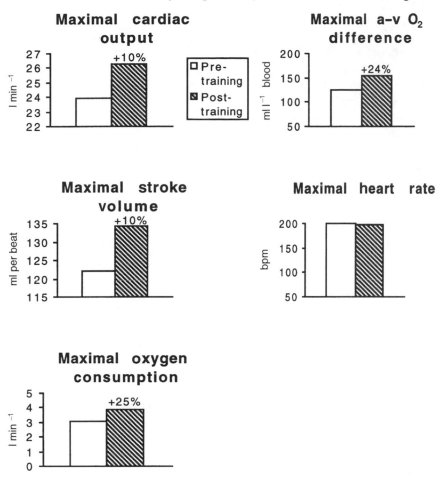

Figure 4.1. Adaptation of cardiovascular parameters to endurance training at maximal intensities

(Tipton *et al.*, 1969). Also, at any given submaximal exercise intensity, endurance training results in a lower HR with a compensatory increase in stroke volume. Thus, compared to an untrained individual, a trained individual during the same physical activity will maintain a lower heart rate.

The mechanism(s) responsible for the training-induced decrease in both resting and submaximal heart rates continues to be investigated. Nonetheless, it appears that endurance training alters the autonomic influence on the heart by increasing the activity of the parasympathetic nervous system (i.e. increased vagal tone) and simultaneously decreasing sympathetic drive (Frick *et al.*, 1967; Hughson *et al.*, 1977; Tipton, 1965, 1969; Winder *et al.*, 1978). Another possible explanation for the decrease in resting and submaximal HR following training is a decreased sensitivity of the myocardium to catecholamines (Badeer, 1975; Smith and El-Hage, 1978). Because sympathetic stimulation of the heart can be modified by peripheral mechanisms, another explanation for training-induced brady-cardia may be modifications in the afferent neural impulses arising from working muscles and joints (Fox *et al.*, 1975; McKenzie *et al.*, 1978). In contrast to adaptations at rest and during submaximal exercise, maximal HR does not typically change in response to endurance training (Rowell, 1986). Thus, changes in maximal HR cannot account for the training-induced improvements in $\dot{V}O_{2\,max}$.

Stroke volume

Following endurance training, both resting and maximal stroke volume (SV) increase. This elevation in SV results from two training-induced cardiovascular adaptations. First, an increase in end diastolic volume (EDV) which occurs primarily due to an augmentation in venous return (i.e. the Frank–Starling mechanism) (Bevegard *et al.*, 1963; Ekblöm *et al.*, 1968). The second factor influencing SV is a decrease in afterload or the peripheral resistance against which the left ventricle must work as it ejects blood into the aorta. Following an endurance-training programme, trained skeletal muscles impose less resistance to blood flow during exercise of maximal intensity. This occurs due to a decrease in sympathetic vasoconstrictor activity in the arterioles of trained muscle, an adaptation facilitating greater muscle blood flow. As we will discuss in the next section, cardiac output increases simultaneously which prevents the decrease in blood pressure that would otherwise result from this reduction in vasoconstriction (Rowell, 1986). It is estimated that increases in SV account for approximately 50 per cent of the training-induced increase in $\dot{V}O_{2\,max}$ which occurs in untrained subjects.

Arterio-venous oxygen difference

While it has been estimated that SV accounts for about 50 per cent of the training-induced increase in $\dot{V}O_{2\,max}$, improvements in extraction of oxygen from the blood, resulting in increases in the arterio-venous oxygen difference (a–v O_2 diff), account for the remaining 50 per cent. This training-induced increase in a–v O_2 diff occurs due to enhanced delivery of blood to the working muscles and an increased number of mitochondria. Circulation of blood is improved via an increase in capillary density in trained muscle; this enhances both oxygen and substrate delivery by reducing the diffusion distance from the blood vessel to the mitochondria (Holloszy and Coyle, 1984).

Maximal cardiac output

Given that during rest and submaximal exercise, HR decreases and SV increases following endurance training, it is intuitive that resting and submaximal cardiac output remain essentially unchanged following training. However, because training induces an increase in maximal SV without changing maximal HR, cardiac output during maximal exercise increases following training. The magnitude of increase in maximal cardiac output has been shown to be directly related to the increase in $\dot{V}O_{2\,max}$ (Ekblöm and Hermansen, 1968).

Cardiac hypertrophy

The size of the heart is larger in trained individuals than in untrained. Using echocardiography, it has been reported that endurance athletes typically have left ventricular hypertrophy that is characterized by a large chamber size with normal thickness of the ventricular walls. This finding is consistent with the increased EDV and SV that are known to result from endurance training. Conversely, individuals trained with high resistance or involved in isometric type activities display normal ventricular chamber size but with thickening of the ventricular walls. These athletes, logically, do not show the increases in EDV and SV typical of endurance-trained athletes (DiMaria et al., 1978; Ehsani et al., 1978; Longhurst et al. 1980; Snoeckx et al., 1982).

Blood volume, haemoglobin content and red blood cells

Plasma volume increases with endurance training (Coyle et al., 1990); two mechanisms are responsible for this adaptation. Firstly, training promotes an increase in plasma proteins which elevates osmotic pressure and thus results in more fluid being retained within the vascular space. Secondly, training is associated with an accelerated release of antidiuretic hormone (ADH) and aldosterone. These hormones act upon the kidneys to reabsorb water and increase blood volume.

In addition to increasing blood volume, training can result in an increase in haemoglobin, the iron-containing portion of red blood cells (RBCs) that binds oxygen. Although RBC volume increases with exercise training, this increase does not match the increase in plasma volume. Because the plasma volume increases to a greater extent than RBC volume, the ratio of RBC volume to total blood volume (haematocrit) decreases, sometimes resulting in apparent anaemia in some trained athletes.

Blood pressure

Endurance training can promote a decrease in resting systolic and diastolic pressure, typically in individuals with mild to moderate hypertension prior to beginning training (Boyer and Kasch, 1970). Blood pressure during submaximal exercise may also decrease slightly when compared to the same absolute workload prior to training (Kilbourn, 1971). However, blood pressure at maximal exercise remains relatively unaffected by training.

Respiratory adaptations to training

Unlike the many training-induced changes in the cardiovascular system, training results in few changes in the respiratory system. Indeed, endurance training does not significantly alter the structure of the lung and therefore does not alter lung volumes and capacities (Clanton *et al.*, 1987). However, endurance training does promote a decrease in ventilation during submaximal exercise (Casaburi *et al.*, 1987). The mechanism to explain this observation continues to be investigated and current evidence suggests that the training-induced reduction in submaximal ventilation is likely to be due to a decrease in afferent feedback from the working muscle (Casaburi *et al.*, 1987; Clanton *et al.*, 1987; Powers and Beadle, 1985). The alveolar–arterial PO_2 gradient and diffusion at the blood–gas interface, however, remain relatively unchanged.

While training does not alter the structure of the lung, training does influence respiratory muscle structure and function. Indeed, respiratory muscle performance improves following endurance training (Vrabas *et al.*, 1995). This improvement in respiratory muscle endurance is linked to increased activity of mitochondrial and antioxidant enzymes in the primary and accessory inspiratory muscles (Moore and Gollnick, 1982; Powers *et al.*, 1990a,b, 1992a,b,c,d, 1994a, 1996, 1997).

Endurance training-induced changes in skeletal muscle bioenergetic pathways

Training-induced adaptations in skeletal muscle combine with the previously described cardiovascular and respiratory changes to allow the athlete to better maintain homeostasis during prolonged submaximal exercise. Endurance training results in skeletal muscle changes that allow for: (1) a more rapid transition from rest to the steady-state metabolic requirement; (2) an increase in fat metabolism; (3) a reduction in lactate and hydrogen ion formation; and (4) an increase in lactate removal. A brief discussion of these issues follows.

Biochemical adaptations

One fundamental adaptation to endurance exercise is the biochemical changes that allow for an increase in the oxidative capacity of skeletal muscle. This adaptation is evidenced by an increase in mitochondrial content which results in increases in the capacity for fatty acid, carbohydrate, ketone and amino acid oxidation and the enzyme pathways required for handling the reducing equivalents. Although the stimuli responsible for this adaptive response remain poorly understood, a number of factors such as exercise intensity, frequency and duration and muscle fibre type influence this response. Investigations into the bioenergetic adaptations to endurance training have provided the exercise scientist with guidelines for exercise training programmes that can provide the maximum skeletal muscle cellular adaptations.

Mitochondrial adaptations

John Holloszy's pioneering work in the 1960s demonstrated that endurance exercise training results in an increase in the mitochondrial content of skeletal muscle (Holloszy, 1967). This was evidenced by an increase in the ability of the mitochondrial oxidization of pyruvate and NADH in treadmill-trained rats. A 3-month training programme increased the mitochondrial enzyme activities two-fold (Holloszy, 1967). Mitochondria from muscles of the trained animals also exhibited a high level of respiratory control and tightly coupled oxidative phosphorylation, providing evidence that the increase in electron transport capacity was associated with a similar rise in the capacity to generate ATP via oxidative phosphorylation. Similar results have been found in subsequent and comparable rodent training studies from our laboratory as well as by others (Davies *et al.*, 1981; Fitts *et al.*, 1975; Powers *et al.*, 1990, 1992a,b,c,d, 1994a,b). In 1971, Morgan *et al.* published data confirming that increases in oxidative capacity and mitochondrial enzyme activities also occur in human skeletal muscle. This, along with electron microscopic studies in rats (Gollnick and King, 1969) and in humans (Hoppeler *et al.*, 1973), have shown that increases in both size and number of mitochondria are responsible for increased mitochondrial content.

Exercise training studies using isolated mitochondria and whole muscle homogenates indicate that rat skeletal muscle undergoes adaptive increases in the capacity to oxidize fatty acids (Baldwin *et al.*, 1972; Mole *et al.*, 1971), ketones (Winder *et al.*, 1974) and pyruvate (Baldwin *et al.*, 1972). Underlying these increases in oxidative capacity are increases in the levels of the enzymes responsible for the activation, transport, and β-oxidation of long chain fatty acids (Baldwin *et al.*, 1972; Mole *et al.*, 1971), the enzymes involved in ketone oxidation (Winder *et al.*, 1974), the enzymes of the Krebs cycle (Holloszy *et al.*, 1970), the components of the respiratory chain involved in oxidation of NADH and succinate

(Holloszy, 1967; Holloszy *et al.*, 1970), and mitochondrial coupling factor 1 (Oscai and Holloszy, 1971). Similar findings have been reported for humans (Costill *et al.*, 1979a,b; Morgan *et al.*, 1971).

Skeletal muscle mitochondria undergo alterations in composition in response to endurance training, with some enzymes increasing two- to three-fold, others increasing 30–60 per cent and some not increasing at all (Holloszy, 1973; Holloszy and Coyle, 1984). The enzymes that do not increase include mitochondrial creatine kinase and adenylate kinase (Oscai and Holloszy, 1971) and mitochondrial α-glycerophosphate dehydrogenase (Holloszy and Oscai, 1969). The absence of an increase in α-glycerophosphate dehydrogenase would be expected to result in a decrease in the ability of muscles to shuttle reduced equivalents of cytoplasmic NADH formed during glycolysis into the mitochondria. However, large compensatory increases in the enzymes of the malate–aspartate shuttle, an alternative pathway for the mitochondrial transfer of NADH, prevent this from occurring (Holloszy, 1975).

Increases in muscle mitochondria with endurance training appear to be mediated by contractile activity rather than by exogenous stimuli. This is supported by the observation that mitochondrial adaptations are limited to the muscle fibres that are recruited during the activity. For example, in runners and cyclists the increase in mitochondria is limited to the muscles of the lower extremities (Gollnick *et al.*, 1972) and when only one lower extremity is trained, the adaptations are limited to the exercised leg (Henriksson, 1977). Little is known, however, regarding the series of events initiated by repeated muscle contractions that lead to the increase in mitochondrial content. Available evidence indicates that increased synthesis, and not decreased degradation, is primarily responsible for increases in mitochondrial proteins (Booth and Holloszy, 1977).

Adaptation of glycolytic enzymes

Endurance training appears to result in only small changes in glycolytic enzyme activity in skeletal muscle (Gollnick *et al.*, 1972). The only major adaptations are an increase in hexokinase activity (Morgan *et al.*, 1971) and a decrease, in some individuals, in total lactate dehydrogenase activity (Sjodin, 1976).

Physiological consequences of biochemical adaptations

The major consequence of the biochemical adaptations is that the same work-rate requires a smaller percentage of maximum aerobic capacity and, therefore, results in less homeostatic disturbance. Other important adaptations include an increase in fatty acid utilization, a proportional decrease in carbohydrate utilization, and smaller increases in muscle and blood lactate concentrations during submaximal exercise. A brief discussion of these issues follows.

Lower blood lactate concentrations

Endurance exercise training results in smaller increases in blood lactate concentration at the same relative exercise intensity. Adaptations also include a considerably higher relative work-rate required to attain a given lactate concentration (Brooks, 1985). Combined, these alterations explain the greater endurance at the same relative exercise intensity in the trained compared with the untrained state (Baldwin *et al.*, 1972) and the ability of trained individuals to maintain a higher relative intensity for a given time period (Astrand and Rodahl, 1986; Baldwin *et al.*, 1972). Decreases in blood lactate can be explained by increases in mitochondrial content which result in lower ADP concentrations and subsequently decreased phosphofructokinase (PFK) activity at the onset of exercise. Decreased PFK activity along with an increased capacity to utilize fats reduces the need for carbohydrate oxidation during prolonged work. If less carbohydrate is used, less pyruvate and, therefore, lactate is formed. In addition, the increase in mitochondrial size and number increases the probability that pyruvate will be taken up by the mitochondria for oxidation in the Krebs cycle, rather than being converted to lactate in the cytoplasm. All of these adaptations favour a lower pyruvate concentration and a reduction in lactate formation (Powers and Howley, 1997).

Glycogen depletion

Studies employing serial muscle biopsies have shown that muscle glycogen is depleted less rapidly in trained human skeletal muscle compared to untrained (Hermanssen *et al.*, 1967). Rodent studies have further revealed that liver glycogen is also depleted less rapidly in the trained state (Fitts *et al.*, 1975). In rats trained at varying levels of intensity, an inverse relationship was found between the oxidative capacity of the leg muscles and the total amount of glycogen utilized during a bout of exercise (Fitts *et al.*, 1975).

Fat oxidation

The most dramatic change in muscle metabolism following training is an increased utilization of fat and subsequent sparing of carbohydrate. This is due to: (1) an improved capacity to mobilize free fatty acids from adipose tissue to muscle; (2) an enhanced ability to transport free fatty acids from the cytoplasm to the mitochondria of the muscle; and (3) an increase in the activity of β-oxidation enzymes needed to degrade free fatty acids to acetyl-CoA for oxidation via the Krebs cycle (Powers and Howley, 1994). These adaptations are reflected in a lower respiratory exchange ratio at both the same absolute exercise intensity and matched relative exercise intensities when individuals are tested before and after endurance training (Holloszy, 1973). There is evidence that depletion of glycogen stores can play a role in the development of fatigue during prolonged strenuous exercise (Holloszy, 1973). The glycogen sparing effect of increased fat oxidation plays a major role in the increase in endurance that occurs with training.

Influence of exercise intensity, frequency and duration on biochemical adaptations

A number of factors affect the biochemical response of skeletal muscle to endurance training. Specifically, the training-induced changes in muscle biochemistry are affected by the force of contraction, the frequency and duration of contraction, and influences of trophic hormones and growth factors (Dudley *et al.*, 1982).

The interaction of intensity and duration of daily exercise on training-induced improvements in citrate synthase activity (Krebs cycle enzyme) of a 'mixed' fibre locomotor muscle (i.e. muscle that contains several fibre types) is illustrated in Figure 4.2. Note the following points. Firstly, the magnitude of the training adaptation is influenced by both the duration and intensity of training. The duration of each exercise bout is important as longer exercise bouts generally bring about larger responses (Dudley *et al.*, 1982; Fitts *et al.*, 1975; Powers *et al.*, 1994). However, there appears to be an upper limit to exercise duration, after which no further increase in oxidative capacity is found (Figure 4.2).

Secondly, the total duration (i.e. number of weeks) of the training programme is also important, since the actual increase in mitochondrial content depends on the length of training (Booth and Holloszy, 1977). In general, it requires 6–8 weeks of training at a given duration/intensity for the adaptation to be complete (Dudley *et al.*, 1982). Thus, it is important to maintain a training programme for a sufficient length of time to permit the cellular adaptation to reach a steady state.

Thirdly, training intensity influences the magnitude of the training adaptation. That is, higher intensity exercise results in a greater training response (Figure 4.2). Although the influence of intensity on muscle adaptation is complicated, this response is probably due, at least in part, to the increased motor unit recruitment during high-intensity exercise (Dudley *et al.*, 1982). That is, higher intensity exercise results in recruitment of more motor units resulting in a greater number of fibres adapting to the activity stimulus.

Endurance exercise and skeletal muscle antioxidant capacity

Radicals (also called free radicals) are highly reactive atoms or molecules which contain an unpaired electron in their outer orbital. Radicals are formed during normal oxidative metabolism (i.e. in the electron transport

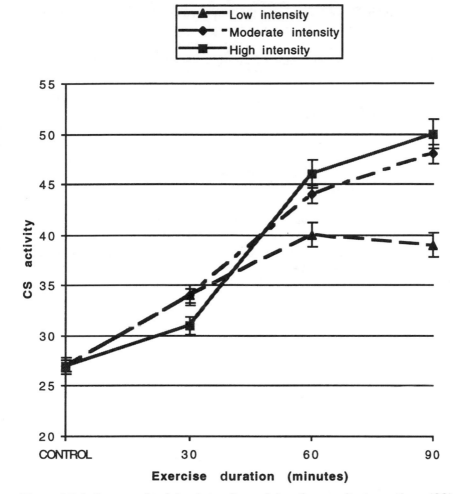

Figure 4.2. Influence of training intensity and duration on citrate synthase (CS) activity (Krebs cycle enzyme) in the plantaris muscle of rats. Daily training duration ranged from 30 to 90 min per day. Training intensity ranged from low ($\sim$50 per cent $\dot{V}O_{2max}$) to high ($\sim$75 per cent $\dot{V}O_{2max}$). Values are means. Enzyme activity units are micromoles of substrate converted per minute per 100 mg of protein. (Data from Powers *et al.*, 1994)

chain) in aerobic organisms. Indeed, it is clear that muscular exercise results in an increased production of radicals and other forms of reactive oxygen species (ROS) (Borzone *et al.*, 1994; Davies *et al.*, 1982; Jackson *et al.*, 1985; Reid *et al.*, 1992a,b). Furthermore, evidence exists to implicate cytotoxic ROS in the underlying aetiology of exercise-induced muscle fatigue and bioenergetic enzyme down-regulation (Barclay, 1991; Ji *et al.*, 1988; Nashawati *et al.*, 1993; Reid *et al.*, 1992a,b; Shindoh *et al.*, 1990). Given the potential role of radicals and ROS in mediating muscular dysfunction, it is not surprising that myocytes contain several naturally occurring defence mechanisms to prevent oxidative injury. In the following section we discuss radical production during muscular activity and briefly explain how endurance training alters the muscle's capacity to remove ROS.

Production of reactive oxygen species

It is now clear that contracting skeletal muscles possess several metabolic pathways which are capable of producing ROS. Specifically, superoxide anions, hydroxyl radicals and nitric oxide are all produced during muscular contractions (Diaz *et al.*, 1993; Kobzik *et al.*, 1994; Reid *et al.*, 1992a). Although the origin of ROS in contracting muscle continues to be investigated, it seems likely that oxygen-derived radicals are produced as a byproduct of oxidative metabolism within mitochondria (Chance *et al.*, 1979). Other potential sites for production of ROS in muscle include membrane oxidoreductases, the cyclo-oxygenase pathway of arachidonic acid metabolism, and cytosolic or endothelial xanthine oxidase (see the review by Halliwell and Gutteridge, 1989).

Reactive oxygen species and skeletal muscle performance

There is growing evidence that during periods of prolonged muscular activity (e.g. endurance exercise), production of ROS contributes to muscle fatigue. Numerous studies suggest that ROS production contributes to muscular fatigue. For example, Novelli *et al.* (1990) and Barclay *et al.* (1991) reported that exogenous antioxidant scavengers reduce the rate of locomotor muscle fatigue both *in vivo* and *in vitro*. These early investigations in locomotor muscles have been followed by numerous studies investigating the effects of ROS on muscle fatigue. Specifically, there are three primary lines of evidence that collectively establish a cause and effect relationship between the production of ROS and muscle fatigue. First, antioxidant treatment (both *in vitro* and *in situ*) attenuates the rate of fatigue development in the contracting muscle (Reid *et al.*, 1992a; Shindoh *et al.*, 1990). Second, exposing contracting muscle to exogenous ROS decreases muscle force production and promotes fatigue (Lawler *et al.*, 1996, 1997). Finally, muscle fatigue is accelerated in diaphragms with reduced levels of glutathione (Anzueto *et al.*, 1992; Borzone *et al.*, 1994; Morales *et al.*, 1993).

Perhaps the strongest experimental support of the notion that ROS actively contribute to muscular fatigue is the experimental finding that fatigue can be inhibited by exogenous antioxidants. This effect was first observed by Shindoh *et al.* (1990) who demonstrated that treatment with the antioxidant *N*-acetylcysteine reduced the development of rabbit diaphragmatic fatigue *in situ*. The results of this early investigation were followed and confirmed by numerous *in vitro* experiments in rodents incorporating a wide variety of antioxidants (e.g. superoxide dismutase, catalase, DMSO) (see Figure 4.3).

Antioxidant protection in skeletal muscles

Two major classes of endogenous protective mechanisms work together to reduce the harmful effects of oxidants in the muscle cell, namely enzymatic and non-enzymatic antioxidants. It seems likely that increased cellular concentrations of one or more of these antioxidants will reduce the risk of cellular injury and muscle fatigue due to radical formation (Barclay, 1990; Ji, 1995; Nashawati et al., 1993; Reid et al., 1992a,b; Shindoh et al., 1990). The role of regular endurance exercise in altering the antioxidant capacity of skeletal muscle has been a topic of research for over two decades. Here we will focus on the effects of endurance training on the activities of primary antioxidant enzymes in muscle. We begin with an overview of the primary antioxidant enzymes.

Overview of antioxidant enzymes

Primary antioxidant enzymes in tissues include superoxide dismutase (SOD), glutathione peroxidase (GPX) and catalase (CAT). All of these enzymes catalyse a one-electron reduction of their ROS. SOD promotes the dismutation of superoxide resulting in the formation of hydrogen

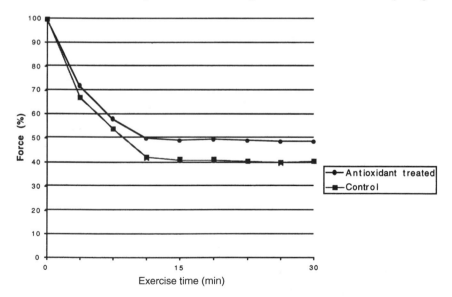

Figure 4.3. Illustration of the effects of antioxidant treatment on muscle fatigue during a 30 min contractile period. Note that the addition of antioxidants to skeletal muscle *in vitro* reduces the rate of fatigue development during prolonged exericse. (Redrawn from Reid *et al.*, 1992)

peroxide (H_2O_2). CAT converts H_2O_2 to water and O_2. GPX, acting with reduced glutathione, can reduce H_2O_2 or hydroperoxides to form oxidized glutathione and alcohol or water. A brief discussion of the cellular location and catalytic function of each of these enzymes follows. For a detailed review of antioxidant enzymes the reader is referred to reviews by Halliwell and Gutteridge (1989) and Ji (1995).

Superoxide dismutase

The primary cellular defence against superoxide radicals ($O_2^{-\bullet}$) is provided by SOD. As mentioned previously, SOD dismutates superoxide radicals to form H_2O_2 and O_2:

$$2O_2^{-\bullet} + 2H^+ \rightarrow H_2O_2 + O_2$$

In mammals, two isozymes of SOD exist in skeletal muscle that vary in both cellular location as well as the metal ion bound to the active site. The Cu-Zn SOD is primarily located in the cytosol whereas the Mn SOD is principally found in the mitochondrial matrix (Halliwell and Gutteridge, 1989). Both enzymes catalyse the dismutation of superoxide anions with similar efficiency (Ohno et al., 1994).

The distribution of the SOD isoforms varies from tissue to tissue. In skeletal muscle, 15–35 per cent of the total SOD activity is in the mitochondria with the remaining 65–85 per cent being in the cytosol. SOD activity is highest in highly oxidative muscles (i.e. high percentage of type I and IIa fibres) compared to muscles with low oxidative capacity (i.e. high percentage of type IIb fibres) (Criswell et al., 1993; Powers et al., 1994a,b).

Glutathione peroxidase

GPX catalyses the reduction of H_2O_2 or organic hydroperoxides to H_2O and alcohol, respectively, using glutathione (GSH) as the electron donor (Halliwell and Gutteridge, 1989):

$$2GSH + H_2O_2 \rightarrow GSSG + H_2O$$

or

$$2GSH + ROOH \rightarrow GSSG + ROH$$

GPX is a selenium-dependent enzyme that exists in one isoform. GPX will reduce a wide variety of hydroperoxides ranging from H_2O_2 to a wide range of complex organic hydroperoxides (Halliwell and Gutteridge, 1989). This favourable characteristic makes GPX an important cellular protectant against ROS-mediated damage to membrane lipids, as well as muscle proteins and nucleic acids.

GPX activity varies across muscle fibre types with type I fibres containing the highest activity and type IIb fibres possessing the lowest activity (Ji *et al.*, 1988; Powers *et al.*, 1994b). In skeletal muscle, approximately 45 per cent of the GPX activity is found in the cytosol whereas the remaining 55 per cent is found in the mitochondria (Ji *et al.*, 1988). The fact that GPX is located in both the mitochondria and cytosol allows it to reach a number of sources of hydroperoxide generation (Ji, 1995).

Catalase
The primary function of CAT is to catalyse the decomposition of H_2O_2:

$$2H_2O_2 \rightarrow H_2O + O_2$$

Although there is some overlap between the function of CAT and GPX, the two enzymes differ in their affinity for H_2O_2 as a substrate. Mammalian GPX has a much greater affinity for H_2O_2 at low concentrations compared to CAT (e.g. GPX $K_m = 1$ μM vs. CAT $K_m = 1$ mM). This means that at low concentrations, GPX plays a more active role in removing H_2O_2 from the muscle cell.

CAT is widely distributed in the cell with high concentrations found in both peroxisomes and mitochondria (Halliwell and Gutteridge, 1989). Similar to SOD and GPX, CAT activity is highest in highly oxidative muscles and lowest in muscle with a large percentage of fast (type II) fibres (Powers *et al.*, 1994b).

Training and muscle antioxidant enzyme activity

The antioxidant capacity of mammalian organ systems is well matched to the rates of oxygen consumption and radical production. Body tissues with the highest oxygen consumption (e.g. liver, brain, heart) have the greatest antioxidant enzyme activity. As discussed earlier, skeletal muscles with high oxidative capacities possess higher antioxidant capacities compared to those muscles with lower oxidative potential.

It is clear that the antioxidant defence systems of many mammalian tissues are capable of adaptation in response to chronic exposure to ROS. Since exercise results in increased production of ROS in skeletal muscle, it seems logical that regular exercise training would up-regulate muscle antioxidant enzyme activities. Indeed, there is growing evidence that endurance exercise training results in an increase in skeletal muscle antioxidant enzyme activity. Specifically, many studies have reported a training-induced increase in total SOD activity (Criswell *et al.*, 1993; Higuchi *et al.*, 1985; Jenkins, 1983; Powers *et al.*, 1994a,b). Further, a survey of training studies reveals that exercise induction of SOD may be fibre type specific with oxidative muscles being most responsive (Criswell *et al.*, 1993; Ji *et al.*, 1988; Laughlin *et al.*, 1990; Powers *et al.*, 1994). It seems likely that differences in fibre recruitment patterns (i.e. the size principle) may account for these differences.

Similar to SOD, it is generally agreed that regular endurance exercise training results in an increase in GPX activity in active skeletal muscles (Criswell *et al.*, 1992, 1993; Ji *et al.*, 1991; Laughlin *et al.*, 1990; Powers *et al.*, 1994a,b; Sen *et al.*, 1992). A review of the literature suggests that: (1) long-duration exercise training is superior to short-duration exercise training in the up-regulation of muscle GPX activity; (2) training-induced up-regulation of GPX activity is generally limited to oxidative skeletal muscles (i.e. type I and IIa fibres); (3) endurance training does not result in parallel and predictable increases in oxidative enzyme activity and GPX activity; and (4) endurance training promotes an increase in both cytosolic and mito-chondrial GPX activity with the greater increase occurring in the mito-chondrial fraction (Ji *et al.*, 1988; Powers, 1994a,b).

There is little evidence to suggest that exercise training promotes an increase in CAT activity in skeletal muscle (Higuchi *et al.*, 1985; Leeuwenburgh *et al.*, 1994; Powers *et al.*, 1994a,b). In fact, several studies have shown that exercise training may result in reduced CAT activity in some locomotor muscles (Laughlin *et al.*, 1990). The explanation for why endurance training may result in lowered CAT activity in muscle remains unclear.

In summary, research indicates that regular endurance training promotes an increase in both total SOD and GPX activity in actively recruited skeletal muscles. Exercise training induced up-regulation of SOD and GPX activity in skeletal muscles may be of physiological significance. Endurance-trained muscles appear to better equipped to eliminate superoxide radicals and hydroperoxides. This means that trained skeletal muscle may be more effective in reducing the oxidative stress caused by an exercise-induced increase in muscle mitochondrial respiration. This could be of particular importance given the recent evidence that free radical formation may promote muscular fatigue.

Skeletal muscle adaptation: contractile proteins

Much of the knowledge regarding skeletal muscle fibre types and contractile properties has been the result of studying the skeletal muscles of animals. While animal research is a valuable tool for expanding the knowledge-base in muscle physiology, clear parallels cannot always be drawn between the results of animal studies and human physiology. In the following discussion, comparisons are made between data obtained from animal research and muscle physiology in humans.

Fibre types and myosin isoforms

The contractile properties of muscle are highly dependent on the fibre-type composition of the muscle. Muscle fibres are frequently identified on the basis of their histochemically determined myofibrillar actomyosin ATPase (mATPase) activity (Brooke and Kaiser, 1970; Guth and Samaha, 1969). Currently, one slow (type I) and three fast (type IIa, type IId/x and type IIb) fibres are delineated in skeletal muscle of small mammals. Single fibre and immunohistochemistry analyses have shown that these fibre types correlate with the expression of correspondingly named myosin heavy chain (MHC) isoforms: MHCI, MHCIIa, MHCIId/x and MHCIIb (Hamalainen and Pette, 1992; Pette and Staron, 1990, 1997; Schiaffino and Reggiani, 1994).

Small animal and human skeletal muscle fibre types differ in that human skeletal muscles appears to contain only three major fibre types. The three myosin heavy chain isoforms in human skeletal muscle are the slow isoform (MHCI) and two fast isoforms (MHCIIa and MHCIIb) (Staron and Johnson, 1993). Recently, human type IIb MHC has been shown to have the greatest degree of homology with the rat mammalian skeletal muscle type IId/x myosin heavy chain (Ennion et al., 1995).

Myosin is known to exist as multiple isoforms in skeletal muscle as a result of expression of both heavy and light chain components. A single myosin molecule contains two identical heavy chains, two alkali or essential light chains, and two regulatory light chains. Both alkali and regulatory light chains have fast and slow isoforms (Pette and Staron, 1997). Combinations of different alkali light chains in a single native myosin molecule yield different isomyosins (Marechal et al., 1989).

Although the light chain composition of single muscle fibres has been shown to correlate with unloaded shortening velocity (Botinelli and Regliani, 1995), the site for ATP hydrolysis is in the head region of the myosin heavy chain of the myosin molecule. Therefore, the activity of mATPase is directly associated with myosin heavy chain type.

Coexpression

In addition to the fibre types presented in Table 4.2, skeletal muscles also contain fibres in which more than one myosin heavy chain isoform is expressed, a phenomenon called coexpression. For example, a coexpression of myosin heavy chains MHCIIb and MHCIId/x, MHCIId/x and MHCIIa, or MHCI and MHCIIa yields three different hybrid fibres. While hybrid fibres that contain a large amount of one type of myosin heavy chain and a very small amount of another may not be distinguishable from pure fibre types, all three myosin heavy chain isoforms have been shown to be coexpressed in a single fibre in humans (Klitgard et al., 1990). Hybrid fibres suggest that a continuum of myosin heavy chain

Table 4.2.   Major MHC and MLC isoforms in adult human skeletal muscle

Gene family	Fast muscles	Slow muscles
MHC*	Type IIa	Type I
	Type IIb	
MLC1 (alkali)	MLC1f	MLC1s
	MLC3f	
MLC2 (alkali)	MLC2f	MLC2s

*Small mammal fast skeletal muscles express three major fast myosin heavy chain isoforms: type IIa, typeIIb and type IId/x. Type IIb in humans is analogous to type IId/x in small mammals.

based fibre types exists that ranges from MHCIIb to MHCI (Aigner *et al.*, 1993; Staron and Pette, 1993).

Alteration of muscle types by endurance exercise training

Skeletal muscle fibres are dynamic structures capable of adapting to altered physiological demands. Although genetic factors play a large role in determining the fibre type distribution in muscle (Komi *et al.* 1997), non-genetic factors also contribute to overall distribution of fast and slow fibres. Neural, humoral and mechanical factors have been shown to play a role in the complex regulation of phenotypic expression of muscle fibres. In this section we discuss exercise training induced changes in skeletal muscle myosin phenotype.

Although once controversial, it now appears clear that endurance exercise training results in a fast-toward-slow shift in skeletal muscle myosin phenotype. Early studies investigating the question of whether endurance training can result in alteration of muscle types suggested that training-induced shifts in fibre types occurred only within type II fibres. For example, several early human endurance training studies reported significant increases in the percentage of type IIa fibres with a concomitant decrease in type IIb fibres (Andersen and Henriksson, 1977; Bauman *et al.*, 1987; Green *et al.*, 1979; Ingjer, 1979; Janson and Kaijer, 1977). Similarly, decreases in the percentage of MHCIIb and increases in the percentage of MHCIIa have been reported in locomotor muscles in rats following endurance training (Demirel *et al.*, 1997; Sugiura *et al.*, 1992). Can endurance training promote a transformation in skeletal muscle phenotype from type II to type I fibres? Chronic low-frequency electrical stimulation studies have clearly shown a sequential fast-to-slow (i.e. IIb →IId/x →IIa →I) fibre-type transformation in rabbit skeletal muscle (Delp and Pette, 1994; Pette and Staron, 1997). Furthermore, several endurance training studies in both humans and rodents have reported increases in type I fibres (Green *et al.*, 1984; Howald *et al.*, 1985; Jansson *et al.*, 1978; Luginbuhl *et al.*, 1984; Simoneau *et al.*, 1985) and in slow isomyosin (Fitzsimons *et al.*, 1990) and MHCI (Demirel *et al.*, 1997). A recent series of experiments demonstrates that increases in daily training duration dictates the magnitude of training-induced fast-to-slow shifts in myosin heavy chain isoforms (see Figure 4.4; Demirel *et al.*, 1997). A fast-to-slow shift in myosin light chains has also been reported following endurance training in humans (Baumann *et al.*, 1987) and in rat skeletal muscle (Green *et al.*, 1984).

Adaptations to resistance training

Resistance exercise training requires the muscles of the body to contract against an opposing force. Resistance-training exercises are generally classified as either isometric (no change in the length of the muscle as it contracts), isotonic (where the muscle is dynamically loaded) or isokinetic (the speed of muscular contraction is kept approximately constant). Isotonic contractions are the most commonly used type of resistance exercises and include lifting free weights and the use of variable-resistance machines.

Physiological adaptations to resistance training occur in many tissues and systems including the nervous system, skeletal muscles, connective tissue and bone. In this section we provide an overview of resistance training induced physiological adaptations.

Magnitude of strength gains

One of the major goals of a resistance-training programme is to increase muscular strength. Strength gains due to resistance-training programmes

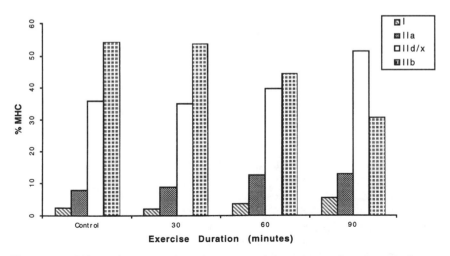

Figure 4.4. Effect of a 10-week endurance-training protocol on myosin heavy chain transformation in rodents. (Unpublished data from Demirel *et al.*)

have been well documented, with the magnitude of gain in strength being inversely related to that of initial strength (Kraemer *et al.*, 1988). Because initial strength varies greatly between individuals, this inverse relationship must be considered when evaluating the effectiveness of different resistance-training programmes (Fleck and Kraemer, 1997). For example, depending upon the initial strength level, resistance training induced increases in one repetition maximal strength (1-RM) for men can range from 7 per cent (Wilmore *et al.*, 1978) to 72 per cent (Allen *et al.*, 1976).

Physiological adaptations to resistance training

Resistance training induced strength gains are due to both muscular and neural adaptations. Skeletal muscle adaptations that have been investigated include changes in myocyte size and number, alterations in fibre type (reviewed in a previous section), adaptations in mitochondrial density, changes in bioenergetic enzyme activities and alterations in fuel supply. A number of other physiological changes have been associated with resistance training and include changes in bone and connective tissue, and alterations in body composition. The relative roles of these physiological adaptations are considered in the following discussion.

Neural adaptations

The initial physiological adaptations that result in strength increases are mainly due to neural factors (Sale, 1992). Neural adaptations are related to improved co-ordination, increased motor learning, improved activation of the prime-mover muscles, increased motor unit recruitment, and an inhibition of the protective mechanisms of the muscle (Sale, 1987). It has been shown that strength gains can be achieved without structural change to the muscle, but not without neural adaptations (Enoka, 1988). Further evidence supporting the importance of neural adaptations is seen when one limb is strength-trained, with strength gains also being observed in the contralateral limb (Kannus *et al.*, 1992).

Muscle hypertrophy

The major long-term adaptation to a resistance training programme is an increase in the size of the major muscles responsible for movement (muscular hypertrophy) (Moritani, 1992). The process of hypertrophy is directly related to the synthesis of cellular material, particularly the protein filaments that constitute the contractile apparatus. Within the muscle cell, myofibrils thicken and increase in number with additional sarcomeres being formed. The time-course of muscular hypertrophy was studied by Staron *et al.* (1994) who found that it typically took more than 16 training sessions for hypertrophy to be evident.

Of interest is whether muscle hypertrophy is selective to fibre type. Research has indicated that high-intensity resistance training results in an increase in the cross-sectional area of both type I and type II fibres, with type II fibres showing a greater response (Gonyea and Sale, 1982; Edgerton, 1978; Tesch, 1988). Interestingly, body builders who train with low-intensity (low-resistance) and large-volume work-outs have smaller type II fibres when compared to power lifters who use high-resistance work-outs (Kraemer, 1988). Therefore, it may be possible to selectively hypertrophy either type I or type II fibres by utilizing either low-intensity/high-volume or high-intensity/low-volume training respectively (Tesch *et al.*, 1984).

Muscle hyperplasia

An ongoing controversy in exercise physiology is whether resistance training results in an increase in the number of muscle fibres (hyperplasia). However, in recent years evidence using both animal models (Gonyea, 1980; Gonyea *et al.*, 1986) and humans (Larsson and Tesch, 1986; MacDougall *et al.*, 1984; Tesch and Karlsson, 1985) strongly suggests that long-term training may result in an increase in the numbers of skeletal muscle fibres. For example, when resistance training resulted in a 24 per cent increase in muscle mass but only an 11 per cent increase in fibre cross-sectional area, it was suggested that hyperplasia may play at least a minor role in muscle enlargement (Mikesky *et al.*, 1991).

Resistance exercise induced changes in muscle fibre types

Chronic resistance exercise training also affects the expression of myosin heavy chain isoforms and fibre types. Investigations utilizing resistance training in humans have revealed a decrease in IIb fibres and an increase in IIa fibres (Colliander and Tesch, 1990; Hather *et al.*, 1991; Adams *et al.*, 1993; Staron *et al.*, 1991, 1994). This IIb to IIa fibre-type shift reversed with detraining and was regained with retraining (Staron *et al.*, 1991). Hence, similar to endurance exercise training, resistance training promotes a shift away from type IIb fibres toward type IIa fibres.

Intramuscular fuel stores

Whether resistance training influences muscle stores of ATP, CP and glycogen is also controversial. In humans, 5 months of resistance training increased the resting intramuscular concentrations of CP, ATP and glycogen by 22 per cent, 18 per cent and 66 per cent respectively (MacDougall *et al.*, 1977). These findings contradict more recent studies (Tesch, 1992, Tesch *et al.*, 1992) which suggest that the training protocol and pre-training condition of the subjects influence the outcome.

In addition to possible adaptations in fuel stores, delivery of nutrients may be altered by resistance training via vascular adaptations. It appears that the intensity and volume of the resistance-training programme dictates whether vascular adaptations occur. For example, power lifters and weight lifters who train using high-intensity and low-volume routines experience no change in the number of capillaries supplying the skeletal muscle (Hurley et al., 1994). However, due to hypertrophy of the muscle fibres these athletes demonstrate a decrease in the capillary density (i.e. the number of capillaries per cross-sectional area) (Tesch et al., 1984). Conversely, body builders who train with low-intensity and high-volume routines have increased muscle capillarization which enhances blood supply and removal of metabolic by-products (Schantz, 1982; Staron et al., 1989).

Bioenergetic adaptations

Isokinetic training in humans has been shown to increase the activity of creatine phosphokinase and myokinase, enzymes involved in the ATP-CP system (Costill et al., 1979a). Similar findings have been reported with isometric training in rodents (Exner et al., 1973). However, other investigations report no adaptation in ATP-PC system enzymes following resistance training (Costill et al., 1979a; Tesch et al., 1992).

Enzymes associated with anaerobic glycolysis are generally unaffected by resistance training (Tesch et al., 1990) with the possible exception of phosphofructokinase which has been reported to increase by 7–18 per cent following isokinetic training (Costill et al., 1979). Interestingly, the mitochondrial volume of the muscle cell decreases with high-resistance training due to an increase in cell volume and a resultant decrease in the ratio of mitochondrial volume to contractile protein (MacDougall et al., 1979). This training response is apparently not harmful to the performance of strength and power athletes due to the anaerobic nature of their events. However, people who train solely with resistance exercises risk a drop in endurance capacity caused by decreasing the aerobic potential per unit muscle mass (Alway et al., 1988).

Cardiovascular adaptations

Resistance-trained athletes have been shown to have greater than normal (absolute) heart wall thickness (Effron, 1989), (absolute) left ventricular mass (Fleck, 1988) and (absolute) left ventricular cavity size (Deligiannis et al., 1988). These adaptations appear to be due to the requirement to pump a relatively small volume of blood against a high pressure (i.e. pressure overload). However, when these two adaptations are expressed relative to body surface area or lean body mass, there are no significant differences (Fleck, 1988). The majority of research indicates that resistance-trained athletes have either average or slightly lower than average resting heart rates, blood pressures and stroke volumes (Effron, 1989; Fleck, 1988).

Alterations in connective tissue and bone

Ligaments and tendons undergo adaptations to resistance training which may assist in the prevention of injury. Load-induced muscular hypertrophy in laboratory animals is associated with increases in the collagen content of the connective tissue sheaths that surround the muscle (Laurent *et al.*, 1978). Resistance training has also been found to increase the thickness of hyaline cartilage on the articular surfaces of bone, which could increase the ability of joints to absorb shock (Ingelmark and Elsholm, 1948).

It appears that the strain and compression imposed during resistance training may result in adaptations which result in increased bone mass. Cross-sectional studies demonstrate that resistance-trained athletes have greater bone mineral content compared to endurance athletes and sedentary individuals (Nilsson and Westkin, 1977). For example, elite junior Olympic weight lifters have significantly higher bone density in the hip and femur regions than age-matched control subjects (Conroy *et al.*, 1993).

Summary

As demonstrated by extensive research conducted over the past 30 years, exercise training results in systemic and cellular adaptations which translate to enhanced homeostasis during submaximal exercise performance. Although a great deal is known regarding exercise-induced adaptations, this body of knowledge is clearly expanding rapidly. As scientists, athletes, coaches, trainers and physicians, we watch with great anticipation as new discoveries unfold.

References

Adams, G.R., Hather, B.M., Baldwin, K.M. *et al.* (1993). Skeletal muscle myosin heavy change composition and resistance training. *J. Appl. Physiol.*, **74**, 911–915.

Aigner, S., Gohlsach, B., Hamalainen, N. *et al.* (1993). Fast myosin heavy chain diversity in skeletal muscles of the rabbit: heavy chain IId, not IIb, predominates. *Eur. J. Biochem.*, **211**, 367–372.

Allemeier, C., Fry, A.C., Johnson, P. *et al.* (1994). Effects of sprint cycle training on human skeletal muscle. *J. Appl. Physiol.*, **77**, 2385–2390.

Allen, T.E., Byrd, R.J. and Smith, D.P. (1976). Hemodynamic consequences of circuit weight training. *Res. Quart.*, **47**, 299–307.

Alway, S.E., MacDougall, J.D., Sale, D.G. *et al.* (1988). Functional and structural adaptations in skeletal muscle of trained athletes. *J. Appl. Physiol.*, **64**, 1114–1120.

Andersen, P. and Henriksson, J. (1977). Training induced changes in the subgroups of human type II skeletal muscle fibers. *Acta Physiol. Scand.*, **99**, 123–125.

Anzueto, A., Andrade, F.H., Maxwell, L.C. et al. (1992). Resistive breathing activates the glutathione redox cycle and impairs performance of the rat diaphragm. *J. Appl. Physiol.*, **72**, 529–534.

Armstrong, R.B. and Laughlin, M.H. (1984). Exercise blood flow patterns within and among rat muscles after training. *Am. J. Physiol.*, **246**, H59–H68.

Astrand, P.O. and Rodahl, K. (1986). *Textbook of Work Physiology*. McGraw-Hill.

Badeer, H.S. (1975). Resting bradycardia of exercise training: a concept based on currently available data. In *The Metabolism of Contraction* (P.E. Roy and G. Rona, eds). University Park Press.

Baldwin, K.M., Klinkerfuss, G.H., Terjung, R.L. et al. (1972). Respiratory capacity of white, red, and intermediate muscle: adaptive response to exercise. *Am. J. Physiol.*, **222**, 373–378.

Barclay, J. and Hansel, M. (1991). Free radicals may contribute to oxidative skeletal muscle fatigue. *Can. J. Physiol. Pharmacol.*, **69**, 279–284.

Baumann, H., Jaggi, M., Solland, F. et al. (1987). Exercise training induces transitions of myosin isoform subunits within histochemically typed human muscle fibres. *Pflugers Arch.*, **409**, 349–360.

Bevegard, S., Holmgren, A. and Jonsson, B. (1963). Circulatory studies in well trained athletes with special reference to stroke volume and the influence of body position. *Acta Physiol. Scand.*, **57**, 26–50.

Blomqvist, C.G. and Saltin, B. (1983). Cardiovascular adaptations to physical training. *Annual Rev. Physiol.*, **45**, 169–189.

Booth, F.W. and Holloszy, J.O. (1977). Cytochrome c turnover in rat skeletal muscle. *J. Biol. Chem.*, **252**, 416–419.

Borzone, G., Zhao, B., Merola, A. et al. (1994). Detection of free radicals by electron spin resonance in rat diaphragm after resistive loading. *J. Appl. Physiol.*, **77**, 812–818.

Botinelli, R. and Reggiani, C. (1995). Force–velocity properties and myosin light chain iso-form composition of an identified type of skinned fibres from rat skeletal muscle. *Pflugers Arch.*, **429**, 592–594.

Bouchard, C., Dionne, F.T., Simoneau, J.-A. and Bonlay, M.R. (1992). Genetics of aerobic and anaerobic performances. *Exerc. Sport Sci. Rev.*, **20**, 27–58.

Boyer, J. and Kasch, F. (1970). Exercise therapy in hypertensive men. *JAMA*, **21**, 1668–1671.

Brooke, M.H. and Kaiser, K.K. (1970). Three 'myosin ATPase' systems: the nature of their pH lability and sulphydryl dependence. *J. Histochem. Cytochem.*, **18**, 670–672.

Brooks, G. (1985). Lactate: glycolytic end product and oxidative substrate during sustained exercise in mammals – the lactate shuttle. In *Circulation, Respiration and Metabolism* (R. Giles, ed.). Springer-Verlag.

Burke, E. (1977). Physiological similar effects of similar training programs in males and females. *Res. Quart.*, **48**, 510–517.

Cadefau, J., Casademont, J., Grau, J.M. et al. (1990). Biochemical and histochemical adaptation to sprint training in young athletes. *Acta Physiol. Scand.*, **140**, 341–351.

Casaburi, R., Storer, T.W. and Wasserman, K. (1987). Mediation of reduced ventilatory response to exercise after endurance training. *J. Appl. Physiol.*, **63**, 1533–1538.

Chance, B., Sies, H. and Boveris, A. (1979). Hydroperoxide metabolism in mammalian organisms. *Physiol. Rev.*, **59**, 527–605.

Clanton, T., Dixon, G.F., Drake, J. and Gadek, J.E. (1987). Effects of swim training on lung volumes and inspiratory muscle conditioning. *J. Appl. Physiol.*, **62**, 39–46.

Colliander, E. B. and Tesch, P. A. (1990). Effects of eccentric and concentric muscle actions in resistance training. *Acta Physiol. Scand.*, **140**, 31–39.

Conroy, B.P., Kraemer, W.J., Maresh, C.M. et al. (1993). Bone mineral density in elite junior weight lifters. *Med. Sci. Sports Exerc.*, **25**, 1103–1109.

Costill, D.L., Coyle, E.F., Fink, W.F. et al. (1979a). Adaptations in skeletal muscle following strength training. *J. Appl. Physiol.*, **46**, 96–99.

Costill, D.L., Fink, W.J. and Pollock, M.L. (1976). Muscle fiber composition and enzyme activities of elite distance runners. *Med. Sci. Sports*, **8**, 96–100.

Costill, D.L., Fink, W.J., Getchell, L.H., Ivy, J.L. and Witzman, F.A. (1979b). Lipid metabolism in skeletal muscle of endurance trained males and females. *J. Appl. Physiol.*, **47**, 787–791.

Coyle, E.F., Hopper, M.K. and Coggan, A.R. (1990). Maximal oxygen uptake relative to plasma volume expansion. *Int. J. Sports Med.*, **11**, 116–119.

Coyle E.F., Martin, W.H., Sinacore, D.R. *et al.* (1984). Time course of loss of adaptations after stopping prolonged intense endurance training. *J. Appl. Physiol.*, **57**, 1857–1864.

Coyle E.F., Martin, W.H., Bloomfield, S.A. *et al.* (1985). Effects of detraining on responses to submaximal exercise. *J. Appl. Physiol.*, **59**, 853–859.

Criswell, D., Powers, S., Dodd, S. *et al.* (1993). High intensity training-induced changes in skeletal muscle antioxidant activity. *Med. Sci. Sports Exerc.*, **25**, 1135–1140.

Davies, C. and Knibbs, A. (1971). The training stimulus: the effects of intensity, duration and frequency of effort on maximum aerobic power output. *Int. Z. Angew Physiol.*, **29**, 299–305.

Davies, K.J.A., Quintanilha, A.T., Brooks, G.A. and Packer, L. (1982). Free radicals and tissue damage produced by exercise. *Biochem. Biophys. Res. Commun.*, **107**, 1198–1205.

Davies, K.J.A., Packer, L. and Brooks, G.A. (1981). Biochemical adaptations of mitochondria, muscle and whole-animal respiration to endurance training. *Arch. Biochem. Biophys.*, **209**, 539–554.

Deligiannis, A., Zahopoulou, E. and Mandroukas, K. (1988). Echocardiographic study of cardiac function in weight lifters and body builders. *Int. J. Sports Cardiol.*, **5**, 24–32.

Delp, M.D. and Pette, D. (1994). Morphological changes during fiber type transitions in low-frequency-stimulated rat fast-twitch muscle. *Cell Tissue Res.*, **277**, 363–371.

Demirel, H.A., Naito, H., Powers, S.K. *et al.* (1997). Influence of endurance training duration on skeletal muscle myosin isoform distribution. *Med. Sci. Sports Exerc.*, **29**, S265.

Diaz, P.T., She, Z.-W., Davis, W.B. and Clanton, T.L. (1993). Hydroxylation of salicylate by the *in vitro* diaphragm: evidence for hydroxyl radical production during fatigue. *J. Appl. Physiol.*, **75**, 540–545.

DiMaria, A.N., Neuman, A., Lee, G. *et al.* (1978). Alterations in ventricular mass and performance induced by exercise training in man evaluated by echocardiography. *Circulation*, **57**, 237–244.

Dudley, G.A., Abraham, W.M. and Terjung, R.L. (1982). Influence of exercise intensity and duration on biochemical adaptations in skeletal muscle. *J. Appl. Physiol.*, **53**, 844–850.

Edgerton, V.R. (1978). Mammalian muscle fiber types and their adaptability. *Am. Zoologist*, **18**, 113–125.

Effron, M.B. (1989). Effects of resistive training on left ventricular function. *Med. Sci. Sports Exerc.*, **21**, 694–697.

Ehsani, A.A., Hagberg, J.M. and Hickson, R.C. (1978). Rapid changes in left ventricular dimensions and mass in response to physical conditioning and deconditioning. *Am. J. Cardiol.*, **42**, 52–56.

Ekblöm, B., Astrand, P., Saltin, B. *et al.* (1968). Effect of training on circulatory response to exercise. *J. Appl. Physiol.*, **24**, 518–528.

Ekblöm, B. (1969). Effect of physical training on oxygen transport in man. *Acta Physiol. Scand.*, **328**, 1–45.

Ekblöm, B. and Hermansen, L. (1968). Cardiac output in athletes. *J. Appl. Physiol.*, **25**, 619–625.

Ennion, S., Pereira, J.S., Sargeant, A.J. *et al.* (1995). Characterization of human skeletal muscle fibers according to the myosin heavy chains they express. *J. Muscle Res. Cell. Motil.*, **16**, 35–43.

Enoka, R.M. (1988). Muscle strength and its development: New perspectives. *Sports Med.*, **6**, 146–168.

Exner, G.U., Staudte, H.W. and Pette, D. (1973). Isometric training of rats – effects upon fast and slow muscle and modification by an anabolic hormone in female rats. *Pflugers Arch.*, **345**, 1–14.

Faria, I. (1970). Cardiovascular response to exercise as influenced by training of various intensities. *Res. Quart.*, **41**, 44–50.

Fitts, R.H., Booth, F.W., Winder, W.W. and Holloszy, J.O. (1975). Skeletal muscle respiratory capacity, endurance, and glycogen utilization. *Am. J. Physiol.*, **228**, 1029–1033.

Fitzsimons, D.P., Diffe, G.M., Herrick, R.E. and Baldwin, K.M. (1990). Effects of endurance exercise on isomyosin patterns in fast- and slow-twitch skeletal muscles. *J. Appl. Physiol.*, **68**, 1950–1955.

Fleck, S.J. (1988). Cardiovascular adaptations to resistance training. *Med. Sci. Sports Exerc.*, **20**, S146–S151.

Fleck, S.J. and Kraemer, W.J. (1997). *Designing Resistance Training Programs*, 2nd Edn. Human Kinetics.

Fox, E.D., McKenzie, D. and Cohen, K. (1978). Specificity of metabolic and circulatory responses to arm or leg interval training. *Eur. J. Appl. Physiol.*, **39**, 241–248.

Frick, M., Elovainio, R., Konttinen, A. and Somer, T. (1967). The mechanism of bradycardia evoked by physical training. *Cardiol.*, **51**, 46–54.

Friman, G. (1979). Effect of clinical bed rest for seven days on physical performance. *Acta Medica Scand.* **205**, 389–393.

Gettman, L.R., Ayres, J.J., Pollock, M.L. *et al.* (1978). The effect of circuit weight training on strength, cardiorespiratory function and body composition. *Med. Sci. Sports Exerc.*, **1**, 171–176.

Gollnick, P.D. and King, W. (1969). Effect of training on enzyme activity and fiber composition of human skeletal muscle. *Am. J. Physiol,.* **216**, 1502–1509.

Gollnick, P.D., Armstrong, R.B., Saubert, C.W. *et al.* (1972). Enzyme activity and fiber composition in skeletal muscle of untrained and trained men. *J. Appl. Physiol.*, **51**, 317–320.

Gonyea, W.J. (1980). Role of exercise in inducing increases in skeletal muscle fiber number. *J. Appl. Physiol.*, **48**, 421–426.

Gonyea, W.J. and Sale, D.G. (1982). Physiology of weight lifting exercise. *Arch. Phys. Med. Rehab.*, **63**, 235–237.

Gonyea, W.J., Sale, D.G., Gonyea, F.B. *et al.* (1986). Exercise induced increases in muscle fiber number. *Eur. J. Appl. Physiol.*, **55**, 137–141.

Green, H.J., Jones, S., Ball-Burnett, M.E. *et al.* (1991). Early muscular and metabolic adaptations to prolonged exercise training in humans. *J. Appl. Physiol.*, **70**, 2032–2038.

Green, H. J., Thomson, J. A., Daub, W. D. *et al.* (1979). Fiber composition, fiber size and enzyme activities in vastus lateralis of elite athletes involved in high intensity exercise. *Eur. J. Appl. Physiol.*, **41**, 109–117.

Green, H.J., Klug, G.A., Reichmann, H. *et al.* (1984). Exercise-induced fibre type transitions with regard to myosin, parvalbumin and sarcoplasmic reticulum in muscles of the rat. *Pflugers Arch.*, **400**, 432–438.

Grimby, L., Bjorntrop, P. *et al.* (1973). Metabolic effects of isometric training. *Scand. J. Clin. Lab. Invest.*, **31**, 301–305.

Guth, L. and Samaha, F.J. (1969). Qualitative differences between actomyosin ATPase of slow and fast mammalian muscle. *Exp. Neurol.*, **25**, 138–152.

Halliwell, B. and Gutteridge, J.M.C. (1989). *Free Radicals in Biology and Medicine*. Clarendon Press.

Hamalainen, N. and Pette, D. (1992). The histochemical profiles of fast fiber types IIB, IID, and IIA in skeletal muscles of mouse, rat, and rabbit. *J. Histochem. Cytochem.*, **41**, 733–743.

Hather, B. M., Tesch, P. A., Buchanan, P. and Dudley, G. A. (1991). Influence of eccentric actions on skeletal muscle adaptations to resistance training. *Acta Physiol. Scand.*, **143**, 177–185.

Henriksson, J. (1977). Training induced adaptations of skeletal muscle and metabolism during submaximal exercise. *J. Physiol. (London)*, 270, 661–675.

Hermansen, L., Hultman, E. and Saltin, B. (1967). Muscle glycogen during prolonged severe exercise. *Acta. Physiol. Scand,.* **71**, 129–139.

Hickson, R.C. (1981). Skeletal muscle cytochrome c and myoglobin, endurance, and frequency of training. *J. Appl. Physiol.*, **51**, 746–749.

Higuchi, M., Cartier, L.J., Chen, M. and Holloszy, J.O. (1985). Superoxide dismutase and catalase in skeletal muscle; adaptive response to exercise. *J. Gerontol.*, **40**, 281–286.

Holloszy, J. O. (1967). Biochemical adaptations in muscle. Effects of exercise on mitochondrial oxygen uptake and respiratory enzyme activity in skeletal muscle. *J. Biol. Chem.*, **242**, 2278–2282.

Holloszy, J. O. (1973). Biochemical adaptations to exercise: aerobic metabolism. In *Exercise and Sport Science Reviews*, (J. Wilmore, ed.), pp. 45–71. Academic Press.

Holloszy, J.O. (1975). Adaptations of skeletal muscle to endurance exercise. *Med. Sci. Sports*, **7**, 155–164.

Holloszy, J.O. and Booth, F.W. (1976). Biochemical adaptations to endurance exercise in muscle. *Ann. Rev. Physiol.*, **38**, 273–291.

Holloszy, J.O. and Coyle, E.F. (1984). Adaptations of skeletal muscle to endurance exercise and their metabolic consequences. *J. Appl. Physiol.: Respir. Environ. Exerc. Physiol.*, **56**, 831–838.

Holloszy, J. O. and Oscai, L.B. (1969). Effect of exercise on alpha-glycerophoshate dehydrogenase activity in skeletal muscle. *Arch. Biochem. Biophys.*, **130**, 653–656.

Holloszy, J. O., Oscai, L.B., Don, I.J. and Mole, P.A. (1970). Mitochondrial citric acid cycle and related enzymes: adaptive response to exercise. *Biochem. Biophys. Res. Commun.*, **40**, 1368–1373.

Holloway, J. and Baeche, T. (1990). Strength training for female athletes: A review of selected aspects. *Sports Med.*, **9**, 216–228.

Hoppeler, H., Luthi, P., Classen, H. *et al.* (1973). The ultrastructure of normal human skeletal muscle. A morphometric analysis of untrained men, women and well trained orienteers. *Pfluegers Arch.*, **344**, 217–232.

Howald, H., Hoppeler, H., Claassen, H., Matieu, O. and Straub, R. (1985). Influences of endurance training on the ultrastructural composition of the different muscle fiber types in humans. *Pflugers Arch.* **403**, 369–376.

Hughson, R.L., Sutton, J.R., Fitzgerald, J.D. and Jones, N.L. (1977). Reduction of intrinsic sinoatrial frequency and norepinephrine response of the exercised rat. *Can. J. Physiol. Pharmacol.*, **55**, 813–820.

Hurley, B.F., Seals, D.R., Ehsani, A.A. *et al.* (1984). Effects of high intensity strength training on cardiovascular function. *Med. Sci. Sports Exerc.* **16**, 483–488.

Ingelmark, B.E. and Elsholm, R. (1948). A study on variations in the thickness of the articular cartilage in association with rest and periodical load. *Uppsala Lakaretorernings Foxhandlingar*, **53**, 61–64.

Ingjer, F. (1979). Effects of endurance exercise on muscle fibre ATPase activity, capillary supply and mitochondrial content in man. *J. Physiol.*, **294**, 419–432.

Jackson, M., Edwards, R. and Symons, M. (1985). Electron spin resonance studies of intact mammalian skeletal muscle. *Biochem. Biophys. Acta*, **847**, 185–190.

Jacobs, I., Esbjornsson, M., Sylven, C., Holm, I. and Jansson, E. (1987). Sprint training effects on muscle myoglobin, enzymes, fiber types, and blood lactate. *Med. Sci. Sports Exerc.*, **19**, 368–374.

Jansson, E. and Kaijser, L. (1977). Muscle adaptation to extreme endurance training in man. *Acta Physiol Scand.*, **100**, 315–324.

Jansson, E., Sjodin, B. and Tesch, P. (1978). Changes in muscle fibre type distribution in man. *Acta Physiol. Scand.*, **100**, 315–324.

Jansson, E., Esbjornsson, M., Holm, I. and Jacobs, I. (1990). Increase in the proportion of fast-twitch muscle fibers by sprint training in males. *Acta Physiol. Scand.*, **140**, 359–363.

Jenkins, R. (1983) The role of superoxide dismutase and catalase in muscle fatigue. In *Biochemistry of Exercise*, Vol. 13 (H. Knuttgen, ed.), pp 467–471. Human Kinetics.

Ji., L. (1995). Exercise and oxidative stress: role of cellular antioxidant systems. In *Exercise and Sport Science Reviews* (J. Holloszy, ed.), pp. 135–166. Williams and Wilkins.

Ji, L.L., Stratman, F. and Lardy, H. (1988). Antioxidant enzyme system in rat liver and skeletal muscle: influence of selenium deficiency acute exercise and chronic training. *Arch. Biochem. Biophys.*, **263**, 150–160.

Ji, L.L., Wu, E. and Thomas, D.P. (1991). Effect of exercise training on antioxidant and metabolic functions in senescent rat skeletal mucle. *Gerontology*, 37, 317–325.

Johnson, B., Babcock, M. and Dempsey, J. (1993). Exercise-induced diaphragmatic fatigue in healthy humans. *J. Physiol. (London)*, **460**, 385–405.

Kannus, P., Alosa, D., Cook, L. *et al.* (1992). Effect of one-legged exercise on the strength, power and endurance of the contralateral leg: A randomized, controlled study using isometric and concentric isokinetic training. *Eur. J. Appl. Physiol.*, **64**, 117–126.

Kilbourn, A. (1971). Physical training with submaximal intensities in women. I: reaction to exercise and orthostasis. *Scand. J. Clin. Invest.*, **28**, 141–161.

Klissouras, V. (1971). Adaptability of genetic variation. *J. Appl. Physiol.*, **31**, 338–344.

Klitgard, H., Mantoni, M., Schiaffino, S. *et al.* (1990). Function, morphology and protein expression of aging skeletal muscle: a cross-sectional study of elderly men with different training backgrounds. *Acta Physiol. Scand.*, **140**, 41–54.

Kobzik, L., Reid, M.B., Bredt, D.S. and Stamler, J.S. (1994). Nitric oxide in skeletal muscle. *Nature*, **372**, 546–548.

Komi, P.V., Viitasalo, J.H.T., Havu, M. *et al.* (1977). Skeletal muscle fibers and muscle enzyme activities in monozygous and dizygous twins of both sexes. *Acta Physiol. Scand.*, **100**, 385–392.

Kraemer, W.J., Deschennes, M.R. and Fleck, S.J. (1988). Physiological adaptations to resistance exercise: Implications for athletic conditioning. *Sports Med.*, **6**, 246–256.

Kraemer, W.J., Marchitelli, L., McCurry, D. *et al.* (1990). Hormonal and growth factor responses to heavy resistance exercise. *J. Appl. Physiol.*, **69**, 1442–1450.

Larsson, L. and Tesch, P.A. (1986). Motor unit fiber density in extremely hypertrophied skeletal muscle in man: electrophysiological signs of muscle fiber hyperplasia. *Eur. J. Appl. Physiol.*, **55**, 130–136.

Laughlin, M.H., Simpson, T., Sexton, W.L. *et al.* (1990). Skeletal muscle oxidative capacity, antioxidant enzymes, and exercise training. *J. Appl. Physiol.*, **68**, 2337–2343.

Laurent, G.J., Sparrow, M.P., Bates, P.C. *et al.* (1978). Collagen content and turnover in cardiac and skeletal muscles of the adult fowl and the changes during stretch-induced growth. *Biochem. J.*, **176**, 419–427.

Lawler, J.M., Cline, C.C., Hu, Z. and Coast, J.R. (1996). Effect of oxidant challenge on contractile function of the aging diaphragm. *Am. J. Physiol.*, **272**(2, Pt 1), E201–E207.

Lawler, J.M., Cline, C.C., Hu, Z. and Coast, J.R. (1997). Effect of oxidative stress and acidosis on diaphragm contractile muscle. *Am. J. Physiol.*, **273**(2, Pt 23), R630–R636.

Leeuwenburgh, C., Fiebig, R., Chandwaney, R. and Ji, L.L. (1994). Aging and exercise training in skeletal muscle: responses of glutathione and antioxidant enzyme systems. *Am. J. Physiol.*, **267**(2, Pt 2), R439–R445.

Longhurst, J.C., Kelley, A.R., Gonyea, W.J. and Mitchell, J.H. (1980). Echocardiographic left ventricular masses in distance runners and weight lifters. *J. Appl. Physiol.*, **48**, 154–162.

Lovind-Andersen, J., Klitgaard, H., Bangsbo, J. and Saltin, B. (1991). Myosin heavy chain expression in human skeletal muscle of elite soccer players: effect of strength training. *Acta Physiol. Scand.*, **143**, 24a.

Luginbuhl, A. J., Dudley, G. A. and Staron, R. S. (1984). Fiber type changes in rat skeletal muscle after intense interval training. *Histochem.*, **81**, 55–58.

MacDougall, J.D., Sale, D.G., Alway, S.E. and Sutton, J.R. (1984). Muscle fiber number in biceps brachii of bodybuilders and control subjects. *J. Appl. Physiol.*, **57**, 1399–1403.

MacDougall, J.D., Ward, G.R., Sale, D.G. *et al.* (1977). Biochemical adaptation of human skeletal muscle to heavy resistance training and immobilization. *J. Appl. Physiol.*, **43**, 700–703.

MacDougall, J.D., Sale, D.G., Moroz, D.G. *et al.* (1979). Mitochondrial volume density in human skeletal muscle following heavy resistance training. *Med. Sci. Sports Exerc.*, **11**, 164–166.

Mador, M., Magalang, U., Rodis, A. and Kufel, T. (1993). Diaphragmatic fatigue after exercise in healthy subjects. *Am. Rev. Resp. Dis.*, **148**, 1571–1575.

Marechal, G., Biral, D., Beckers-Bleukx, G. and Colson-Van Schoor, M. (1989). Subunit composition of native myosin isoenzymes of some striated mammalian muscles. *Biomed. Biochim. Acta*, **48**, S417–S421.

McArdle, W.D., Magel, J.R., Delio, D.J. *et al.* (1978). Specificity of run training on $\dot{V}O_{2\,max}$ and heart rate changes during running and swimming. *Med. Sci. Sports*, **10**, 16–20.

McKenzie, D.C., Fox, E.L. and Cohen, K. (1978). Specificity of metabolic and circulatory responses to arm or leg interval training. *Eur. J. Appl. Physiol.*, **39**, 241–248.

Mikesky, A.E., Giddings, C.J., Mathews, W. *et al.* (1991). Changes in muscle fiber size and composition in response to heavy-resistance exercise. *Med. Sci. Sports Exerc.*, **23**, 1042–1049.

Misner, S.E., Broileau, R.A., Massey, B.H. *et al.* (1974). Alterations in the body composition of adult men during selected physical training. *J. Am. Geriatric Soc.*, **22**, 33–38.

Mole, P.A., Oscai, L.B. and Holloszy, J.O. (1971). Adaptation of muscle to exercise. Increase in levels of palmityl CoA synthetase, carnitine palmityltransferase, and palmityl CoA dehydrogenase and in the capacity to oxidize fats. *J. Clin. Invest.*, **50**, 2323–2330.

Moore, R.L. and Gollnick, P.D. (1982). Response of ventilatory muscles of the rat to endurance training. *Pflugers Arch.*, **392**, 268–271.

Morales, C.F., Anzueto, A., Andrade, F. *et al.* (1993). Diethylmaleate produces diaphragmatic impairment after resistive breathing. *J. Appl. Physiol.*, **75**, 2406–2411.

Morales-Lopez, J. L., Aguera, E., Miro, F. and Diaz, A. (1990). Variations in fibre composition of the gastrocnemius muscle in rats subjected to speed training. *Histol. Histopathol.*, **5**, 359–364.

Morgan, T.E., Cobb, L.A., Short, F.A. *et al.* (1971). Effects of long term exercise on human muscle mitochondria. In *Muscle Metabolism During Exercise* (B. Pernow and B. Saltin, eds), pp. 87–95. Plenum.

Moritani, T. (1992). Time course of adaptations during strength and power training. In *Strength and Power in Sport* (P.V. Komi, ed.), pp. 266–278. Blackwell Scientific.

Morrow, J. and Hosler, W. (1981). Strength comparisons in untrained men and trained women. *Med. Sci. Sports Exerc.*, **13**, 194–198.

Nashawati, E., DiMarco, A. and Supinski, G. (1993). Effect of a free radical generating solution on diaphragm contractility. *Am. Rev. Respir. Dis.*, **147**, 60–65.

Neufer, P.D., Costill, D.L., Fielding, R.A. *et al.* (1987). Effect of reduced training on muscular strength and endurance in competitive swimmers. *Med. Sci. Sports Exerc.*, **19**,486–490.

Novelli, G.P., Bracciotti, G. and Falsini, S. (1990) Spin trappers and vitamin E prolong endurance to muscle fatigue in mice. *Free Rad. Biol. Med.*, **8**, 8–13.

Ohno, H., Suzuki, K., Ffujii, J. *et al.* (1994). Superoxide dismutases in exercise and disease. In *Exercise and Oxygen Toxicity* (C. Sen, L. Packer and O. Hanninen, eds), pp.127–161. Elsevier.

Oscai, L.B. and Holloszy, J. O. (1971). Biochemical adaptations in muscle II. Response of mitochondrial adenosine triphosphatase, creatine phosphokinase, and adenylate kinase activities in skeletal muscle to exercise. *J. Biol. Chem.*, **246**, 6969–6972.

O'Shea, J. and Wegner, J. (1981). Power weight training in the female athlete. *Physician Sports Med.*, **9**, 109–114.

Pechar, G.S., McArdle, W.D., Katch, F.I. *et al.* (1974). Specificity of cardiorespiratory adaptation to bicycle and treadmill training. *J. Appl. Physiol.*, **36**, 753–756.

Penpargkul, S. and Scheuer, J. (1970). The effect of physical training upon the mechanical and metabolic performance of the rat heart. *J. Clin. Invest.*, **49**, 1859–1868.

Pette, D., Muller, W., Leisner, E. and Vrbova, G. (1976). The time dependent effects on contractile properties, fibre population, myosin light chains, and enzymes of energy metabolism in intermittently and continuously stimulated fast twitch muscles of rabbit. *Pflugers Arch.*, **364**, 103–112.

Pette, D. (1984). Activity-induced fast to slow transitions in mammalian muscle. *Med. Sci. Sports Exerc.*, **16**, 517–528.

Pette, D. and Staron, R.S. (1997). Mammalian skeletal muscle fiber type transitions. *Int. Rev. Cytol.*, **170**, 143–221.

Pette, D. and Staron, R.S. (1990). Cellular and molecular diversities of mammalian skeletal muscle fibers. *Rev. Physiol. Biochem. Pharmacol.*, **116**, 1–76.

Pierce, E.F., Weltman, A., Seip, R.L. and Snead, D. (1990). Effects of training specificity on the lactate threshold and $\dot{V}O_2$ peak. *Int. J. Sports Med.*, **11**, 267–272.

Poehlman, E.T., Melby, C.L. and Goran, M.I. (1991). The impact of exercise and diet restriction on daily energy expenditure. *Sports Med.*, **11**, 78–101.

Pollock, M.L. (1973). Quantification of endurance training programs. In *Exercise and Sport Science Reviews* (J. Wilmore, ed.), pp.155–188. Williams and Wilkins.

Pollock, M.L., Ward, A., Ayers, J.J. *et al.* (1977). Cardiorespiratory fitness: response to differing intensities and durations of training. *Arch. Phys. Med. Rehab.*, **58**, 467–473.

Powers, S. and Beadle, R.E. (1985). Onset of hyperventilation during incremental exercise: A brief review. *Res. Quart. Exerc. Sport*, **56**, 352–360.

Powers, S.K. and Howley, E.T. (1997). *Exercise Physiology: Theory and Applications to Fitness and Performance.* Brown and Benchmark.

Powers, S., Lawler, J., Criswell, D. *et al.* (1990). Endurance training-induced cellular adaptations in respiratory muscles. *J. Appl. Physiol.*, **68**, 2114–2118.

Powers, S.K., Criswell, D., Lieu, F.K. *et al.* (1992a). Diaphragmatic fiber type specific adaptation. *Resp. Physiol.*, **89** 195–207.

Powers, S.K., Criswell, D., Lieu, F.K. *et al.* (1992b). Exercise-induced cellular alterations in the diaphragm. *Am. J. Physiol.*, **263**, R1093–R1098.

Powers, S., Lawler, J., Criswell, D. *et al.* (1992c). Aging and respiratory muscle metabolic plasticity: effects of endurance training. *J. Appl. Physiol.*, **72**, 1068–1073.

Powers, S., Grinton, S., Lawler, J. *et al.* (1992d). High intensity exercise training-induced metabolic alterations in respiratory muscles. *Resp. Physiol.*, **89**, 169–177.

Powers, S., Criswell, D., Lawler, J. *et al.* (1994a). Regional training-induced alterations in diaphragmatic oxidative and antioxidant enzymes. *Resp. Physiol.*, **95**, 227–237.

Powers, S., Criswell, D., Lawler, J. *et al.* (1994b). Influence of exercise and fiber type on antioxidant enzyme activity in rat skeletal muscle. *Am. J. Physiol.*, **266**, R375–R380.

Powers, S., Farkas, G., Criswell, D. *et al.* (1994c). Metabolic characteristics of primary inspiratory and expiratory muscles in the dog. *J. Appl. Physiol.*, **77**, 2188–2193

Powers, S.K. and Criswell, D. (1996). Adaptive strategies of respiratory muscles in response to endurance training. *Med. Sci. Sports Exerc.*, **28**, 1115–1122.

Powers, S. K., Coombes, J. and Demirel, H. (1997). Exercise training-induced changes in respiratory muscles. *Sports Med.*, **24**,120–131.

Quintanilha, A.T. (1984). The effect of physical exercise and/or vitamin E on tissue oxidative metabolism. *Biochem. Soc. Trans.*, **12**, 403–404.

Reid, M., Haack, K., Franchek, K. *et al.* (1992). Reactive oxygen in skeletal muscle. I. Intracellular oxidant kinetics and fatigue *in vitro*. *J. Appl. Physiol.*, **73**, 1797–1804.

Reid, M., Shoji, T., Moody, M. and Entman, M. (1992). Reactive oxygen in skeletal muscle. II. Extracellular release of radicals. *J. Appl. Physiol.*, **73**, 1805–1809.

Rowell, L.B. (1986). *Human Circulation Regulation During Physical Stress.* Oxford University Press.

Sale, D.G. (1988). Neural adaptation to resistance training. *Med. Sci. Sports Exerc.*, **20**, S135–S145.

Sale, D.G. (1992). Neural adaptation to strength training. In *Strength and Power in Sport* (P.V. Komi, ed.), pp. 249–265. Blackwell Scientific.

Salmons, S. (1994). Exercise, stimulation and type transformation of skeletal muscle. *Int. J. Sports Med.*, **15**, 136–141.

Saltin, B. and Gollnick, P.D. (1983). Skeletal muscle adaptability: Significance for metabolism and performance. In *Handbook of Physiology: Skeletal Muscle* (L.D. Peachy, R.H. Adrian and S.R. Geiger, eds). Williams and Wilkins.

Saltin, B., Henriksson, J., Nygaard, E. *et al.* (1977). Fiber types and metabolic potentials of skeletal muscles in sedentary man and endurance runners. *Ann. N.Y. Acad. Sci.*, **301**, 3–29.

Saltin, B., Blomqvist, G., Mitchell, J.H. *et al.* (1968). Response to exercise after bed rest and after training. *Circulation*. **38**, 1–78.

Saltin, B., Nazar, K., Costill, D.L., *et al.* (1976). The nature of the training response: peripheral and central adaptations to one–legged exercise. *Acta Physiol. Scand.*, **96**, 289–305.

Salmons, S. and Henriksson, J. (1981). The adaptive response of skeletal muscle to increased use. *Muscle Nerve*, **4**, 94–105.

Schiaffino, S. and Reggiani, C. (1994). Myosin isoforms in mammalian skeletal muscle. *J. Appl. Physiol.*, **77**, 493–501.

Schantz, O. (1982). Capillary supply in hypertrophied human skeletal muscle. *Acta Physiol. Scand.*, **114**, 635–637.

Seals, D. and Victor, R. (1991). Regulation of muscle sympathetic nerve activity during exercise in humans. In *Exercise and Sport Science Reviews* (J. Holloszy, ed.), pp. 313– 350. Williams and Wilkins.

Sen, C., Marin, E., Kretzschmar, M. and Hanninen, O. (1992). Skeletal muscle liver glutathione homeostasis in response to training, exercise and immobilization. *J. Appl. Physiol.*, **73**, 1265–1272.

Sharkey, B. (1970). Intensity and duration of training and the development of cardiorespiratory endurance. *Med. Sci. Sports*, **2**, 197–202.

Shindoh, C., DiMarco, A., Thomas, A. *et al.* (1990). Effect of *N*-acetylcysteine on diaphragm fatigue. *J. Appl. Physiol.*, **68**, 2107–2113.

Simoneau, J.A., Lortie, G., Boulay, M.R., Marchotte, M., Thibault, M.C. and Bouchard, C. (1985). Human skeletal muscle type alteration with high-intensity intermittent training. *Eur. J. Appl. Physiol.*, **54**, 250–253.

Sjodin, B. (1976). Lactate dehydrogenase in human skeletal muscle. *Acta Physiol. Scand. Suppl.*, **436**, 9–18.

Smith, D.C. and El-Hage, A. (1978). Effect of exercise training on the chronotropic response of isolated rat atria to atropine. *Exp.*, **34**, 1027–1028.

Snoeckx, L.H., Abeling, E.H., Lanbreghts, J.A.C. *et al.* (1982). *Med. Sci. Sports Exerc.*, **14**, 428– 434.

Staron, R.S. and Johnson, P. (1993). Muscle polymorphism and differential expression in adult human skeletal muscle. *Comp. Biochem. Physiol.*, **106**, 463–475.

Staron, R.S., Karapondo, D.L., Kraemer, W.J. *et al.* (1994). Skeletal muscle adaptations during the early phase of heavy resistance training in men and women. *J. Appl. Physiol.*, **76**, 1247– 1255.

Staron, R.S., Malicky, E.S., Leonardi, M.J. *et al.* (1989). Muscle hypertrophy and fast fiber type conversions in heavy resistance-trained women. *Eur. J. Appl. Physiol.*, **60**, 71–79.

Staron, R.S. and Pette, D. (1993). The continuum of pure and hybrid myosin heavy chain-based fiber types in rat skeletal muscle. *Histochem.*, **100**, 149–153.

Suguira, T., Morimoto, A. and Murakami, N. (1992). Effect of endurance training on myosin heavy-chain isoforms and enzyme activity in rat diaphragm. *Eur. J. Physiol.*, **421**, 77–81.

Terjung, R.L. (1976). Muscle fiber involvement during training of different intensities and durations. *Am. J. Physiol.*, **230**, 946–950.

Terjung, R.L. (1979). The turnover of cytochrome c in different skeletal muscle fibers of the rat. *Biochem. J.*, **178**, 569–574.

Termin, A. and Pette, D. (1990). Electrophoretic separation by an improved method of fast myosin HCIIb-, HCIId-, HCIIa-based isomyosins with specific alkali light-chain combinations. *FEBS Lett.*, **275**, 165–167.

Termin, A. and Pette, D. (1992). Changes in myosin heavy-chain isoform synthesis of chronically stimulated rat fast-twitch muscle. *Eur. J. Biochem.*, **204**, 569–573.

Tesch, P.A. (1988). Skeletal muscle adaptations consequent to long term heavy resistance exercise. *Med. Sci. Sports Exerc.*, **20**, S132–S134.

Tesch, P.A. (1992). Short- and long-term histochemical and biochemical adaptations in muscle. In *Strength and Power in Sport* (P.V. Komi, ed.), pp. 239–248. Blackwell Scientific.

Tesch, P.A., Thorsson, A. and Kaiser, P. (1984). Muscle capillary supply and fiber type characteristics in weight and power lifters. *J. Appl. Physiol.*, **56**, 35–38.

Tesch, P.A. and Karlsson, J. (1985). Muscle fiber types and size in trained and untrained muscles of elite athletes. *J. Appl. Physiol.*, **59**, 1716–1720.

Tesch, P.A., Dudley, G.A., Duvoisin, M.R. *et al.* (1990). Force and EMG signal patterns during repeated bouts of concentric or eccentric muscle actions. *Acta Physiol. Scand.*, **138**, 263–271.

Thorstensson, A., Sjodin, B. and Karlsson, J. (1975). Enzyme activities and muscle strength after sprint training in man. *Acta Physiol. Scand.*, **94**, 313–318.

Thorstensson, A, Hulten, B., vonDobeln, N.W. and Karlsson, J. (1976). Effect of strength training on enzyme activities and fiber characteristics in human skeletal muscle. *Acta Physiol. Scand.*, **96**, 392–398.

Thorstensson, A., Larsson, L., Tesch, P.A. and Karlsson, J. (1977). Muscle strength and fiber composition in athletes and sedentary men. *Med. Sci. Sports*, **9**, 26–30.

Tipton, C. (1965). Training and bradycardia in rats. *Am. J. Physiol.*, **209**, 1089–1094.

Tipton, C., Barnard, RJ. and Tcheng, K.T. (1969). Resting heart rate investigations with trained and nontrained hypophysectomized rats. *J. Appl. Physiol.*, **26**, 585–588.

Tipton, C.M., Matthes, R.D., Maynard, J.A. and Carey, R.A. (1975). The influence of physical activity on ligaments and tendons. *Med. Sci. Sports Exerc.*, **7**, 165–175.

Tsika, R.W., Herrick, R.E. and Baldwin, K.M. (1987). Interaction of compensatory hypertrophy and hindlimb suspension on myosin isoform expression. *J. Appl. Physiol.*, **62**, 2101–2110.

Vanhelder, W.P., Radomski, M.W. and Goode, R.C. (1984). Growth hormone responses during intermittent weight lifting exercise in men. *Eur. J. Appl. Physiol.*, **53**, 31–34.

Weiss, L.W., Cureton, K.J. and Thompson, F.N. (1983). Comparison of serum testosterone and androstenedione responses to weight lifting in men and women. *Eur. J. Appl. Physiol.*, **50**, 413–419.

Wenger, H.A. and Bell, G.J. (1984). The interactions of intensity, frequency, and duration of exercise training in altering cardiorespiratory fitness. *Sports Med.*, **3**, 346–56.

Wilmore, J.H., Parr, R.B., Girandola, R.N. *et al.* (1978). Physiological alterations consequent to circuit weight training. *Med. Sci. Sports Exerc.*, **10**, 79–84.

Winder, W.W., Hagberg, M., Hickson, R.C. *et al.* (1978). Time course of sympathoadrenal adaptation to endurance exercise training in man. *J. Appl. Physiol.*, **45**, 370–374.

Winder, W.W., Baldwin, K.M. and Holloszy, J.O. (1974). Enzymes involved in ketone utilization indifferent types of muscle: adaptation to exercise. *Eur. J. Biochem.*, **47**, 461–467.

Wong, T.S. and Booth, F.W. (1990). Protein metabolism in rat tibialis anterior muscle after stimulated chronic eccentric exercise. *J. Appl. Physiol.*, **69**, 1718–1724.

Further reading

Abernathy, P.J., Jurimae, J., Logan, P.A., Taylor, A.W. and Thayer, R.E. (1994). Acute and chronic response of skeletal muscle to resistance exercise. *Sports Med.*, **17**, 22–38.

Booth, F.W. and Thomason, D.E. (1991). Molecular and cellular adaptation of muscle in response to exercise: perspectives of various models. *Physiol. Rev.*, **71**, 541–585.

Enoka, R.M. (1988). Muscle strength and its development: new perspectives. *Sports Med.*, **6**, 146–168.

Fleck, S.J. and Kraemer, W.J. (1997). *Designing Resistance Training Programs*, 2nd Edn. Human Kinetics.

Holloszy, J.O. (1973). Biochemical adaptations to exercise: aerobic metabolism. In *Exercise and Sport Science Reviews* (J. Wilmore, ed.), pp. 45–71. Academic Press.

Pette, D. and Staron, R.S. (1997). Mammalian skeletal muscle fiber type transitions. *Int. Rev. Cytol.*, **170**, 143–223.

Pette, D. and Staron, R.S. (1990). Cellular and molecular diversities of mammalian skeletal muscle fibers. *Rev. Physiol. Biochem. Pharmacol.*, **116**, 1–76.

Powers, S.K. and Howley, E.T. (1997). *Exercise Physiology: Theory and Applications to Fitness and Performance*. Brown and Benchmark.

Yu, B. (1994). Cellular defences against reactive oxygen species. *Physiol. Rev.*, **74**, 139–162.

5

The biomechanics of human movement

Henryk K.A. Lakomy

Biomechanics is often described as the study of the effects produced by the internal and external forces acting on the body. This chapter will focus on those factors which affect the maximum force that a muscle, or muscle group, can generate and how this force is transmitted to the external environment. Some of the effects that these forces have on the external environment will then be examined.

Factors which affect the maximum force or tension that a muscle can generate

The speed and type of muscle action

When stimulated, all the fibres of the motor units recruited attempt to shorten. Despite the unreserved force produced by the myosin heads pulling the actin filaments towards the centre of the sarcomere within each active muscle fibre, there are three possible outcomes of this muscle activation (Figure 5.1):

- **Concentric muscle action.** If the tension generated within the muscle exceeds the load resisting movement then shortening of the muscle occurs.
- **Isometric muscle action.** If the load is matched by the muscle tension (or the load is immovable) then no movement of the limb occurs and there is, therefore, no overall change in muscle length.
- **Eccentric muscle action.** If the external load exceeds the tension created within the muscle the muscle will be forced to lengthen, despite the attempt being made by the active fibres to shorten.

Often the term 'contraction' is used to descibe the action of a muscle. This term is inappropriate when the muscle may shorten, lengthen or remain the same length as active and, consequently the term muscle action has been adopted to describe the result of muscle force production (Cavanagh, 1988).

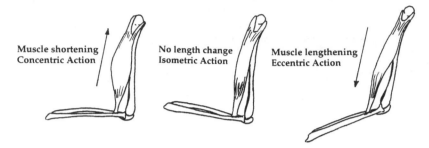

Figure 5.1. Examples of the three types of actions muscles can perform

The maximum tension that is created within a fully activated muscle is not a constant. During a concentric muscle action the maximum tension generated decreases in a curvilinear fashion with increasing speed of shortening. This relationship was first described by Fenn and Marsh (1935). Hill (1938) described the relationship mathematically for isolated muscle fibres *in vitro*. It has been found that although muscle *in vivo* does not behave according to Hill's equation exactly the general characteristic of declining force with increasing speed of shortening is evident. Each cross-bridge, created by the myosin heads attaching to the actin filaments, can be regarded as an independent force generator (Huxley, 1957). It is the combined effect of the cross-bridges acting at any instant which determines the total tension created within the muscle. More particularly the cross-bridge should be regarded as independent **impulse**, rather than force, generators as it is not only the magnitude of the force created within each cross-bridge which influences the overall muscle tension, but also the duration for which this force is applied. As the speed of muscle shortening increases the number of cross-bridges attached at any instant decreases (Huijung, 1992). As the overall tension is dependent on the number of active cross-bridges then the net effect is a reduction in maximum muscle tension with increasing shortening speed. There is a theoretical maximum speed of shortening (usually termed V_0 or V_{max}) at which the force created by the cross-bridges has become so small that it only just matches the internal resistance within the muscle resulting in no external muscle tension being produced. This maximum speed is thought to be closely linked to the maximum rate at which cross-bridges are able to cycle (Edman *et al.*, 1988). This speed is not achievable during concentric muscle actions *in situ* due to the additional resistance caused by the inertia of the limbs which must be overcome by a positive net muscle tension which can be produced only at speeds slower than V_{max}. It is important to note that the inverse relationship between maximum tension and speed of shortening only describes concentric and isometric muscle actions. The relationship is very different for eccentric actions in which the muscle is being forced to lengthen.

During slow eccentric muscle actions a small increase in the speed of lengthening results in a disproportionately large increase in maximum muscle tension (Joyce *et al.*, 1969). In this action some of the myosin heads complete a full cross-bridge cycle releasing in the normal manner at the end of the cycle, but others are probably being torn from the binding sites on the actin filament. Tearing of the cross-bridges results from the actin filaments being forced to move away from the centre of the sarcomere, in a direction opposite to that which would result from the conformational change in the myosin head. The myosin heads are forced back until the limit of possible extension in this direction is reached. The external forces on the muscle create forces on the cross-bridge which exceed the strength of the bond between the myosin head and the actin filament breaking the bond and lengthening of the muscle continues. As the speed of lengthening of the muscle is increased the proportion of cross-bridges in which the cycle is completed diminishes. More myosin heads are being torn from the actin filaments before they are able to complete a cycle. The force required to tear the bond of a cross-bridge is large, compared with that produced during a normal cross-bridge cycle. The duration of the cross-bridge attachment is probably longer for one in which conformational change is not achieved as extension of the elastic structures will occur before the myosin head is torn away from the binding site. The resulting impulse is substantially larger for a torn cross-bridge than for one which goes through a normal cycle. The number of cross-bridges being created at any instant during an eccentric action is greater than for concentric actions. Consequently, the combined increase in impulse per cross-bridge and the number of active cross-bridges results in a maximum eccentric muscle tension which is greater than that which could be created during a concentric muscle action. A comparison of the maximum muscle tensions generated by the three types of muscle action (Figure 5.2) shows that:

Eccentric maximum tension > Isometric maximum tension >
Concentric maximum tension

Not only do the type and speed of muscle action affect the maximum tension generated but these factors also markedly influence the **power** produced by the muscle.

Muscular power, measured in watts (W), is the product of muscle tension and the speed at which the length of the muscle is changing.

Power (W) = Force (N) × Speed (m s^{-1})

During an isometric muscle action there is no overall change in muscle length. The speed of length change is, therefore, zero and no external power can be produced, despite the high forces being produced within the muscle. In a concentric action the muscle is shortening. Figure 5.3

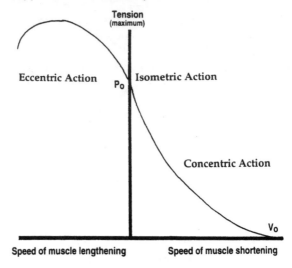

Figure 5.2. The relationship between maximum tension and speed of muscle shortening and lengthening (P_0 = maximum isometric tension; V_0 = maximum speed of shortening)

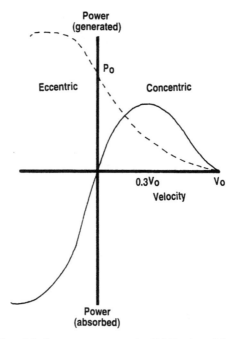

Figure 5.3. The relationship between power (solid line) and force (dashed line) and speed of muscle length change

shows how the power output produced by the muscle rises with increasing shortening speed to a peak level, which occurs in the region of $0.3V_0$ (Wickiewicz *et al.*, 1984). If the speed of shortening continues to rise then power output falls until at the theoretical maximum speed of shortening (V_0) no force can be developed by the muscle and consequently no power can be produced.

In contrast to concentric actions, during eccentric actions the muscle is being lengthened (negative speed of shortening). During eccentric activity work is being done by the external load to overcome the resistance created by the muscle. The muscle is thereby absorbing the work being done by the external load power, expressed as negative power. As the maximum muscle tension of an eccentric action has been shown to be greater than that produced during a concentric action so the maximum power that a muscle can absorb is also greater for an eccentric action.

Force–length relationship of muscle

In addition to the number of cross-bridges created and the impulse produced by each cross-bridge, it has been shown that the elastic structure of the muscle can contribute to the overall tension that can be produced by the muscle. The cross-bridges can be regarded as *active* tension producers whilst the elastic structures generate *passive* tension. The number of cross-bridges that can be formed is dependent on the extent of the overlap between the actin and myosin filaments (Gordon *et al.*, 1966; Edman and Reggiani, 1987). The natural resting length of the muscle sarcomere (I_s) is approximately 2.85 μm. At this length there is near optimal overlap of the filaments for maximum cross-bridge formation, and at this length the muscle will be able to generate maximum muscle tension from the active cross-bridges. If the muscle shortens then the actin filaments start to overlap each other. At a sarcomere length of less than 2.6 μm this overlap reduces the number of sites available for cross-bridge formation thereby reducing the active contribution to muscle tension. If, however, the muscle is stretched, then the actin filaments are pulled away from the myosin heads nearest to the centre of the sarcomere such that they cannot create cross-bridges. This results in a reduction in both the total number of cross-bridges formed and the tension produced by these active elements. At a sarcomere length of approximately 4.2 μm (150 per cent of I_s) there can be no cross-bridges formed at all. Figure 5.4 shows the muscle tension that would result from the active component i.e. the cross-bridges as muscle length varies.

Muscle tension is not produced exclusively from the active cross-bridges. As the muscle is stretched beyond its natural resting length (I_s) the physical structure of the muscle is put under tension. This structure is highly elastic, and the more the muscle is stretched the greater will be the tension created within these passive elastic structures. Overall muscle tension results from adding together the contributions being made by both the active and the passive components, as shown in Figure 5.4. At

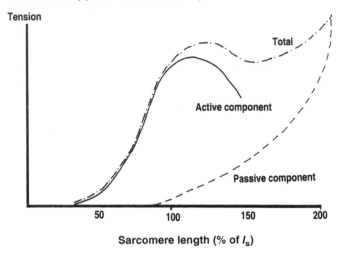

Figure 5.4. The relationship between muscle length and maximum tension, showing the contribution to the total tension made by the active and passive components

sarcomere lengths less than I_s little tension is being created in the passive elements consequently the overall muscle tension is influenced by the only the active components. Above I_s the contribution being made by the passive elements increases substantially with increasing muscle stretch (Sodeberg, 1986).

When muscle is being stretched not all the sarcomeres are being lengthened to the same extent. Rarely are the length changes of the sarcomere such that the extremes of possible shortening or lengthening are reached. During normal activity the average length of muscle sarcomere ranges between approximately 80 and 120 per cent of I_s, which corresponds to the relatively flat response area of the force–length relationship as shown in Figure 5.4 (Edman, 1992). This is beneficial as the maximum tension in a muscle is relatively independent of the joint angle which in turn influences the length of the muscle.

Angle of pennation

Fibres of a number of muscles lie parallel to the long axis of the muscle, acting directly along the line of pull of the muscle, a line passing through the point of muscle attachment to the bone. However, in some muscles the fibres are arranged such that they are angled away from the line of pull of the muscle. The angle created between the fibre direction and the line of pull of the muscle is called the angle of pennation.

The number of fibres (n) within a fixed volume of muscle increases with the angle of pennation, with a proportional decrease in average fibre length (Josephson, 1975; Edgerton *et al.*, 1987). The maximum tension that can be generated by a muscle reflects the number of fibres that can be recruited. Pennation of fibres would, therefore, appear to be an advantage. In pennate muscle the net tension produced by the muscle via the tendons to the bones is, however, not simply the sum of the forces produced by the individual fibres. Only a proportion of the force created within each fibre is transmitted along the line of pull of the muscle. Some of the force produced is wasted. If F_f is the force produced within a fibre, and θ is the angle of pennation, then the contribution (F_t) made to the overall muscle tension in the desired direction by each fibre is:

$$F_t = F_f \cos \theta$$

The total tension created by the muscle (T) in the desired direction is given by

$$T = n \cdot F_t$$

As the angle of pennation increases n is also increasing while the proportion of the useful tension being created per fibre is decreasing (Alexander and Vernon, 1975). However, these changes occur at different rates. At small angles of pennation the loss in useful tension per fibre is less than the relative increase in the number of fibres and the resultant muscle tension in the desired direction increases (Figure 5.5). At large angles the loss of useful tension per fibre exceeds the rate of increase in fibre number resulting in a rapid fall off of muscle tension. There should be an optimum angle of pennation at which the greatest level of tension will be developed by the muscle during force development. A specific angle, however, cannot be defined for muscle as not all the fibres in a pennate muscle have the same angle of pennation and as this angle does not remain constant. The architecture of the muscle changes on activation which results in an angle of pennation which is varying (Otten, 1988). A range of optimum angles of pennation have been found for different muscles, but these are usually $30°$ or less (Alexander, 1981).

It would appear that all muscles should be pennated. However, although maximum tension can be improved with pennation, the range of shortening of the muscle is reduced. The average length of the muscle fibres of pennate muscle is shorter than for fusiform (non-pennate) muscle, reducing the magnitude of possible shortening. The possible length change is further attenuated due to the fibres being at an angle to the line of shortening of the muscle further reducing the effective length of the fibres. Muscles which need to have large changes in length without the need for very high forces, for example the sartorius, do not have pennate muscle fibres. In contrast, pennate fibre arrangements have evolved in many muscles in which a high capacity for force generation, and not the range of movement, is the primary requirement.

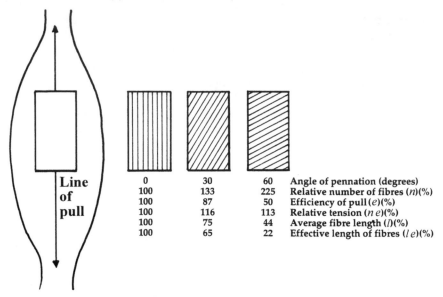

	0	30	60	Angle of pennation (degrees)
	100	133	225	Relative number of fibres (n)(%)
	100	87	50	Efficiency of pull (e)(%)
	100	116	113	Relative tension ($n\,e$)(%)
	100	75	44	Average fibre length (l)(%)
	100	65	22	Effective length of fibres ($l\,e$)(%)

Figure 5.5. The effect of pennation on average fibre number and length, and on the effective muscle tension generated

It is interesting to note that a consequence of pennation of muscle fibres allows muscle to operate over a greater range of length change whilst staying within the most effective range of the force–length relationship discussed earlier (Muhl, 1982).

Angle of insertion

So far some of the factors which affect the maximum tension created within a muscle have been examined. This tension acts on limbs and is manifested as the force, or torque, produced by the limbs. There are two factors which modify the efficiency of converting the muscle tension to external limb force. These are the distance of the muscle tendon insertion on the bone from the joint axis and the angle of insertion. The angle of insertion of a muscle is the angle the tendon makes with the bone to which it is attached.

As the tendon is permanently attached to the bone its distance from the joint axis can usually be regarded as being constant. Movement of the limb can sometimes affect this distance by either causing a shift in the position of the joint axis or the 'apparent' point of tendon insertion, e.g. the 'apparent' distance of the insertion of the biceps brachii from the elbow joint is reduced by pronation of the radio-ulnar joint due to the tendon wrapping itself around the radius bone.

The tension created by the muscle causes the limb to rotate around its joint axis, and the magnitude of this rotation is a function of the moment

or torque created (Figure 5.6). Torque is defined as the product of the force
(F) and the perpendicular distance it is acting from the axis of rotation (d):

Torque (N m) $= F(N) \times d(m)$

In the limb the force is the component of the muscle tension acting per-
pendicularly to the limb and the distance is that from the point of insertion of the tendon to the centre of axis of the joint.

If T_t is the muscle tension then $T_t \sin\theta$ is the perpendicular component
of force acting on the limb, where θ is the angle of insertion. This angle of
insertion is not a constant but varies during limb movement. If x is the
distance from the tendon insertion to the joint centre then the torque (T)
produced is

$T = T_t \sin\theta x$

The external perpendicular force produced by the limb (F_1) is given by

$F_1 = (T_t \sin\theta x)/d_1$

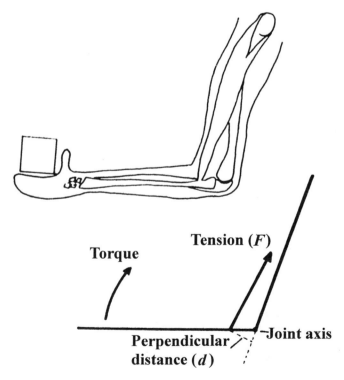

Figure 5.6. The torque created by muscle tension (F) acting at a perpendicular
distance (d) from the joint axis

where d_1 is the distance of the point of external force application by the limb and the joint centre.

If the tension created by a muscle were to remain constant throughout the range of limb motion then, as a consequence of the changing angle of insertion, the external force would also be changing. Optimum torque would be produced when the angle of insertion was at 90°, as shown in Figure 5.7. It has already been shown that the actual tension generated by a muscle is affected by its length and the speed of length change, both of which are changing during dynamic movements. The resulting change in maximum muscle tension linked with a changing angle of insertion results in varying external forces during dynamic actions.

The limbs, acting as levers, transmit the muscle tension to external loads. The bone is the lever arm moving about the joint axis or fulcrum. There are three possible lever arrangements depending on the relative position on the lever arm of the joint axis, the muscle insertion and the resistance. Examples of the two most common lever types are shown in Figure 5.8. In general, although the arrangements of the muscle insertion, lever arm and joint axis vary, the further the muscle insertion is

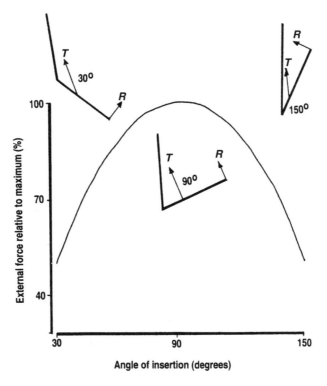

Figure 5.7. The influence of the angle of muscle insertion on the relative magnitude of the external force (R) produced by a constant muscle tension (T)

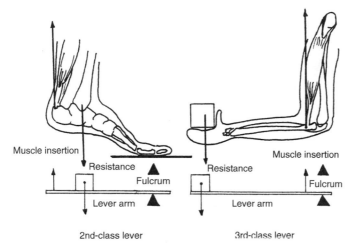

Figure 5.8. Examples of the two common lever arrangements found in the body, showing the relative positions of the fulcrum, resistance and muscle insertion

from the joint axis the greater the torque or leverage produced. However, although torque increases with increasing distance of muscle insertion from the joint axis, there is a proportional decrease in the speed of limb movement.

Not only are muscles required to move bones but a component of the force produced is needed to maintain the integrity of the joints. Depending on their characteristics and location muscles are sometimes described as being either spurt or shunt (MacConaill, 1949). Spurt muscles are characterized by having their insertions close to the joint axis of the bone being moved. In this arrangement the greatest component of the tension produced by the muscle causes limb movement. In contrast shunt muscles insert some distance from the joint axis, so that most of the muscle tension produced acts to compress the joint. If we examine the elbow joint, for example, the biceps brachii produces a large turning affect due to its insertion being close to the joint axis (Figure 5.9). The brachioradialis muscle, however, inserts close to the wrist joint with the muscle fibres lying almost parallel with the forearm, acting to maintain the elbow joint during activity. The classification of muscles into spurt and shunt is often criticized as some muscles which act on more than one joint have spurt characteristics at one joint and shunt characteristics at the other.

So far the only internal forces described have resulted from muscle tension. There are a number of other forces which act on the body. The branch of mechanics which deals with forces that act on a system is called kinetics. Gravitational forces, for example, act on the body to create the

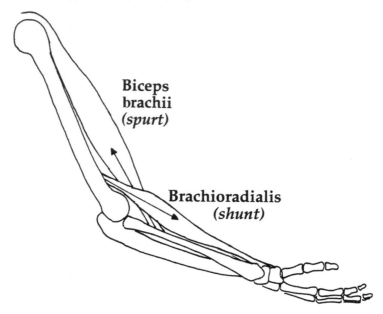

Figure 5.9. An example of a spurt (biceps brachii) and shunt (brachioradialis) muscle acting at the elbow joint

force of weight. Weight acts, internally, to compress or extend muscles, tendons, bones and joints as well as creating forces against the external environment.

It is important to understand that mass and weight are not the same thing. Mass is a fixed quantity, measured in kg, upon which gravity acts to create a force. For example an athlete of 75 kg mass (M) on earth is subjected to a gravitational force (g) attempting to accelerate him downwards at approximately 10 m sec^{-2} (more exactly 9.81 m sec^{-2}). The force created by the athlete against the ground upon which he is standing is $M g = 750$ N, known as his weight (W).

An example of an internal force required to overcome gravitational forces is an athlete (75 kg mass) standing on the toes of one foot. As the body is in static equilibrium the reaction force (R) of the ground contact must be equal to the weight of the athlete.

$$R = 750 \text{ N}$$

As there is no rotation by the foot about the joint axis of the ankle joint then the moment around the ankle created by the force (F) in the tendon must be equal to that caused by the ground reaction. For this athlete the tendon inserts on the calcaneus 0.035 m from the ankle joint (x) (Figure

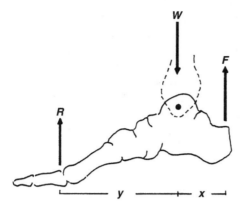

Figure 5.10. Example of the forces created in the foot when standing on the toes (*W* = weight acting through the ankle joint; *F* = tension on Achilles tendon; *R*= ground reaction force)

5.10) and the point of contact of the toes with the ground is 0.10 m from the ankle (y). Then:

$$F\,x = R\,y$$

$$\therefore\ F = R\,y/x = 750 \times 0.1/0.035 = 2143\ \text{N}$$

The force in the ankle joint (J_f) is also very large and is given by:

$$J_f = F + R = 2893\ \text{N}$$

The internal forces acting on the muscles, tendons and joints, illustrated in this example, are very much greater than those acting on the external environment (reaction force). This is the most common relationship between these forces.

The unit for force is the newton. It is sometimes useful, however, to use units of body weight (BW) to describe the magnitude of a force. One BW is not a fixed force but is dependent on the mass of the individual. In the above example the mass of the athlete was 75 kg, giving a body weight of 750 N. The force in the achilles tendon was just under three times body weight.

Kinematics

So far in this chapter only forces have been considered. The forces acting on a body are often difficult to measure. Useful information can be obtained by examining the spatial and temporal components of motion without measuring the applied forces. This branch of mechanics is called kinematics. Analysis of kinematic factors can be numerical (quantitative) or non-numerical (qualitative). Kinematics analysis can be made using direct observation or measurement systems from which only position, velocity and acceleration data can be obtained, such as cine or video.

Before giving an example of a kinematic analysis, the behaviour of objects will be examined briefly. Motion results from an object being moved from its initial location. This movement can be either linear (translational) or angular (rotational), or a combination of the two.

Linear motion

Distance and displacement

Distance (*l*) is the path actually covered whilst displacement (*d*) is the length in a straight line from the start to the finish point, both measured in metres. In a 100 m track race, for example, the path actually covered is the same as the linear distance from the start to end of the race, both being 100 m. In a 400 m track race, however, although the path covered was 400 m (distance) the start and finish points are coincident, and therefore the displacement was zero.

Velocity and speed

Speed is calculated by dividing the distance actually covered by the time taken. If the time involved was so short that no significant change in speed was possible then the value obtained is that of **instantaneous speed**. If, however, speed changes were possible during the event then the value obtained is called **average speed**.

The velocity of an object is calculated by dividing the displacement by the time taken. As with speed a value for **instantaneous velocity** is obtained if the time involved was so short that no change in velocity could occur, with **average velocity** being obtained for longer durations. Thus we have:

$$\text{Speed, } S = l/t \quad \text{and} \quad \text{Velocity, } V = d/t$$

Both speed and velocity are measured in metres per second (m s^{-1}).

If the time taken to cover 400 m on a track is 47 s then the average speed was $400/47 = 8.51$ m s^{-1}, whereas the average velocity was $0/47 = 0$ m s^{-1}.

Acceleration

Due to the forces being applied to objects, such as the body, the velocities at which they are moving are often changing. Acceleration is a measure of the rate at which the velocity of the object is changing with respect to time. The change in velocity is given by (final velocity (V_f) – initial velocity (V_i)) and average acceleration is the change in velocity divided by the time taken, i.e.:

$$a = (V_f - V_i)/t$$

Acceleration is measured in metres per second per second ($m\ s^{-2}$).

For example in a 40 m sprint from a stationary start the initial velocity of the sprinter is $0\ m\ s^{-1}$ in contrast to $10.8\ m\ s^{-1}$ when crossing the line. If it takes 4.8 s (t) then the average acceleration was:

$$a = (V_f - V_i)/t = (10.8 - 0)/4.8 = 2.25\ m\ s^{-2}$$

Acceleration is the result of an increase in velocity. When there is a decrease in velocity the resultant negative acceleration is often termed deceleration.

Vector and scalar quantities

Both speed and distance are completely described by their magnitude only, and are called **scalar** quantities. However, acceleration, velocity and displacement are **vector** quantities which require the direction in which they act to be described in addition to their magnitude.

Vector quantities are often represented by arrows with the length of the arrow representing its magnitude and the arrowhead showing its direction.

Angular motion

The linear kinematic factors have corresponding angular counterparts. When all parts of an object move through the same angle, without being displaced by the same amount, angular motion is said to have taken place.

The **angular distance** is the angle between the initial and final position, of a body, measured following the path covered. Thus to throw a heavy object the arm is initially swung backwards (extension of the shoulder joint) through 30°. Shoulder flexion then follows, swinging the arms forward through 60° before the object is released (see Figure 5.11). At the point of release the angular distance moved will be the sum of the two movements, namely 30° + 60° =90°. The angular displacement will be the

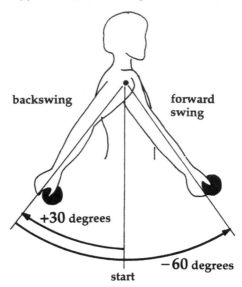

Figure 5.11. The angular distance and angular displacement of the shoulder joint in an underarm throw.

smallest angular distance between the initial and final positions. In this example the angular displacement will, therefore, be −30°. The direction of angular displacement must be specified and often the terms clockwise and anticlockwise (counter-clockwise) are used for this purpose. The clockwise direction is usually deemed to be the positive direction and so the negative sign indicates that the displacement was anticlockwise.

Average **angular speed** and **angular velocity** are determined by dividing the angular distance and angular displacement, respectively, by the time taken, so that angular speed = angular distance/time taken and angular velocity = angular displacement/time taken.

If in the above example if it took 0.5 sec to swing the arm back and 0.7 s to complete the forward swing, the total time taken would have been 1.2 s. The average angular speed would therefore have been 90°/1.2 s = 75° s^{-1}. In contrast the average angular velocity was −30°/1.2 s = −25° s^{-1}, the negative sign indicating the anticlockwise direction of the angular velocity.

In human performance maximum angular velocities are approximately 1000° s^{-1} but are more usually 60° s^{-1} or less.

Dividing the change in angular velocity by the time taken gives average **angular acceleration**.

In the above example the arm was stationary at the end of the back swing. If at the point of release the angular velocity was −140° s^{-1} then the change in angular velocity was −140° s^{-1}−0° sec$^-$1=−140° s^{-1}. As the time taken was 0.7 s then the average angular acceleration was −140°/0.7 s = −200 s^{-2}.

During some sporting activities an angular movement of a limb results in contact with an object which then travels with linear motion. Consider the action of kicking a ball. Angular movement at the hip joint results in foot contact with the ball imparting velocity to the ball. At the point of contact between the foot and the ball the relationship between the angular velocity of the limb and the linear velocity of the ball can be determined (Figure 5.12). The equation of the relationship is:

$$V = \omega\, r$$

where V is the velocity of the ball, ω is the angular velocity of the limb and r is the distance from the point of contact at the foot to the axis of rotation at the hip joint.

To correctly link linear and angular kinematics (and kinetics) mathematically, angular velocity needs to be expressed not in degrees per second but in radians per second. A radian is the angle subtended by an arc on the circumference of a circle equal to the length of its radius. This angle turns out to be approximately $57.3°$ and, therefore, the conversion requires the angular velocity (in ° $\sec^{-1}$) to be divided by 57.3 to obtain the correct units (rad s^{-1}).

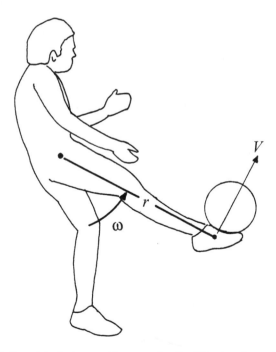

Figure 5.12. Relationship between linear velocity (V), angular velocity (ω) and limb length (r) during the action of kicking a football

An example of a kinematic analysis

The velocity of a runner is determined by two kinematic factors, namely stride length and stride frequency. Stride length is the distance travelled between two successive contacts with the ground by the same foot. Stride rate is the number of such contacts made every minute, whilst stride frequency is stride rate expressed per second (stride rate divided by 60). The average running speed is given by:

$$\text{Running speed (m s}^{-1}) = \text{Stride length (m)} \times \text{Stride frequency (Hz)}$$

Running speed can be altered by changing either stride length or frequency, or both. At slow running speeds, both variables increase, but a change in stride length is the predominant factor. It is not possible to keep increasing stride length indefinitely. At high running speeds, further speed increases result mainly from increases in stride frequency (Hoshikawa *et al.*, 1973).

Further information can be obtained by subdividing the stride into its flight phase, in which there is no contact with the ground, and the support phase, during which the foot is in ground contact. Kinematic analysis shows that the proportion of the stride spent in the support phase decreases with increasing running speed (Bates and Haven, 1974).

More subtle analysis enables us to discover what is happening during the support phase. Even when running at a constant average pace there are substantial changes in velocity taking place. Following heel contact there is a decline in velocity which is reversed near mid-contact. By the time toe-off is reached the velocity has increased such that it is the same as at initial heel contact. Figure 5.13 shows the pattern of velocity changes and acceleration occurring during the support phase of constant pace running.

Kinetics and related variables

Kinetics is the area of mechanics which deals with the causes of motion and is, therefore, concerned primarily with the forces which have already been discussed. There are, however, other variables which influence movement.

Inertia

A stationary object appears reluctant to move and once moving continues moving at constant velocity unless acted upon. This reluctance by the object to change its state of motion is called inertia.

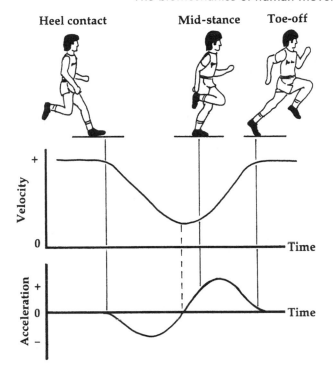

Figure 5.13. Changes in velocity and acceleration during the foot contact in constant pace running

Mass

The measure of the inertia of an object is its mass, which describes the quantity of matter from which it is made. Mass is measured in kilograms (kg). An increase in the mass of an object is reflected by an equal increase in its reluctance to change its motion, its inertia.

Force

The quantity which acts on an object to change its motion is called a force. Examples of internal and external forces have already been discussed in this chapter. Forces are vector quantities which must be described by both magnitude and direction.

Momentum

The product of the mass and velocity of an object is known as its momentum (P). To change the momentum of an object force has to be applied to it. If the force results in acceleration of the object then its momentum increases. Conversely, deceleration decreases its momentum. Momentum is different from inertia in so far as the magnitude of an object's momentum is a function of its velocity whilst its inertia is constant. The units of momentum are kg m s^{-1}.

Impulse

The product of the average exerted force (F) and the duration (t) of the exertion is called impulse (J). Impulse and momentum are strongly linked. The change in momentum of an object is equal to the impulse applied to it.

$$J = F\,t = m\,V_f - m\,V_i$$

where m is the mass, and V_i and V_f are the initial and final velocities of the object, respectively. The units of impulse are N sec.

Kinematic knowledge of the movement of an object can give us information about the forces acting on it. For example, if a ball of 0.5 kg mass is thrown straight up into the air from an initial position of rest in the hand, video analysis could be used to determine the velocity at the point of release. In this example it was found to be 9.6 m s^{-1}, and the time to ball release from the start of the movement was 0.12 s. The change in momentum of the ball is given by:

$$m\,V_f - m\,V_i = m\,(V_f - V_i) = 0.5\,(9.6 - 0) = 4.8 \text{ kg m s}^{-1}$$

This change in momentum is equal to the applied impulse; therefore

$$F\,t = 4.8 \text{ kg m s}^{-1}$$

The average applied force was

$$F = 4.8 \text{ kg m s}^{-1}/0.12 = 40 \text{ N}$$

As with kinematics all the linear kinetic variables discussed have angular counterparts. For a more complete description refer to texts such as that by Hamill and Knutzen (1995).

The impulse–momentum relationship is a manipulation of Newton's Second Law which states that force equals mass times acceleration ($F = m\,a$) and is the backbone of the analysis of activity. This is the fundamental law which links kinetic to kinematic parameters. This law holds equally for linear and rotational motion. For the latter, torque is substituted for force, with moment of inertia and angular acceleration replacing mass and acceleration, respectively. This Law, also known as the Law of Acceleration, is the foundation upon which the mechanics of human movement is based.

'Physical exercise and sport performance are made possible by means of forces developed by the voluntary muscles of the body acting through lever systems of the skeleton' (Knuttgen and Komi, 1992). It is clear that a knowledge of the factors affecting force production is central to biomechanics. Application of biomechanical principles enables an increase in our understanding of human movement, essential if performance is to be enhanced, teaching is to be improved or the risk of injury reduced. This chapter has given only a brief introduction to some of the key elements which influence movement and some of the mechanical factors affecting performance.

References

Alexander, R.M. and Vernon, A. (1975). The dimensions of knee and ankle muscles and the forces they exert. *J. Human Movement Studies*, **1**, 115–123.

Alexander, R.M. (1981). Mechanics of skeleton and tendons. In *Handbook of Physiology*, Vol. 4 (V.B. Brooks, ed.), p. 17. American Physiological Society.

Bates, B.T. and Haven, B.H. (1974). Effects of fatigue on the mechanical characteristics of highly skilled female runners. In *Biomechanics IV* (R.C. Nelson and C.A. Morehouse, eds), pp. 119–125. University Park Press.

Cavanagh, P.R. (1988). On 'muscle action' vs. 'muscle contraction'. *J. Biomechanics*, **22**, 69.

Edgerton, V.R., Bodine, S.C. and Roy, R.R. (1987). Muscle architecture and performance: Stress and strain relationships in a muscle with two compartments arranged in series. In *Medicine and Sport Sciences: Muscular Function in Exercise and Training*, Vol. 26 (P. Marconnet and P.V. Komi, eds), pp. 12–23.

Edman, K.A.P. and Reggiani, C. (1987). The sarcomere length–tension relation determined in short segments of intact muscle fibres of the frog. *J. Physiol.*, **385**, 709–732.

Edman, K.A.P., Reggiani, C., Schiaffino, S. and te Kronnie, G. (1988). Maximum velocity of shortening related to myosin isoform composition in frog skeletal muscle fibres. *J. Physiol.*, **395**, 679–694.

Edman, K.A.P. (1992). Contractile performance of skeletal muscle fibres. In *Strength and Power in Sport* (P. Komi, ed.), pp. 96–114. Blackwell Scientific Publications.

Fenn, W.O. and Marsh, B.S. (1935). Muscular force at different speeds of shortening. *J. Physiol.*, **85**, 277–297

Gordon, A.M., Huxley, A.F. and Julian, F.J. (1966). The variation on isometric tension with sarcomere length in vertebrated muscle fibres. *J. Physiol.*, **184**, 170–192.

Hamill, J. and Knutzen, K. (1995). *Biomechanical Basis of Human Movement*. Williams and Wilkins.

Hill, A.V. (1938). The heat of shortening and dynamic constants of muscle. *Proc. Royal Soc. London, B*, **126**, 136–195.

Hoshikawa, T., Matsui, H. and Miyashita, M. (1973). Analysis of running patterns in relation to speed. In *Medicine and Sport Vol. 8: Biomechanics III*, pp. 342–348. University Park Press.

Huijung, P.A. (1992). Mechanical muscle models. In *Strength and Power in Sport* (P. Komi, ed.), pp. 130–150 Blackwell Scientific Publications.

Huxley, A.F. (1957). Muscle structure and theories of contraction. *Progr. Biophysics Biophysical Chem.*, **7**, 255–318.

Josephson, R.K. (1975). Extensive and intensive factors determining the performance of striated muscle. *J. Exp. Zoology*, **194**, 135–154.

Joyce, G.C., Rack, P.M.H. and Westbury, D.R. (1969). The mechanical properties of cat soleus muscle during controlled lengthening and shortening movements. *J. Physiol.*, **204**, 461–474.

Knuttgen, H.G. and Komi, P.V. (1992). Basic definitions for exercise. In *Strength and Power in Sport* (P. Komi, ed.), pp. 3–6. Blackwell Scientific Publications.

MacConaill, M.A. (1949). The movement of bones and joints. 2. Function of the musculature. *J. Bone Joint Surg. (British)*, **31**, 100–104.

Muhl, Z.F. (1982). Active length–tension relation and the effect of muscle pinnation on fiber lengthening. *J. Morphology*, **173**, 285–292.

Otten, E (1988). Concepts and models of functional architecture in skeletal muscle. *Exerc. Sports Sci. Rev.*, **16**, 89–137.

Sodeberg, G.L.(1986). *Kinesiology: Application to Pathological Motion.* Williams and Wilkins.

Wickiewicz, T.L., Roy, R.R., Powell, P.L., Perrine, J.J. and Edgerton, V.R. (1984). Muscle architecture and force–velocity relationships in humans. *J. Appl. Physiol.*, **57**, 435–443.

6

Nutritional demands of training and competition

Louise M. Burke and Elizabeth M. Broad

In ancient times athletes searched for special foods and potions that might enable them to achieve great sporting feats. As we approach a new century, sports nutrition has become a credible science, offering the athlete a powerful tool in the achievement of their sporting potential. It has developed from a random and elusive search for a magic food into the systematic application of nutritional goals underpinned by rigorous research. These goals are summarized in Table 6.1. Of course, the relevance and priority of each goal varies with the individual athlete and their type and level of sporting activity. Importantly, the interest of sports nutrition lies equally with its *practice*. Athletes are often required to meet nutrient intake targets that are beyond their appetite, gastrointestinal comfort or access to food. Finding creative ways to provide athletes with their nutrient needs in a variety of unusual situations is part of the challenge of sports nutrition.

In this chapter we will overview the general science and practice of sports nutrition. The goals summarized above fall into four basic themes:

1. Meeting energy requirements, and achieving the physique (especially body mass, body fat and muscle mass) that promotes good performance in the athlete's sport.
2. Meeting special or increased needs for nutrients arising from a regular exercise programme.
3. Undertaking acute strategies before, during and after each exercise session to optimize performance and ensure efficient recovery.
4. Knowing how and when to incorporate the use of special sports supplements into the athlete's nutrition programme.

Energy balance and physique

One of the fundamental requirements for life, and for exercise, is energy. Energy, or fuel, can be described in many ways, with the combustible energy from food being measured in kilocalories (kcal), or kilojoules (kJ). The energy intake of athletes is important in determining their potential

Table 6.1.   The goals of sports nutrition (Burke, 1997)

During training, the athlete must aim to:
1. Keep healthy – especially by looking after the increased needs for some nutrients resulting from a heavy training programme.
2. Get into ideal shape for their sport – achieve a level of body mass, body fat and muscle mass that is consistent with good health and good performance.
3. Refuel and rehydrate well during each training session so that they perform their best at each session.
4. Practise any intended competition eating strategies so that beneficial practices can be identified and fine-tuned.
5. Enhance adaptation and recovery between training sessions by providing all the nutrients associated with these processes.
6. Eat for long-term health by paying attention to community nutrition guidelines.
7. Continue to enjoy food and the pleasure of sharing meals.

For competition, the athlete must:

1. In the case of weight-classed sports, achieve the weigh-in target without sacrificing fuel stores and body fluid levels.
2. 'Fuel up' with adequate body carbohydrate stores prior to the event.
3. Minimize dehydration during the event by using opportunities to drink fluids before, during and after the event.
4. Supply additional carbohydrate during events 1 h in duration or other events where body carbohydrate stores become depleted.
5. Achieve pre- and during event strategies without causing gastrointestinal discomfort or upsets.

for intake of nutrients, as well as playing a role in determining or modifying body composition and physique. Alterations to body shape and composition will depend upon the balance between intake and output. The effects of a change in energy balance over 1 day will be insignificant – noticeable changes in body composition will tend not to occur unless the balance has been altered for a period of time.

The components of energy balance

The components of energy expenditure include (McArdle *et al.*, 1991):

1. Resting metabolic rate (RMR) which typically accounts for ~ 60–75 per cent of energy expenditure, and is affected by muscle mass, genetics and energy intake.
2. Thermogenesis including thermic effect of feeding (~ 10 per cent).
3. Growth, pregnancy and lactation where applicable.
4. Exercise and physical activity which typically account for ~ 15–30 per cent of total energy expenditure.

The total amount of energy used during exercise and the source of that fuel varies according to the duration and intensity of exercise, environmental conditions and the level of fitness of the individual. Most sedentary adults aged 18–50 years have daily energy expenditures of around 10 500–12 500 kJ (2500–3000 kcal) for men and 8400–10500 kJ (2000–2500 kcal) for women (Deakin and Brotherhood, 1995), with lower levels generally seen in older populations. Regular exercise increases this expenditure by around 30 per cent, whereas the energy cost of the training or competition schedules of some elite athletes may double their total energy expenditure. Training itself increases the efficiency of activity; hence trained individuals will generally expend less energy at a specific speed than an untrained individual. Furthermore, children expend more energy per kg body mass (BM) than adults and may therefore have higher than expected energy requirements if they are fairly active (Saris and van Baak, 1994). The increased energy output incurred by exercise extends beyond the actual exercise period – exercise may increase RMR and the thermic effect of feeding for up to 24 hr after the actual exercise period.

Energy intake is the total amount of energy derived from the food we eat. The four nutrients providing energy to the body are protein (17 kJ or 4 kcal per g), carbohydrate (16 kJ/4 kcal per g), fat (36 kJ/9 kcal per g) and alcohol (27 kJ/7 kcal per g). These nutrients differ not only in energy density, but in the way that they are metabolized by the body. For example, fat is easily converted to body fat stores in adipocytes when not immediately required for fuel, whereas carbohydrate (CHO) is stored as muscle or liver glycogen, or used as an immediate source of glucose by the body. Any excess can be converted to body fat stores; however, this process requires energy in itself and hence approximately 25 per cent of the CHO is oxidized in the process.

Overall energy intake is therefore dependent upon the composition of the diet and the volume of food consumed. Due to the energy density of fats, high fat diets can become excessive in total energy if the volume of food consumed (or total energy intake) is not adjusted. Fat is not as satiating as proteins or fibre-rich CHO foods, making it easier to overconsume. Therefore, increasing the CHO:fat ratio in a diet can assist in preventing body fat gains.

Ideal body composition in athletes

The ideal body composition of athletes will vary immensely depending on the activity they are undertaking. The relationship between physique and sporting performance can be divided into five separate patterns:

1. No obvious special body composition requirements except general health requirements. Examples of sports which fit this category include archery, shooting, bowling and golf. Being within a healthy

weight range will benefit these sports people in terms of minimizing the likelihood of heat stress and maintaining optimum health.

2. A requirement for high muscle mass, but low body fat levels are not necessary. Examples include throwing events and 'heavyweight' categories in combat sports and weight lifting. As with the first group, it is still important to prevent obesity (excess body fat) for general health reasons.

3. General benefit from lower body fat levels, but very low levels are not directly correlated with improved performance. Examples include team sports and swimming. It may be more important for certain players in a team sport to carry lower body fat levels (such as the running players in football teams) and therefore the range of body compositions can vary widely within a team or sport.

4. Strong requirement for low body fat levels, and moderate to high muscle mass for maximal performance. This requirement may be to improve power-to-weight ratio, reduce the 'dead weight' that must be transported, or to improve appearance in subjectively judged sports. Athletes will generally sustain their physique throughout a full training and competition season. This group includes distance runners, triathletes, road and mountain cyclists, gymnasts, divers, skaters, skiers, sprint runners and cyclists, jumping and track event athletes and rowers. Athletes in these sports may require extra support when injured or taking a break from training in order to prevent large increases in body fat levels.

5. Weight-matched sports. In some sports, athletes compete in weight divisions that are designed to match opponents of similar size and strength. These include lightweight rowing, combative sports and weight lifting. Typically these athletes reduce their weight just prior to competition, by drastic energy restriction or by dehydration, in order to compete at a body weight that is considerably lower than their training or natural levels.

Athletes achieve their physique as a result of their genetics as well as the conditioning effect of training and diet. Hopefully they have chosen a sport to which they are suited, and then use appropriate strategies of training and nutrition to fine-tune levels of body fat and muscle mass. It is inappropriate that athletes are prescribed, or prescribe themselves, a rigid body composition goal since there is immense individual variability in the capacity to develop muscle mass and lose body fat. More importantly, the relationship between body physique and performance applies to populations and groups rather than individuals (for review, see Wilmore, 1992). An athlete's ideal level of body fat and muscle mass is unique to them, and one must safeguard optimal health and adequate nutritional intake as well as promoting good performance. Measurement of body composition and physique should be undertaken as one issue in the assessment of the nutritional status of the athlete. It is preferable that a

```
     #661  01-31-2017 1:52PM
Item(s) checked out to p18030804.

LE: ACSM's resources for clinical exe
CODE: 33015001195782
  DATE: 02-21-17

LE: Sports medicine : prevention, ass
CODE: 33015001113116
  DATE: 02-21-17

LE: Women and exercise : physiology a
CODE: 31927002934484
  DATE: 02-21-17

LE: Basic and applied sciences for sp
CODE: 33015001166403
  DATE: 02-21-17

merville Public Library - West Branch
       617-623-5000, x2975
```

series of measurements is made over time to determine the range of levels within which the athlete might achieve their goals.

Assessing body composition

Currently, there is no highly reliable or accurate method of assessing whole body composition which is inexpensive and convenient. Many new methods are reaching the market-place; however, all have inherent assumptions and larger degrees of technical errors of measurement than is ideal (for review, see Kerr, 1994). A few comments on common techniques used in the athletic world should be made at this point:

- Body mass and body mass index (BMI) are inappropriate to monitor body composition since they cannot differentiate between body fat, muscle, fluid and other components. Scales are most appropriately used by athletes to measure short-term alterations in body mass to indicate changes in fluid balance (e.g. dehydration occurring during a training or competition session).
- Anthropometry (including skin-fold and limb circumference measurements) is a quick and practical method of body fat assessment, suitable for field-work. If used appropriately it is sufficiently reliable to indicate changes in body fat levels over time in an individual. Anthropometric measurements should be taken by technicians trained to international standards, over a selection of body sites (typically at least seven sites). It is now common and preferable to interpret body fatness in terms of a sum of skin-fold measurements (in mm) rather than to introduce considerable error by using an equation to convert to an estimation of percentage body fat. Repeat measurements over time in an individual athlete should be done by the same technician.
- New electrical techniques of body fat measurement such as bioelectrical impedence (BIA) have entered the market-place over the last few years. To date, attempts to validate the reliability and validity of these measures have proven to be unsuccessful due to the inherent assumptions of body compartment densities on which they are based.
- Other techniques such as underwater weighing or dual energy X-ray absorptiometry (DEXA) are often labelled as the 'gold standard' for measuring body composition. In general, these are expensive and impractical for field-work with athletes; instead they belong in the realms of research. In any case, these methods still suffer from errors related to reliability and validity.

Modifying energy balance to lose or gain body mass/fat

A common reason for an athlete to consult a sports nutrition or medical professional is for advice to gain body mass (e.g. muscle mass) or lose body fat to improve their athletic performance (for review, see Burke, 1994a). Firstly it is important to fully assess whether the changes they wish to achieve are practical and relevant to the sport in which they are competing. Athletes have the same misconceptions about body weight and are just as prone to radical diets and inappropriate weight loss methods as the general population. Similarly, the world of body building and muscle development is well known for promoting unscientific and exaggerated claims for strategies that purport to increase muscle mass and strength.

Advising clients can be difficult. The counsellor requires a full understanding of the athlete's current eating habits, the issues that restrict change (such as their lifestyle, finances or family pressures), their attitude about food, and their sport-specific requirements. A sports dietitian has particular expertise in this area. However, some basic advice has been summarized in Table 6.2.

Making weight

It is the goal of weight divisions in sports to match competitors of similar size and strength. This is a feature of sports such as judo, boxing, wrestling and taekwondo, weight lifting, lightweight rowing, and for the jockeys in horse racing. Whilst it is ideal to advise individuals to compete in a division that is commensurate with their 'natural' or training weight, most athletes ignore this advice in favour of having a larger weight advantage over their opponent(s). The common pattern is to lose weight equivalent to ~2–10 per cent of total body mass (BM) in the day(s) leading up to the weigh-in, and then to recover some of this between the weigh-in and the competition (Steen and Brownell, 1990).

The time between weigh-in and competition, and the number of times that an athlete must weigh-in during a competition, varies between the sports. For example, lightweight rowers and weight lifters only have 2 h between the weigh-in and event, wrestlers often weigh in once only the evening before competition begins, while professional boxers have to weigh in up to 12 hr before each fight. Hence, a number of different strategies are used by athletes to 'make weight' and then to recover, many of which can have severe health consequences. Common methods used to 'cut weight' include food restriction, fluid restriction, dehydrating by undertaking saunas and heavy training in specialized 'sweat suits', diuretic abuse and even purgative substances or behaviours (Steen and Brownell, 1990). The process of making weight can leave the athlete with inadequate glycogen stores, dehydration, weakness, chronic malnutrition and feelings of anxiety and irritability. As a result, many athletes will

Table 6.2.   Practical tips for eating to change body physique and composition

A. **Assess what you currently eat**
1. Keep a food record for 4–7 days to provide an honest overview of what foods and fluids are consumed.
2. Look at eating patterns:
   - Is food consumed regularly over the day or are large time gaps left between eating?
   - Is breakfast eaten regularly?
   - Are you eating 'on the run'?
   - Is there a heavy reliance on high fat take-away or convenience foods?
   - Is food consumed because you are bored, upset or stressed?

B. **Set realistic goals**
1. Set realistic short- and long-term goals. Generally gains or losses of over 0.5 kg per week are unlikely in the short term, and changes tend to be lower over the longer term.
2. Base muscle gain goals on likely genetic potential and past experience.

C. **Dietary changes to achieve loss of body fat**
1. Look at ways to reduce fat and/or alcohol intake where possible. It is unnecessary to eliminate fat from the diet totally: it has important functions in providing essential fatty acids and fat soluble vitamins, as well as providing texture and flavour to foods. However, by reducing intake of fats and oils you can reduce total energy intake while preserving a meal plan that is filling and nutritionally adequate.
   - Minimize obvious sources of fat, such as by trimming fat off meat and skinning poultry, reducing spreads of butter or margarine, using reduced fat or low fat dairy products and salad dressings, and avoiding the consumption of 'greasy' or fried foods.
   - Use cooking and food preparation techniques that require minimum or no added fats and oils.
   - Become aware of hidden fats in foods. Read food labels to find where fats have been hidden in foods such as processed meats, cheese, crisps, biscuits, chocolate, processed foods, ice cream and other foods.
   - Drink alcohol in moderation – aim to have at least three alcohol-free days each week and limit alcohol to one to two drinks on any day.
2. Eat breakfast and spread the food intake over the day to prevent excessive hunger.
3. Find your appetite again – learn to eat in response to hunger signals rather than because it's meal time or the food is there.
4. Consider your current training programme or general activity level to see if energy expenditure can be increased. For elite competitors, this will be very difficult and should only be undertaken in consultation with the coach. However, some athletes engaged in skill-based sports may be able to undertake some aerobic exercise training.

Table 6.2. (Continued)

5. Don't over-restrict food intake. There is evidence that many athletes, particularly females, chronically over-restrict food intake (i.e. are restrained eaters). Energy intake should be no more than 2000–4000 kJ per day (500–1000 kcal per day) lower than estimated requirements. Some athletes may actually respond well to a small increase in their food intake instead of seeking further reductions. This can boost 'energy levels' and training performance, and kick-start loss of body fat.

D. **Dietary changes to increase energy intake**
1. Ensure that the athlete has a suitable training programme designed to stimulate muscle development and growth (see Chapter 11).
2. Increase energy intake by:
   - Eating small regular meals and snacks over the day (six to eight times) rather than infrequent large meals
   - Making use of carbohydrate- and nutrient-dense snacks, such as low fat muesli bars/cakes/muffins, dried fruit, and extra sugar, jam or honey on toast, pancakes, cereals and in drinks.
   - Utilizing fluids as an energy source. For example, instead of water, or tea and coffee, substitute fruit juices, soft drinks, fruit smoothies, hot milk drinks and liquid meal supplements. Use sports drinks during and immediately after exercise.
   - Avoiding excessive intakes of high fibre foods as they can be overly filling and reduce the capacity to increase total energy intake.
3. Be organized. Between two to three training sessions each day, and work, study and other commitments, there is little time for eating and resting. Think ahead to carry sufficient fluids and snacks with you all day rather than leaving their intake 'to chance'.

perform poorly since they will not have sufficient time to recover fully from the effort made to cut weight. In some instances, success in competition may be unrelated to skill and training, but rather reflect the ability to survive weight-making techniques.

Athletes competing in weight-category sports should be encouraged to achieve a healthy training weight that is close to their competition weight (i.e. within 2 per cent). This requires the selection of an appropriate competition division, as well as safe and effective weight-loss techniques undertaken well in advance of competition. The sporting organizations which run these sports should support these ideals with rule changes and other strategies to deter athletes from severe weight-making practices. Some simple guidelines for safer and healthier practices for the athlete are summarized in Table 6.3.

Table 6.3.   Guidelines for making weight safely

- Choose a weight division that you can reach by a combination of long-term loss of body fat and light last minute 'fine-tuning'.
- Begin 'cutting' weight early by losing excess body fat. Body fat loss should commence at least 2–3 weeks out from competition by restricting daily energy intake by around 2000 kJ (500 kcal) per day. Allow sufficient time to lose 0.5 kg of body fat per week.
- In the few days before competition, restrict intake of salt and salty foods in order to minimize fluid retention.
- Reduce fibre intake and use a low-residue diet in the 1–2 days before competition. Some meals can be replaced by a liquid meal supplement to limit the amount of undigested food remnants in the lower intestine.
- Restrict fluid intake over the last day if body mass is still above competition weight.
- Avoid using heavy exercise, or laxatives or diuretics, to achieve dehydration.
- After weigh-in, gradually resume food and fluid intake to aid rehydration and store glycogen. Some athletes make the mistake of consuming excessive amounts after the weigh-in. This can lead to vomiting and severe gastrointestinal discomfort, particularly when the event is within 1–2 h. Aggressive rehydration strategies involve replacing sodium as well as fluid (see Chapter 7).

Possible consequences of restricted energy intake and low body fat levels

There is some evidence that some athletes aim to reach minimum levels of body fat levels rather than their natural body fat levels, believing that this will improve their athletic performance. This is common among female athletes, particularly among those involved in endurance sports and sports where appearance is also important in the performance outcome (e.g. gymastics). Chronic restriction of energy intake and/or very low body fat levels may have negative outcomes both to health and performance. An area in which this has emerged as a potential key risk factor is menstrual dysfunction (oligomenorrhoea, or amenorrhoea) in female athletes.

Delay in menarche (primary amenorrohea) is not considered to have major health consequences. It occurs most commonly in gymnasts together with delayed growth and development. Studies of bone mineral density in gymnasts have shown higher levels of bone density than counterparts of the same age, probably due to the high loading on bone resulting from gymnastics training. In contrast, amenorrhoea (absence of menses) and oligomenorrhoea (irregular menses) can have serious consequences if it is prolonged for greater than 6 months. Several potential causes of menstrual dysfunction have been studied, including high volumes of high intensity exercise, stress, low energy intakes, eating disorders and unnaturally low body fat levels. Generally the existence of one factor alone is insufficient to cause dysfunction, whereas a combination of two or more, can produce sufficient physiological stress to reduce oestrogen levels (for review, see Highett, 1989). Due to the chronic reduction in oestrogen levels, one major medical concern is bone mineral density and the risk of stress fractures. Studies in long-distance runners have shown low bone mineral density in amenorrhoeic athletes which can be reversed upon resumption of menses. However, if amenorrhoea is long term (over 3 years), there is evidence that the loss of bone density from trabecular bone cannot be completely reversed, and may result in an increased risk of stress fractures and early osteoporosis (for review, see Drinkwater, 1992).

Menstrual function can resume with slight increases in energy intake (as small as 500 kJ per day increase) combined with a small reduction in the volume of high intensity exercise undertaken. Unfortunately, the elite athlete (and coach) is often resistant to this treatment due to the risk of body fat gain or comparatively insufficient training. It is often difficult to convince an athlete or coach that their performance may actually improve. A 3–4 week trial of dietary and training changes should be undertaken in agreement with the athlete and coach (where appropriate).

The spectrum of disordered eating among athletes is far wider than anorexia nervosa or bulimia nervosa (Gilchrist and Burke, 1995) and can occur both in males and females. The number of people with a distorted perception of food is so great that it is now increasingly difficult for many to define 'normal' eating behaviours. Some view the problem as being greater for the 'sub-elite' athlete who is struggling to improve the final step to compete against their peers. There appears to be a greater prevalence of disordered eating among athletes in sports in which weight or body fat levels are considered important for performance, than among those who participate in sports in which physique and body composition are not stressed (for review, see Brownell and Rodin, 1992).

Eating disorders are not directly caused by energy imbalance, but rather by a complex interaction of psychological, social and physiological factors. However, some common elements in the development of an eating disorder include pressure from coaches and others to lose weight, or failed attempts to lose body fat or mass (for review, see Sundgot-Borgen, 1994). Apparently low energy intakes or a complete avoidance of dietary fat, along with a distorted body image, intense fear of gaining weight and low self-esteem, can be early signals of a disordered view of food. This can result in the athlete losing sight of their true nutritional needs and training goals. The issues relating to the causes and treatment of eating disorders are complex and generally require a team approach to counselling and treatment.

Meeting nutrient requirements

Athletes or active individuals require an adequate balance of nutrients for general health and optimization of performance. Most athletes will be able to fulfil these nutrient needs within a varied diet, especially since they are often consuming more food than the general population. Theoretically, there is an increased need for many nutrients in those who are training regularly due to increased excretion in sweat, increased turnover and other biochemical adaptations to exercise. However, there is little scientific evidence available to substantiate these theories or the existence of widespread vitamin deficiencies in athletes (van der Beek, 1991). Furthermore, in Western societies, the consumption of a variety of nutritious foods in a high energy diet would reduce any risk of deficiency. In contrast, it is recommended that athletes who consume low energy diets or diets with restricted food variety should take a broad spectrum, low dose, multivitamin supplement in order to prevent any likelihood of a nutrient deficiency. Since restricted food variety and irregular meal patterns are a common feature of international travel, many travelling athletes might also consider multivitamin supplementation. Of course, the preferred strategy to achieve nutrient needs is by increasing the amount and variety of dietary intake to more appropriate levels.

Carbohydrate (CHO)

Specific guidelines for CHO intake before, during and after exercise have been set to optimize fuel availability for the session and to enhance recovery afterwards. These will be discussed below. The integration of these issues into a recommendation for the everyday carbohydrate requirements of the athlete has caused some confusion and debate. Historically, population dietary guidelines have considered CHO as an 'energy filler', making up energy requirements after protein requirements have been met and fat intake has been moderated. Population guidelines in Westernized countries generally recommend an increase in CHO intake, particularly from nutritious CHO-rich foods, to provide at least 50–55 per cent of total dietary energy. These recommendations are appropriate to address the health needs and fuel requirements of athletes undertaking a moderate training load.

Some authorities have suggested that athletes undertaking prolonged daily exercise sessions should increase CHO intakes to 65–70 per cent of dietary energy (American Dietetic Association, 1993). However, the rigid interpretation of this guideline may prove unnecessary and unfeasible for some athletes. Athletes with very high energy intakes (e.g. 4000–5000 kcal per day or 16 000–20 000 kJ per day) will achieve absolute CHO intakes of over 700–800 g CHO per day with such a dietary prescription. This may exceed their combined requirement for daily glycogen storage and training fuel, and furthermore, be bulky to consume. Athletes with such high energy intakes may be able to meet their daily needs for glycogen recovery with a diet where 50–60 per cent of energy is from CHO. Therefore, it is preferable to provide CHO intake recommendations in grams (relative to the BM of the athlete) and allow flexibility for the athlete to meet their requirements within the context of their energy needs and other dietary goals. Female athletes, who have lower energy intakes than might be expected, may need to devote a greater proportion of their dietary intake (e.g. up to 65–70 per cent of energy) to CHO intake, and even then may fail to meet the absolute CHO intakes suggested for optimal daily glycogen recovery (for review, see Burke, 1999).

The current debate about CHO intake recommendations is caused by the observation that studies fail to show clear-cut benefits to training adaptation and performance with high CHO intakes compared to moderate CHO diets (for review, see Sherman and Wimer, 1991). Studies show that higher CHO intakes allow better recovery/maintenance of muscle glycogen levels during periods of heavy training. However, there is no consistent evidence of significantly enhanced performance in the high CHO group at the end of the study period, nor impairment of performance in the moderate CHO group. It has been suggested that athletes may adapt to the lower CHO intake and muscle glycogen depletion. However, it is also possible that the protocols used to measure performance in these studies were not sufficiently sensitive to detect the differences between the groups and that the studies were not conducted over sufficiently long periods to elicit clear differences in performance. In any case, there is clear proof from studies of acute dietary manipulation that endurance and performance are enhanced when body CHO stores are optimized, and that carbohydrate depletion causes an impairment of performance (see below). Furthermore, there is anecdotal evidence, including comments from the studies above, that athletes complain of 'tiredness' and 'muscle fatigue' during training when dietary carbohydrate is insufficient. Therefore, the recommendation that athletes should consume a high CHO diet to cover the fuel cost of their training loads and recovery remains prudent. Further long-term studies are awaited to adequately test the benefit of this strategy (Burke, 1999). Practical guidelines for carbohydrate intake are summarized in Table 6.4.

Protein

Protein requirements of athletes are greater than those of the sedentary population. Additional protein is needed as a source of fuel during exercise, for repair and recovery of damaged muscle following training, and for the generation of new muscle mass (see Lemon, 1995). In general, the protein needs of athletes in heavy training are approximately double those of the non-active population, whilst those who exercise less regularly (i.e. three to five sessions per week) have only slightly elevated requirements. Although the underlying reasons for higher protein needs

Table 6.4.   Guidelines for carbohydrate intake for athletes

- Base meals and snacks around nutritious carbohydrate foods such that these take up at least half of the room on the plate. Examples include breads and breakfast cereals, rice, pasta, fruits, starchy vegetables, legumes and sweetened dairy products (e.g. fruit flavoured yoghurt).
- When maximal muscle glycogen storage is required, ensure that carbohydrate intake reaches the goal of 7–10 g per kg body mass each day. Situations include recovery between prolonged daily training or competition sessions, or loading in preparation for a competition. Special dietary counselling may be needed to achieve these levels of fuel intake.
- Be aware of low fat eating strategies. Many foods commonly believed by athletes to be carbohydrate-rich are actually high fat foods (e.g. cakes, take-away foods, chocolates and pastries).
- When carbohydrate and energy needs are high, the athlete should increase the number of meals and snacks that they eat, rather than the size of meals. This requires organization to have snacks on hand in a busy day.
- Lower fibre choices of carbohydrate-rich foods may be useful when energy needs are high, or when the athlete needs to eat just before exercise.
- Consider carbohydrate drinks (e.g. fruit juices, soft drinks, fruit/milk smoothies) and high sugar foods as a compact fuel source for special situations or high carbohydrate diets. This category includes many of the supplements made specially for athletes (e.g. sports drinks, liquid meal supplements).
- Before exercise, choose meals based on high carbohydrate, low fat eating. Experiment to find the type, amount and timing of food that suits you. Athletes usually have their own special pre-competition strategies. Popular choices include toast, breakfast cereal, pasta with low fat sauces, pancakes, fruit and special sports supplements (bars, drinks).
- To enhance recovery of muscle fuel stores after training or competition, eat a high carbohydrate meal or snack containing at least 1g of CHO per kg within 15–30 min. Nutritious carbohydrate-rich foods and drinks can provide protein and other nutrients that may also be useful in recovery. Examples include sandwiches, fruit smoothies, breakfast cereal, sports bars and liquid meal supplements.
- Consume carbohydrate during training and competition sessions, especially when the event is longer than 1 h, or there has been inadequate recovery from the previous session. Sports drinks and other sugary drinks will look after fluid and carbohydrate needs simultaneously, with sports drinks being specially designed to rapidly deliver these nutrients.

differ between strength- and endurance-training athletes, the estimated requirements are the same, at 1.2–1.8 g kg^{-1} BM daily (Lemon, 1995), with those who train twice a day or in heavy phases of competition requiring the most. Adolescent athletes who are growing may have slightly higher requirements again (up to 2.0 g kg^{-1} BM daily). Inadequate energy or carbohydrate intake will also increase protein requirements. Many studies which have estimated higher requirements than these recommendations have often not ensured energy or carbohydrate balance, or have not translated a positive nitrogen balance into gains in muscle mass or strength. There remains insufficient evidence of gender or age differences in protein requirements (Lemon, 1995).

Few athletes in Western societies are at risk of inadequate protein intake since the increased requirements are easily met within a varied diet, particularly if overall energy intake is increased. Dietary intake studies of athletes frequently report protein intakes greater than 1.8 g kg^{-1} BM daily, and very few have reported intakes below the recommended range (Burke and Inge, 1994). Even vegetarian athletes are not at risk provided they replace animal sources of protein with dairy products, eggs or nuts and legumes. Those who may be at risk of insufficient protein intakes are restrictive eaters or those who have low energy intakes; however, education on suitable food choices will usually rectify suboptimal intakes. Individual amino acid or protein powder supplements are considered unnecessary and expensive.

Iron

Iron is required for the transport of oxygen in the blood stream and within the muscle, and is a component of cytochromes and ferro-enzymes involved in energy production. It is therefore an important requirement for aerobic exercise performance. The iron requirements of active people are increased above those of the sedentary population due to increased losses through haemolysis, sweat and gastrointestinal bleeding, as well as increased blood volume requiring greater red blood cell production (for review, see Deakin, 1994). Iron needs are estimated to vary from 7 to 17 mg per day among male athletes and from 13 to 23 mg per day in female athletes. Iron deficiency is more common in females, endurance athletes in heavy training, pregnant and lactating women, rapidly growing adolescent athletes, and vegetarian athletes. This reflects increased iron needs, poor dietary iron intake or both. Common symptoms of iron deficiency are fatigue, pallor and ineffective training. Athletes in high-risk groups should be screened at least every 6 months for iron status, whereas those who are generally active should be screened when symptoms appear. The blood parameters typically considered important to screen are haemoglobin and ferritin, with ferritin levels below 30 mg ml^{-1} in conjunction with symptoms of fatigue often responding well to iron therapy. Further research is required to identify a more precise measure of low iron status in athletes since currently used indicators may show spurious results. For example, a transient low level may occur in response to a large increase in training volume. This may be due to a rapidly increased plasma volume and/or greater red blood cell destruction, rather than a true iron deficiency (Deakin, 1994).

Evaluation and management of iron status is best done on an individual basis by a sports medicine expert. Prevention and treatment of iron deficiency may include iron supplementation. However, this should be considered as a part of the overall management plan along with dietary counselling to increase the intake of bioavailable iron and appropriate strategies to reduce iron loss. Mass supplementation of athletes with iron and self-diagnosis of iron deficiency are to be avoided since they exclude the opportunity for a more holistic plan. Dietary guidelines for increasing iron intake should be integrated with the other nutritional goals of the athlete, so that goals of high CHO intakes or reduced energy intake to reduce body fat can be met simultaneously. This is where the expertise of a sports dietitian is most useful. Food sources of iron, together with advice on iron-rich meals, are summarized in Table 6.5.

Calcium

The calcium requirements for athletes mirror those of the sedentary population (800–1000 mg per day) except for amenorrhoeic female athletes who require approximately 20 per cent more (i.e. 1000–1500 mg). Increased calcium requirements are found among pregnant and breast-feeding athletes, and adolescents undergoing growth spurts. A small proportion of athletes are at risk of low calcium intakes, such as restricted energy consumers, vegans and those avoiding dairy products due to allergies or food fads (for review, see Burke, 1994b). Wherever possible, dietary sources of calcium should be encouraged. Guidelines are summarized in Table 6.5.

Zinc

Zinc serves as a cofactor of many enzymes, including those involved in energy metabolism and recovery processes. Studies of the zinc status of athletes have provided conflicting results. Difficulties in measuring body zinc content have arisen since plasma zinc levels are generally not correlated with dietary zinc intake (Clarkson, 1995). Plasma zinc concentrations tend to fall post-exercise but appear to return to normal within hours, and hence are therefore not likely to be reflective of a chronic deficiency. Zinc intake is at risk of being lower than recommendations in those individuals who reduce their meat (or meat alternative) intake in order to reduce fat intake or those who consume a low energy intake. It is important to educate athletes on the overall nutritional benefits of all food types in order to minimize potential deficiencies.

Table 6.5.   Guidelines for consuming iron and calcium

- Foods containing well-absorbed haem sources of iron include liver and liver pâté, red meat, shellfish and dark cuts of poultry. 'White' meats such as the breast cuts of poultry and fish provide only a fair source of this iron.
- Food containing moderate to high amounts of non-haem iron include iron-fortified breakfast cereals, wholegrain cereal foods, eggs, soya products and legumes, green leafy vegetables, nuts and dried fruit. Unfortunately, this form of iron is poorly absorbed and the availability is further reduced when it is mixed with tannins (tea), oxalates (spinach and silver beet), phosphates (dairy products) and phytates (wholegrain cereals).
- Include haem iron-containing foods in your carbohydrate-rich meals – for example, beef kebabs with rice, roast lamb in a sandwich, bolognaise sauce on pasta. The presence of these foods increases total iron absorption from the meal as well as providing its own iron contribution.
- Increase the absorption of non-haem iron by matching iron foods with a vitamin C source – for example, omelet with parsley and tomato, breakfast cereal consumed with orange juice.
- Dairy products are the major source of dietary calcium. Eat three to four servings each day, where one serving is equivalent to a cup of milk or yoghurt, or 30 g of cheese. Add these to carbohydrate-rich meals – for example, milk on breakfast cereal, cheese on toast, flavoured yoghurt with fresh fruit.
- Alternative sources of calcium include soya products (e.g. fortified soya milk, tofu) and fish eaten with bones (e.g. salmon, sardines).
- Where the athlete is unable or unwilling to consume iron- and calcium-rich foods in suitable amounts, a consultation with a sports dietitian is recommended. This will allow the athlete to optimize dietary potential and then assess the need for supplementation.

Antioxidants

Although regular exercise is beneficial to overall health, exercise has been shown to increase the production of free radicals which play an important role as mediators of skeletal muscle damage and inflammation after strenuous exercise (Dekkers *et al.*, 1996). Many individual nutrients have been investigated for their antioxidant potential, the benefit not being directly related to performance but to a reduction in injury severity. Training itself increases the activity of several major antioxidant enzymes and improves overall antioxidant status (Dekkers *et al.*, 1996), thereby providing a protective effect to those who exercise regularly. The methods currently used to determine the occurrence of lipid peroxidation are often difficult to interpret in the view of other consequences of exercise and may not be reliable. Despite this, a combination of vitamin C (ascorbic acid), vitamin E and β-carotene has been successfully used in research to reduce the indicators of free radical damage following exercise. The optimal doses of these vitamins, and whether they can actually be obtained through improving dietary choices such as increasing fresh fruit and vegetable intake and maintaining a wide variety of food choices, are yet to be elucidated.

Nutritional strategies before, during and after exercise

Fatigue during exercise performance, particularly prolonged exercise, is often related to depletion of body fluid and carbohydrate levels. Nutritional strategies to optimize fuel availability during exercise, and to maintain hydration by replacing sweat losses, are important in reducing or delaying the effects of fatigue. An enhanced rate of recovery after exercise is important for athletes who are undertaking several training sessions each day, or competing in progressive stages or games in a tournament. Issues relating to fluid replacement during and after exercise will be discussed in Chapter 7; therefore this section will focus on strategies for optimizing CHO status, with guidelines being summarized in Table 6.4.

Carbohydrate is the predominant source of energy for muscle metabolism during short (60 sec) bouts of supramaximal work and the preferred fuel for muscle for prolonged, moderate-intensity exercise lasting up to 4 h (Hawley and Hopkins, 1995). Unfortunately, however, the total body stores of CHO are limited, and are often substantially less than the fuel requirements of many athletic events. Strategies to match CHO availability to the requirements of training and competition are cyclical.

Post-exercise CHO ingestion must promote muscle and liver glycogen resynthesis in order to maximize body CHO stores for the subsequent exercise. Pre-exercise CHO meals are used to 'top up' fuel stores, while CHO intake during exercise may be needed to provide additional fuel as body stores become depleted.

Preparation for competition

Before competition an athlete should ensure that liver and muscle glycogen stores are matched to the anticipated fuel needs of the event. Normalized glycogen stores can be achieved by a high carbohydrate intake, in conjunction with a reduction in exercise volume and intensity for the 24–36 h pre-event. This is considered sufficient for most sports events, particularly events lasting less than 60 min. Athletes who compete in events longer than this (particularly events longer than 90 min) may try to maximize their muscle glycogen stores by undertaking an exercise–diet programme known as glycogen (or carbohydrate) loading.

The original CHO loading protocol, as described by Scandinavian researchers in the late 1960s, used extremes of diet and exercise to first deplete then supercompensate glycogen stores. Recent research suggests that trained athletes do not need to undertake the severe depletion phase to subsequently achieve an increase in glycogen stores. Instead, they need only to taper their training and ensure a high (8–10 g kg^{-1} BM per day) carbohydrate intake over the 72 h prior to an event to achieve similar increases in muscle glycogen to those reported in the more extreme regimens (for review, see Coyle, 1992). Some studies have reported that athletes do not have sufficient practical nutrition knowledge to achieve such carbohydrate intakes and may require dietary counselling.

The pre-event meal

The pre-event meal offers a last chance to fine-tune fluid and fuel levels prior to the event, as well as to ensure gastrointestinal comfort. An athlete who is well tapered and has been consuming high carbohydrate meals over the last 2–3 days may already have optimized muscle CHO stores. In this case, the major concern is to top up liver glycogen stores after an overnight fast should the event be early in the day. Conversely, if preparation for the event has been less than optimal due to inadequate recovery from the last exercise session, food eaten in the pre-event meal (1–4 h pre-event) may significantly contribute to muscle fuel stores (see Coyle, 1992).

Pre-exercise meal choices vary between individual athletes, and are determined by personal preferences, the time of day of competition and the degree of importance of this preparation. The ideal meal should include high carbohydrate, low fat foods, with reduced fibre and protein content being an additional recommendation for those who experience gastrointestinal discomfort. Fluid intake is also important, especially in preparation for events carried out in hot conditions. Some athletes can comfortably consume a larger meal or snack 3–4 h prior to competition. However, those involved in early morning events, or competing in a number of events with a short gap in between, may prefer to consume a smaller snack 1–2 hours beforehand. In the training situation some athletes with early morning sessions (e.g. swimmers) may not consume any food at all. Liquid meals such as commercially available supplements or fruit smoothies provide a practical alternative for athletes who find it difficult to consume solid foods prior to exercise, or where the time interval is small. The athlete is advised to experiment with various pre-event routines during training to define the optimal strategy.

Sugar prior to the event?

The consumption of CHO in the 30–60 min prior to exercise causes a pronounced elevation in plasma glucose and insulin concentrations at the onset of exercise. This will reduce the availability and oxidation of fatty acids during exercise and increase reliance on carbohydrate fuel. In the late 1970s one study found that feeding glucose 30 min prior to exercise actually impaired cycle time to exhaustion. They observed a rapid drop in blood glucose concentration during the first 10 min of exercise after subjects had been fed CHO, but suggested that the major factor in fatigue was an accelerated use of muscle glycogen (Foster *et al.*, 1979). Unfortunately, the results of this study have been so well publicized that warnings to avoid CHO intake during the hour prior to endurance exercise have become part of many sports nutrition guidelines. However, a review of the literature reveals that this is the *only* study to find reductions in performance after the ingestion of CHO in the hour before exercise. Other investigations have found either no detrimental effect or improvements in performance ranging from 7 to 20 per cent (for review, see Hawley and Burke, 1997).

A few individuals may experience an exaggerated and detrimental response to the hyperinsulinaemia associated with pre-exercise feedings. Such athletes complain of rapid and overwhelming fatigue. However, these symptoms may be overcome by manipulating the timing of CHO feedings, or by choosing CHO sources that produce a lower glycaemic response. For the majority of athletes, any metabolic alterations associated with the intake of CHO in the hour prior to exercise are transient, of little physiological significance, and are compensated by the increased CHO availability. Hence, the benefits and the practical issues associated with pre-exercise feedings should be judged according to the situation and the individual athlete (Hawley and Burke, 1997).

CHO intake during exercise

There is now strong evidence that increasing the availability of CHO during prolonged, moderate-intensity exercise can improve work capacity. The majority of well controlled trials of either prolonged cycling or treadmill running (> 90 min) have shown significant improvements in exercise performance with CHO ingestion. Even when there was no significant positive effect of CHO ingestion on exercise capacity, neither was performance adversely affected by CHO intake. The major effects of CHO feedings during prolonged exercise are to maintain plasma glucose concentration, sustain high rates of CHO oxidation and spare liver glycogen (Coggan and Coyle, 1991).

Recent studies have shown that carbohydrate ingestion also enhances the performance of sustained high-intensity exercise of ~ 1 h duration (Jeukendrup *et al.*, 1997). Since fuel availability is unlikely to be limiting in this type of exercise, another mechanism is needed to explain these findings. Perhaps athletes receive a 'central' boost or reduced perception of effort following carbohydrate ingestion. Further research is needed to support and explore these findings. Although it is more difficult to undertake performance studies in team and racket sports, it is reasonable to assume that athletes in these sports will also benefit from CHO intake during training and competition sessions. Fuel stores may become depleted during prolonged games, particularly in the case of 'mobile' players. Furthermore, in tournaments and during daily training there may be inadequate time to fully restore glycogen levels between games. The central effects of carbohydrate ingestion are also likely to benefit skill and cognitive function.

Typically, intakes of 30–60 g of CHO per hour are required to provide performance benefits. Tracer studies estimate that only small amounts of ingested CHO are oxidized during the first hour of exercise; thereafter oxidation rates peak at ~ 1 g hr^{-1}. Carbohydrate intake promotes greater performance benefits when consumed throughout exercise, and certainly in advance of fatigue, rather than when the athlete waits for the onset of symptoms of fuel depletion (for review, see Hawley and Burke, 1997). Both solid and liquid forms of CHO have been used by athletes to provide these intakes. However, fluids such as commercially available sports drinks are tailor-made for the needs of sport, since they can provide appropriate amounts of fluid and CHO simultaneously (see Chapter 7).

Of course, practical considerations may dictate the timing and frequency of an athlete's feeding. During endurance events, energy replacement occurs while the athlete is literally 'on the run', and might only be limited by consideration of the time lost in stopping or slowing down to consume food or fluid, or the impact of such ingestion on gastrointestinal discomfort (Coyle and Montain, 1992). On the other hand, in many team sports the opportunity to ingest fluid is governed by the official rules of the sport and is limited to formal breaks or during informal injury stoppages (Burke and Hawley, 1997).

Post-exercise glycogen recovery

Rapid recovery of fuel stores is important when the athlete has to train or compete within 8–24 h. This is a common issue in the training schedules of elite athletes, but may also occur in competition settings for athletes who compete in weekly or biweekly fixtures, tournaments or multi-stage events. The most important determinant of muscle glycogen storage is the amount of carbohydrate consumed. Studies have shown that an optimal rate of refuelling occurs when approximately 1 g of CHO per kg body mass is consumed immediately after exercise, towards a total intake of 7–10 g kg^{-1} over the next 24 h. Higher CHO intakes may be useful to compensate partially for reduced storage rates in damaged muscles, or to provide the fuel needs of further exercise. There is evidence that the rate of glycogen storage is enhanced during the first couple of hours of post-exercise recovery. However, the main reason for recommending CHO intake early in the recovery period is that substantial storage does not occur until CHO substrate is provided. Thus early feeding maximizes the length of effective recovery between exercise sessions.

Although practical issues such as appetite and food availability may dictate the eating patterns of athletes during the recovery period, the total amount of CHO consumed is more important than whether food is eaten in large meals or as a series of smaller snacks. There is some evidence that high glycaemic index CHO foods (e.g. potato, glucose, bread) promote more efficient rates of carbohydrate storage than foods with a low glycemic index (e.g. lentils, oatmeal, pasta). However, athletes are guided to eat a variety of CHO-rich foods and drinks to meet their total fuel needs (for review, see Hawley and Burke, 1997).

Dietary supplements and nutritional ergogenic aids

The sports world is filled with supplements that promise to make the athlete leaner, faster, stronger, quicker to recover or otherwise better perform. Many of these products are supported by testimonials of athletes and advertising hype rather than well-conducted research trials. These supplements might be viewed as falling into two categories: dietary supplements for athletes, and nutritional ergogenic aids (Burke and Heeley, 1994). Dietary supplements share the characteristics of providing nutrients in amounts typical of dietary intake, in a form that is practical and appropriate for use by athletes. These products are most useful for allowing an athlete to meet nutrient intake goals in a situation where everyday foods are impractical or unsuitable. This is particularly the case for nutritional goals immediately before, during or after exercise. Some common examples of dietary supplements used by athletes are summarized in Table 6.6. When the dietary supplement is used by an athlete to achieve a particular nutritional goal it may directly enhance performance or at least assist with long-term performance goals.

By contrast, nutritional ergogenic aids typically contain nutrients or food components in amounts much greater than typical dietary intake. They often claim to 'supercharge' physiological systems to provide a performance lift. The vast majority of these supplements and their claims are untested, and those that have been subjected to scientific research have failed to show evidence of significant performance improvements. The exceptions to this are creatine, caffeine and bicarbonate. Each of these substances has been found to enhance exercise performance under specific circumstances (for reviews, see Spriet, 1999; McNaughton, 1999; Greenhaff, 1999). However, it is important to recognize that some athletes do not respond to these supplements, and that some may even suffer performance impairment or negative side-effects. Furthermore, laboratory studies of recreationally or mildly trained subjects do not necessarily relate to performances of elite and well-trained athletes in real competition.

Table 6.6. Types of sports supplements (taken from Hawley and Burke, 1998)

Supplement	Forms	Composition	Major uses
Sports drinks Gatorade, Powerade, Lucozade Sport, Isostar	Drink or powdered form for making into drink	• 5–8 per cent carbohydrate • 10–25 mmol l^{-1} sodium	• Fluid and/or carbohydrate replacement during exercise • Post-exercise rehydration and refuelling
High carbohydrate source (= carbohydrate loaders) Gatorload, Maxim	Powder (for making into drink or adding to foods) or ready-made drink	• carbohydrate powder – usually glucose polymers. • Drinks usually made up at 20–25 per cent carbohydrate concentration. • Sometimes with B vitamins added	• Supplement to high carbohydrate diet • Carbohydrate loading or 'fuelling up' • Concentrated carbohydrate drink during exercise • Post-exercise refuelling
Gels Gu, Power Gel, Ultragel, Leppin Squeezy, Relode,	30–40 g sachets, or larger tubes of thick syrup for a 'quick squeeze' of carbohydrate	• 60–70 per cent carbohydrate gel • Provides ~ 25 g carbohydrate per sachet	• Concentrated form of carbohydrate during exercise

Table 6.6. (Continued)

Supplement	Forms	Composition	Major uses
Liquid meal supplements Sustagen Sport, Gator Pro, Exceed	Ready-made drink, or powder for mixing in water or milk to make drink	When made as drink: • $1–1.5$ kcal ml^{-1} • $50–70$ per cent carbohydrate • $15–20$ per cent protein • low–moderate fat • 100 per cent RDI of vitamin/minerals in $\sim 500–1000$ ml	• Compact energy and nutrient supplement for a high energy diet • Pre-event meal • Post-event recovery • Nutrition for the travelling athlete
Sports bars 1. Power Bar, VO2 max bar, Maxim bar 2. PR bar, Balance bar	$50–70$ g bar – chewy or 'muesli bar' consistency	1. $40–50$ g CHO + $5–10$ g protein. Usually low in fat. Often fortified with $50–100$ per cent RDI of vitamins and minerals 2. 40:30:30 ratio of CHO, fat and protein for 'zone diet'	• Supplement to a high carbohydrate diet • Pre-exercise meal or snack • Carbohydrate source during exercise • Post-exercise refuelling

Summary

Sports nutrition encompasses issues related to the health of the athlete, as well as nutritional practices aimed at improving training and performance. In the competition setting, dietary strategies before, during and after the event can reduce the detrimental effects of fatigue, thereby enhancing performance. While these factors are important considerations for elite athletes, they apply equally to the much larger number of highly motivated recreational athletes. The practice of sports nutrition can improve the performance and enjoyment of sporting activities undertaken by many people.

References

American Dietetic Association and Canadian Dietetic Association (1993). Position stand on nutrition for physical fitness and athletic performance for adults. *J. Am. Diet. Assoc.*, **93**, 691–696.

Brownell, K.D. and Rodin, J. (1992). Prevalence of eating disorders in athletes. In *Eating, Body Weight and Performance in Athletes*. (K.D. Brownell, J. Rodin and J.H. Wilmore, eds), pp. 128–145. Lea and Febiger.

Burke, L.M. (1994a). Sport and body fatness. In *Exercise and Obesity* (A.P. Hills and M.L. Wahlqvist, eds), pp. 217–231. Smith-Gordon.

Burke, L.M. (1994b). Sports amenorrhea, osteopenia, stress fractures and calcium. In *Clinical Sports Nutrition* (L.M. Burke and V. Deakin, eds), pp. 200–226. McGraw-Hill.

Burke, L.M. (1999). Dietary carbohydrates. In *IOC Encyclopaedia of Sports Medicine: Nutrition in Sports* (R.J. Maughan, ed.). Blackwell Science.

Burke, L.M. and Heeley, P. (1994). Dietary supplements and nutritional ergogenic aids in sport. In *Clinical Sports Nutrition* (L.M. Burke and V. Deakin, eds), pp. 227–284. McGraw-Hill.

Burke, L.M. and Hawley, J.A. (1997). Fluid balance in team sports: Guidelines for optimal practices. *Sports Med.*, **24**, 38–54.

Burke, L.M. and Inge, K. (1994). Protein requirements for training and bulking up. In *Clinical Sports Nutrition* (L.M. Burke and V. Deakin, eds), pp. 124–150. McGraw-Hill.

Clarkson, P.M. (1995). Micronutrients and exercise: Antioxidants and minerals. *J. Sports Sci.*, **13**, S11–S24.

Coggan, A.R. and Coyle, E.F. (1991). Carbohydrate ingestion during prolonged exercise: effects on metabolism and performance. In *Exercise and Sports Science Reviews*, Vol. 19 (J. Holloszy, ed.), pp. 1–40. Williams and Wilkins.

Coyle, E.F. (1992). Timing and method of increased carbohydrate intake to cope with heavy training, competition and recovery. In *Food, Nutrition and Sports Performance* (C.Williams and J.T. Devlin, eds), pp. 35–62. E. and F. Spon.

Coyle, E.F. and Montain, S.J. (1992). Benefits of fluid replacement with carbohydrate during exercise. *Med. Sci. Sports Exerc.*, 24 (Suppl.), S324–S330.

Deakin, V. (1994). Iron deficiency in athletes: identification, prevention and dietary treatment. In *Clinical Sports Nutrition* (L.M. Burke and V. Deakin, eds), pp. 174–199. McGraw-Hill.

Deakin, V. and Brotherhood, J.R. (1995). Nutrition and energy sources. In *Science and Medicine in Sport* (J. Bloomfield, P.A. Fricker and K.D. Fitch, eds), pp. 97–128. Blackwell Science.

Dekkers, J.C., van Doornen, L.J.P. and Kempe, H.C.G. (1996). The role of antioxidant vitamins and enzymes in the prevention of exercise-induced muscle damage. *Sports Med.*, **21**, 213–238.

Drinkwater, B.L. (1992). Amenorrhea, body weight and menstrual function. In *Eating, Body Weight and Performance in Athletes* (K.D. Brownell, J. Rodin and J.H. Wilmore, eds), pp. 235–247. Lea and Febiger.

Foster, C., Costill, D.L. and Fink, W.J. (1979). Effects of pre-exercise feedings on endurance performance. *Med. Sci. Sports*, **11**, 1–5.

Gilchrist, P.N. and Burke, L. (1995). Eating disorders. In *Science and Medicine in Sport* (J. Bloomfield, P.A. Fricker and K.D. Fitch, eds), pp. 665–673. Blackwell Science.

Greenhaff, P. (1997). Creatine. In *IOC Encyclopaedia of Sports Medicine: Nutrition in Sports* (R.J. Maughan, ed.). Blackwell Science.

Hawley, J.A. and Hopkins, W.G. (1995). Aerobic glycolytic and aerobic lipolytic power systems. A new paradigm with implications for endurance and ultra-endurance events. *Sports Med.*, **19**, 240–250.

Hawley, J.A. and Burke, L.M. (1997). Effect of meal frequency and timing on physical performance. *Sports Med.*, **77** (Suppl.), S91–S103.

Hawley, J.A. and Burke, L.M. (1998). *Peak Performance: Training and Nutrition Strategies for Sport*. Allen and Unwin.

Highet, R. (1989). Athletic amenorrhea: an update on aetiology, complications and management. *Sports Med*, **7**, 82–108.

Jeukendrup, A.E., Brouns, F., Wagenmakers, A.J.M. and Saris, W.H.M. (1997). Carbohydrate–electrolyte feedings improve 1 h time-trial cycling performance. *Int. J. Sports Med.*, **18**, 125–129.

Kerr, D. (1994). Kinanthropometry. In *Clinical Sports Nutrition* (L.M. Burke and V. Deakin, eds), pp. 74–103. McGraw-Hill.

Lemon, P.W.R. (1995). Do athletes need more dietary protein and amino acids? *Int. J. Sports Nutr.*, 5 (Suppl.), S39–S61.

McArdle, W.D., Katch, F.I. and Katch, V.L. (1991). Human energy expenditure during rest and physical activity. In *Exercise Physiology. Energy, Nutrition and Human Performance* (W.D. McArdle, F.I. Katch and V.L. Katch, eds), pp. 158–173. Lea and Febiger.

McNaughton, L. (1999). Bicarbonate and citrate. In *IOC Encyclopaedia of Sports Medicine: Nutrition in Sports* (R.J. Maughan, ed.), Blackwell Science.

Saris, W.H.M. and van Baak, M.A. (1994). Consequences of exercise on energy expenditure. In *Exercise and Obesity* (A.P. Hills and M.L. Wahlqvist, eds), pp. 85–102.Smith-Gordon.

Sherman, W.M. and Wimer, G.S. (1991). Insufficient dietary carbohydrate during training: does it impair athletic performance? *Int. J. Sports Nutr.*, **1**, 28–44.

Spriet, L. (1999).Caffeine. In: *IOC Encyclopaedia of Sports Medicine: Nutrition in Sports* (R.J. Maughan, ed.). Blackwell Science.

Steen, S.N. and Brownell, K.D. (1990). Patterns of weight loss and regain in wrestlers: has the tradition changed? *Med. Sci. Sports Exerc.*, **22**, 762–768.

Sungdot-Borgen, J. (1994). Risk and trigger factors for the development of eating disorders in female elite athletes. *Med. Sci. Sports Exerc.*, **26**, 414–419.

Van der Beek, E.J. (1991). Vitamin supplementation and physical exercise performance. In *Foods, Nutrition and Sports Performance* (C. Williams and J.T. Devlin, eds), pp. 95–112. E. and F. Spon.

Wilmore, J.H. (1992). Body weight standards and athletic performance. In *Eating, Body Weight and Performance in Athletes* (K.D. Brownell, J. Rodin and J.H. Wilmore, eds), pp. 315–329. Lea and Febiger.

Further reading

Burke, L.M. (1995). *The Complete Guide to Food for Sports Performance,* 2nd Edn. Allen and Unwin.

Maughan, R.J. (ed.) (1999). *IOC Encyclopaedia of Sports Medicine: Nutrition in Sports*. Blackwell Science.

7

Fluid requirements and exercise in the heat

R.J. Maughan

Many of the major sporting events of recent years have been held during the summer months in countries where high heat and humidity are common. Many military, industrial and occupational situations also call for men and women to perform hard physical work at extremes of environmental conditions. In environments with a combination of high heat and humidity, not only is working capacity seriously compromised, but health and well-being are also at risk. In occupational settings, there are clearly defined limits to the severity and duration of heat exposure that are considered acceptable, but sporting events are seldom if ever cancelled because of hot weather conditions, even though the intensity and duration of effort involved in sports competition may far exceed anything encountered in an occupational situation. The peripheral tissues of the body can function normally over a wide temperature range, and the temperature of the skin and subcutaneous tissues will generally follow the ambient temperature. The deeper tissues, and especially the brain, however, must be maintained within a few degrees of the normal body temperature of 37°C if normal function is to be maintained and irreversible damage prevented. Exposure to a high ambient temperature threatens the body's ability to keep its temperature within the optimum working range.

Factors reducing the effects of heat

Many different factors can contribute to a reduction of the risk of heat illness, and the adaptational changes in the physiological and biochemical characteristics of the individual that result from repeated exposure to the stressful environment are undoubtedly of crucial importance. A second crucial factor is replacement of water loss and the prevention of dehydration. It is equally clear, however, that fatigue and system failure remain the inevitable outcome when exercise is undertaken in hot, humid conditions. The question of what limits the capacity of humans to adapt to the homeostatic threat imposed by exercise performance in the heat is intimately linked with a more fundamental question which asks what sets the limitation to exercise heat tolerance.

Several different lines of evidence give some indications as to where the limitation might lie. It is apparent, firstly, that exercise capacity is reduced at high ambient temperatures, and this is generally accepted as evidence of a thermoregulatory limitation to exercise performance (Brown *et al.*, 1982; Febbraio *et al.*, 1996). This effect, however, is seen even at rather moderate ambient temperatures: Galloway and Maughan (1997) showed a significant reduction in exercise time to fatigue at 21°C relative to 11°C (Figure 7.1). This calls into question the generally accepted idea that performance of prolonged exercise is limited by the availability of muscle glycogen as a metabolic substrate in exercise of this type and duration (Hargreaves, 1994). Perhaps more importantly for many athletes and team doctors, these results also indicate that thermoregulatory factors – and a strategy for dealing with them – may be important in temperate climates, and thus may affect far more athletes than previously thought. Sportsmen and women may be particularly at risk on a warm spring day when they have been accustomed to cool weather. It is also apparent that fluid balance has a strong influence on exercise tolerance and that the significance of this factor increases as ambient temperature rises. If an individual begins to exercise in a state of hypohydration, then performance is impaired relative to the euhydrated condition, whether the fluid deficit is induced by sweat loss during exercise, by sauna exposure or by diuretics. Armstrong *et al.* (1985) showed this rather convincingly in a field trial where a modest level (1.5–2 per cent of body mass) of fluid loss induced by administration of a diuretic agent caused a reduction in running times

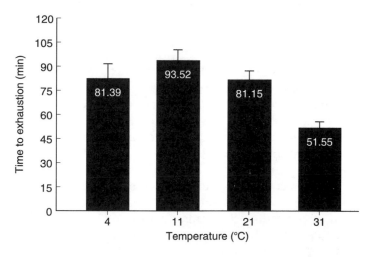

Figure 7.1. Exercise time to exhaustion during cycling exercise in a climatic chamber maintained at temperatures of 4, 11, 21 and 31°C. Exercise time was greater at 11°C than in any of the other trials and was lowest at 31°C. Values are mean and SEM for eight subjects. (Based on the data of Galloway and Maughan, 1997)

in simulated races over distances of 1500–10 000 m: the effects on performance were dramatic, with the reduction in speed in the 10 000 m race corresponding to about 1.5 laps (600 m). Many studies have shown that the administration of fluids during exercise can attenuate the rise in core temperature that occurs and can improve exercise performance (see Maughan, 1994a, for a review of these studies). Although most of these studies have used fluids of varying composition and few have investigated the effects of ingestion of plain water, it is apparent that drinking water itself can extend exercise time during a prolonged exercise test (Maughan *et al.*, 1996). Below *et al.* (1995) have shown that the ingestion of water and carbohydrate have independent and additive effects on exercise performance. These results again suggest a thermoregulatory component to the fatigue process in prolonged exercise, even when the heat stress appears not to be high.

The observation that a period of acclimatization led to improvements in endurance performance but that exercise was terminated at the same core temperature, led Nielsen *et al.* (1993) to conclude that 'the high core temperature *per se*, and not circulatory failure, is the critical factor for the exhaustion during heat stress'. While this statement may prove to be true, it provides no insight into possible mechanisms by which core temperature may cause individuals to terminate exercise. It is also apparent that, if we cannot understand the factors that limit exercise tolerance in the heat, there is little chance of identifying the limitations of man's capacity to adapt and of developing the most effective strategies for coping with exercise in the heat.

An alternative approach to the problem, which has been adopted by Nielsen (1996), is to calculate the effects of environmental heat stress on the thermoregulatory responses of an exercising athlete. When the thermal load exceeds the capacity of the individual for heat dissipation, body heat storage must occur as dictated by the heat balance equations described below. Body temperature will continue to rise until the rate of heat storage is reduced because of either an increased rate of heat loss or a reduced rate of heat production, or system failure occurs. The key factors are the total heat load, consisting of the rate of metabolic heat production plus the thermal load imposed by the environment, and the capacity for heat loss. The endurance athlete, and especially the marathon runner, is a good example on which to base the calculations. In most real situations, however, the picture is far more complex as the energy demand is rarely constant: even in constant-pace running, variations in the terrain or in running technique will influence the energy cost and therefore the heat production.

Heat exchange with the environment

The calculations normally used to quantify heat exchange with the environment involve a number of assumptions and simplifications. Failure to recognize the significance of some of these factors has sometimes led to conclusions that are not supported by everyday experience. At its simplest, the heat balance equation can be described as:

$$S = M \pm R \pm K \pm C - E \pm Wk$$

This indicates that the rate of body heat storage (S) is equal to the metabolic heat production (M) corrected for the net heat exchange by radiation (R), conduction (K), convection (C) and evaporation (E). A further correction must be applied to allow for work (Wk) done: this may be positive in the case of external work done, or negative when eccentric exercise is performed.

Ignoring the negligible exchange via conduction, which becomes significant only in the case of exercise carried out in water, the avenues of heat exchange can be quantified as follows:

Convective loss	$C = 8.3\ (T_{sk}\ T_a)\sqrt{v}$	$W\ {}^\circ C^{-1}\ m^{-2}$
Radiant loss	$R = 5.2\ (T_{sk}\ T_{mrt})$	$W\ {}^\circ C^{-1}\ m^{-2}$
Evaporative loss	$E = 124\ (P_{sk}\ P_a)\sqrt{v}$	$W\ kPa^{-1}\ m^{-2}$

Where: T_{sk} = mean skin temperature (${}^\circ C$); T_a = ambient temperature (${}^\circ C$); T_{mrt} = mean radiant temperature (${}^\circ C$); P_{sk} = mean skin water vapour pressure (kPa); P_a = ambient water vapour pressure (kPa); and v = mean air velocity (m s^{-1}).

Even a superficial consideration of these thermal balance equations reveals several interesting aspects, bearing in mind that the rate of heat production by a runner in the speed range that can be sustained for prolonged periods is an approximately linear function of running speed. Convective heat loss is proportional to the temperature gradient from skin to environment, and is also related to the square root of air velocity. As ambient temperature rises, the gradient from skin to environment falls, and above about 35°C the gradient is reversed so that heat is gained from the environment. As running speed increases, the metabolic rate increases more rapidly than convective heat exchange. Convective heat exchange is also a function of body surface area, whereas, for any given speed, the energy cost of running is a function of body mass. Body surface area increases as the square of body mass: this has the consequence that, where the temperature gradient from skin to environment is positive, meaning that heat is being lost by convection, the bigger runner is at an advantage. However, when the temperature gradient is reversed, and the body is gaining heat by convection, the heavier runner will gain more heat. The same considerations apply to radiant heat exchange.

Convection and radiation are effective methods of heat loss when the skin temperature is high and ambient temperature is low: under these conditions, these two processes will account for a major part of the heat loss even during intense exercise. As ambient temperature rises, the thermal gradient from skin to environment decreases, and evaporation becomes increasingly important for heat loss. The increased rate of heat loss by evaporation balances rather precisely the reduced heat loss by physical transfer as ambient temperature increases. Nielsen (1938) showed that the steady-state core temperature achieved during exercise was closely related to the power output but independent of ambient temperature in the temperature range from about 10 to 25°C. The core temperature is more closely related to the relative work-rate, expressed as a fraction of maximum oxygen uptake (VO_{2max}), than it is to the absolute power output (Astrand, 1960), but there is a large variation between individuals, and the factors accounting for this variability are not well understood.

A high rate of evaporative heat loss is clearly essential when the rate of metabolic heat production is high and where there is little or no loss possible by other means. Although the potential for heat loss by evaporation of water from the skin is high, this will not be the case if the sweating rate is insufficient to wet the skin surface, or if the vapour pressure gradient between the skin and the environment is low. This latter situation will arise if the skin temperature is low or if the ambient water vapour pressure is high. Insulative clothing that restricts air flow will restrict the evaporation of water from the skin surface (Gonzalez, 1988). A similar effect will occur if the evaporation of large amounts of sweat from the skin causes a large increase in the salt concentration of water on the skin surface: this will decrease the vapour pressure at any given skin temperature. A large body surface area and a high rate of air movement over the body surface are also factors that will have a major impact on evaporative heat loss, but these same factors will also promote heat gain by convection and radiation when the ambient temperature is higher than skin temperature (Leithead and Lind, 1964).

It was the likelihood of extreme environmental conditions occurring in Atlanta on the occasion of the 1996 Summer Olympic Games that led Nielsen (1996) to estimate the potential effect on marathon running performance. Nielsen's calculations involved a 67 kg athlete with a body surface area of 1.85 m^2 running at a speed of 19.4 km h^{-1} (5.4 m s^{-1}) which would give a finishing time of about 2 h 10 min. The weather records from the Atlanta area indicated that a combination of high heat and humidity was likely to occur (Figure 7.2) and Nielsen's calculations assumed an ambient temperature of 35°C and a relative humidity of 80 per cent. Calculations were performed for a mean skin temperatures of 37°C, and radiant and convective heat exchange were considered to be negligible. A constant running speed at an average oxygen cost of 4.3 l min^{-1} was also assumed, giving a rate of metabolic heat production

Average summer climatic conditions

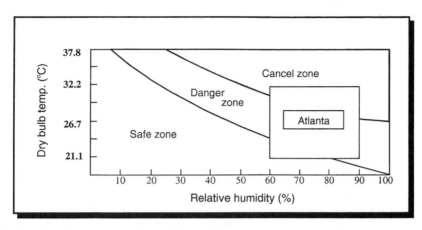

Figure 7.2. Anticipated weather conditions during the period of the 1996 Olympic Games held in Atlanta. The combination of high temperature and humidity leads to a situation where heat loss is sufficiently restricted that sustained hard exercise poses a significant risk to the individual. Many other major sporting events are held in similar conditions. (Reproduced with permission from Lamb, 1984)

of 1440 W if the mechanical efficiency was 25 per cent. The mean air velocity over the body surface was taken to be the same as the running speed, and the maximum possible rate of evaporative heat loss was calculated as follows.

Consider a 67 kg runner, BSA 1.85 m^2, running speed 19.4 km h^{-1} (5.4 m s^{-1}), running a 2 h 10 min marathon:

Heat production = 1440 W (VO$_2$ = 4.3 l min^{-1})

Assume 35°C, 80 per cent RH, wind velocity equal to running speed and T_{sk} of 37°C:

Evaporative capacity = 124$\sqrt{5.4}$(6.27 − 4.42) × 1.85 W
$$= 995 \text{ W (1.475 g sweat h}^{-1})$$

Thus the balance between heat production and evaporative capacity is given by (1440 − 995) W = 445 W. Taking the heat capacity of the human body to be 3.47 kJ °C^{-1} kg^{-1}, the body temperature would rise by 1°C every 8.7 min.

The evaporative capacity of the environment would be reached with the evaporation of 1475 g of sweat per hour, which is well within the sweating rates that have been reported for athletes in various sports (Rehrer and Burke, 1996). The metabolic heat production, however, will exceed the evaporative capacity of the environment by 445 W, leading to heat storage in the body and an inevitable rise in body temperature. Assuming the heat capacity of human tissue to be 3.47 kJ °C^{-1} kg^{-1}, body temperature would rise by 1°C every 8.7 min as outlined above, and the runner would exceed the upper limit of the tolerable core temperature before completing even one-third of the race distance. This suggests that the running speed will be limited by the capacity to dissipate heat. By an extension of these same calculations, Nielsen predicted that the fastest time that would be possible in these environmental conditions would be about 3 h 20 min.

This conclusion is manifestly incorrect. Even in more extreme environmental conditions, the surprising thing is not that performance is impaired but how closely elite runners are able to approach their best performance achieved in cooler conditions. Marathon runners have demonstrated many times in championship events held in adverse conditions that they are capable of times that come within a few minutes of their best performance achieved in temperate or cool conditions. As the conclusion is wrong, there must be an error in the assumptions, and an examination of the possible sources of error requires a careful consideration of the factors that allow the elite endurance athlete to perform so well in these conditions. A detailed consideration of the factors involved in thermal balance is provided by Santee and Gonzalez (1988) and Gonzalez (1988). Such a consideration is beyond the scope of this chapter, but some of the more important points can be highlighted.

Body mass is an important factor in the calculations as this will have a strong influence on the energy cost of running and hence on the metabolic heat load. Marathon runners typically have a rather low body mass, primarily as a consequence of the low body fat content (Maughan, 1994b), giving a high power to mass ratio. A more reasonable estimate of the body mass of an elite runner capable of completing the distance in 2 h 10 min would be about 60 kg. This would reduce the oxygen consumption required to meet the energy cost of running at 19.4 km h^{-1} from 4.3 l min^{-1} to 3.9 l min^{-1}, assuming that the oxygen cost remained constant at 64 ml kg^{-1} min^{-1}. This would reduce the rate of metabolic heat production from 1440 W to 1290 W. With height remaining unchanged, there would be some reduction in body surface area (from 1.85 m^2 to 1.80 m^2) with the reduced body mass, with a corresponding reduction in the capacity for heat exchange with the environment: the 10 per cent reduction in mass, however, has reduced surface area by less than 3 per cent. A reduction in body mass will also decrease the heat storage capacity of the body.

It seems likely that an elite runner would have a higher than normal running economy, allowing any given speed to be achieved at a lower than normal energy cost. The issue of running economy has been the subject of some debate, but there is good evidence of an inverse relationship between the energy cost of running and the best performance that an individual can achieve (Maughan, 1994b). It seems reasonable, therefore, to assume a further reduction in the energy cost: a 10 per cent reduction in the rate of metabolic heat production would give a value for the average rate of heat generation of 1160 W.

Using these revised values, the evaporative capacity of our modified runner now becomes:

Evaporative capacity $= 124\sqrt{5.4}\ (6.63 - 4.42) \times 1.80$ W
$$= 1146 \text{ W}$$

This means that the rate of heat storage, the imbalance between heat production and heat loss, is now reduced to (1160 − 1146 W), or 14 W. Body temperature would rise by 1°C after 248 min. It is clear that this runner can reach the end of the race with a tolerable thermal load. Experience suggests, however, that most marathon runners will experience a rise in body temperature of between 1 and 3°C (Maughan, 1994b) even in temperate conditions. This therefore calls for a further re-examination of the assumptions on which these calculations are based. At least three further factors must be considered. These are the effects of the sweat electrolyte content on the latent heat of vaporization of sweat, an enhanced air flow over the limbs caused by the movements involved in running, and the restriction placed on evaporative loss by the clothing worn. For none of these variables are there sufficient data available to allow realistic calculations to be made. The most reliable information available relates to the change in body temperature, and this can do no more than set the outer limits for the sum of the heat exchange mechanisms.

It is also necessary to take account of one factor ignored by Nielsen: this is the cardiovascular demand imposed by the skin blood flow that is necessary to convect the heat load from the body core to the skin surface. With a skin temperature of 37°C and a core temperature of 39.5°C, the gradient for heat transfer is rather small (2.5°C) and a high flow rate will be required. Here is the dilemma: a lower skin temperature (or a higher core temperature) will increase the core–skin temperature gradient, reducing the skin blood flow that is necessary to convect heat from the core to the periphery, thus decreasing the cardiovascular demand, but will reduce the water vapour pressure at the skin surface, reducing the evaporative capacity. Raising the skin temperature will increase the vapour pressure gradient between skin and environment, increasing evaporative capacity, but at the expense of an increased requirement for skin blood flow. This may be especially important where the cardiovascular capacity is compromised, as happens with hypohydration.

A crucial factor is the effect of increasing skin temperature on water vapour pressure at the skin surface, as shown in Table 7.1. In the example of the modified runner quoted above, it is possible to calculate the effects of varying the skin temperature on the evaporative capacity, and hence the implications for thermal balance. Thermal balance is achievable even when ambient temperature and humidity are high if the skin temperature can be maintained at a high enough level. However, it is not possible to provide sufficient cutaneous blood flow to maintain skin temperature at this level. When the limit of skin blood flow is reached, at a flow rate of about 7–8 l min^{-1}, the transit time must be reduced, otherwise the entire blood volume would be accommodated in the capacitance vessels of the

Table 7.1. Effect of variations in skin temperature on the saturation pressure of water (kPa) at the skin surface, and on the vapour pressure gradient (ΔVP) between skin and environment at 35°C and 80 per cent relative humidity

Temperature (°C)	Vapour pressure (kPa)	ΔVP (kPa)
25	3.17	0
30	4.24	0
35	5.62	1.20
40	7.38	2.96

skin (Rowell, 1986). Rowell suggested that a point is reached where further increasing skin blood flow would reduce the rate of heat loss because of the reduction in transit time through the vascular bed of the skin. There is experimental evidence that skin blood flow is actually reduced when the skin temperature is raised to 38°C or higher (Brengelmann, 1983), perhaps as a consequence of the need for peripheral vasoconstriction to maintain central venous pressure.

Correcting for the heat storage that would result if an increase in body temperature of 3°C was allowed makes little difference to the outcome and conclusions. This clearly suggests that the ability to maintain a high skin blood flow, and hence a high vapour pressure gradient between skin and atmosphere, is a crucial factor. This leads to the inescapable conclusion that the ability to maintain cardiac output will ultimately limit performance of endurance exercise in the heat.

It is clear from the picture described above that the athlete competing in a warm environment is in an extremely precarious situation with regard to thermal balance. Even small changes in heat gain or heat loss may make the difference between successful completion of the event and hospitalization.

Acclimatization strategies for exercise in the heat

Acclimatization or acclimation involving repeated exposures to exercise in the heat results in marked improvements in exercise time to fatigue (Montain et al., 1996). These two terms are sometimes confused and are often used interchangeably: acclimation refers to the process of adaptation carried out in a controlled laboratory setting, and acclimatization refers to the same process carried out in a natural setting of warm weather. For convenience, acclimatization is often used to describe both processes. Increased tolerance to exercise in the heat is achieved by lowering the temperature threshold for the onset of sweating and increasing the sensitivity of the sweating mechanism so that a greater sweat rate is achieved for any given level of body temperature. There is also a more even distribution of sweating over the body surface, ensuring an effective rate of evaporation while minimizing the amount of sweat that drips from the body surface without evaporating. The salt content of the sweat is reduced, allowing conservation of electrolytes to occur and allowing the preferential maintenance of the plasma volume. These adaptations appear within 1 or 2 days of exposure to the heat, and the degree of adaptation is related to the amount of heat strain experienced. Adaptations occur more rapidly and more completely if exercise is performed during periods of heat exposure. Adaptation appears to be largely complete after about 10–15 consecutive days of exposure to exercise in the heat, but it must be remembered that the studies on which this statement is based relate largely to industrial workers, military personnel and student volunteers: these studies have not been done with well-trained athletes. After adaptation, heart rate will be lower at any given level of thermal stress and exercise tolerance is greatly increased.

Even after a comprehensive programme of heat acclimatization, however, exercise performance remains impaired relative to that which can be achieved in cool conditions. The major changes that are generally thought to be responsible for the improved work capacity include an expansion of the plasma volume, a reduced temperature threshold for the onset of sweating and increased sensitivity of the sweat glands to increasing temperature, and a reduced sweat sodium content. These adaptations provide for an earlier and more effective initiation of the sweating response and allow a greater cardiovascular reserve for provision and maintenance of skin blood flow without compromising central venous pressure (Rowell, 1986).

There is little evidence in man for an improved ability to tolerate increased core temperatures in response to heat acclimation (Figure 7.3; Nielsen et al., 1993). There is also no evidence for an improved thermal tolerance in endurance-trained individuals (Sawka et al., 1992). Furthermore, the energy cost of work, and therefore the rate of heat production, is not significantly affected by acclimatization, and there is little evidence for major improvements in mechanical efficiency in response to training, although some small change may occur. If the rate of heat generation is the same and there is not an increased heat tolerance, the improvements in exercise time to exhaustion that are normally observed after training or acclimatization must be a consequence of an increased capacity for heat dissipation causing a slower rate of rise in core temperature.

Factors leading to acclimatization

There is no doubt that regular exposure to hot humid conditions results in a number of adaptations which together reduce the negative effects of these conditions on exercise performance and reduce the risk of heat injury. The magnitude of the adaptation to heat that occurs is closely related to the degree of heat stress to which the individual is exposed.

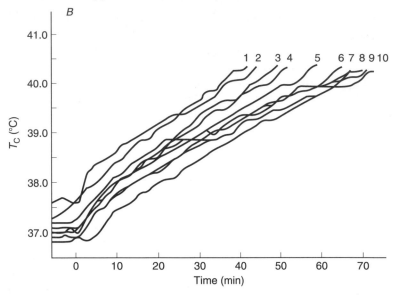

Figure 7.3. A period of acclimation results in an improved exercise capacity during work in a hot environment, but the core temperature at which the subject is forced to stop exercising is not changed. (Reproduced from Nielsen *et al.*, 1993 by permission of the authors and publishers)

The two primary determining factors for adaptation to hot humid conditions are:

1. The rise in body temperature that occurs.
2. The sweating response that is induced.

Adaptation therefore depends largely on the intensity and duration of exercise and on the environmental conditions, and there is clearly an optimum set of conditions for the most effective acclimatization. Some adaptation is seen within the first few days of exposure to exercise in the heat, and even a few sessions of exercise in the heat are beneficial (Lind and Bass, 1963). Adaptation is more or less complete for most individuals within about 7–14 days and so there may be no advantage of living for prolonged periods in a hot climate (Montain *et al.*, 1996): too much time spent in the heat may limit the amount of training that can be completed. It is equally clear that regular endurance training in temperate conditions confers some protection (Piwonka and Robinson, 1967) as trained subjects are already partially adapted. And it has to be admitted that we do not know how complete this process is for highly trained Olympic athletes. The endurance athlete who trains wearing extra clothing to induce sweating even in a cool climate will also show some degree of heat acclimation, but this can be further enhanced by a period of training in the heat (Dawson, 1994). There can be no doubt that a period of acclimatization is necessary for all athletes if they are to achieve optimum performance in hot weather conditions. This probably becomes even more important when repeated rounds or events have to be completed. In sports where a high level of aerobic fitness is not normally required, and for team officials and support staff who may be older or less fit, this may be a good reason for undertaking an endurance exercise programme in the weeks and months prior to a major championship. The idea of arriving shortly before competition in order to minimize the effects of living in these conditions prior to competition is to be *strongly discouraged*. Except for a few exceptional situations, such a practice will lead to a decrement in performance. The coach and athlete must decide together whether this risk is worth taking, and this judgement can only be made on the basis of individual experience.

Prior to competition

There are two ways of acclimatizing for competitions in the heat. One is to live and train in a climate similar to that expected at the competition venue, while the other approach is to live at home and adapt by training in an artificial climate. There are positive and negative aspects to both approaches. Because exercise capacity is reduced so much in the heat, training intensity and volume must be reduced for at least the first few days of the acclimatization process. This effect may be minimized if the athlete lives at home and is exposed to heat only during training, or during one of two daily training sessions, allowing some quality training to be continued in the other session. If two training sessions per day are carried out, whether at home or in a hot weather camp, it seems sensible for the quality session to be done first, with the heat acclimatization session coming later in the day. The quality training session should be outdoors if at home, or in the early morning while it is still cool if at a hot weather venue.

The weather is notoriously unpredictable and the acclimatization venue selected may not provide suitable conditions for optimum acclimatization, whereas these can easily be simulated at home. If the heat acclimatization training is one of two sessions per day, the athlete is generally happier to adopt a less drastic regimen: the heat training can be gradually phased in, beginning with short (perhaps 30–60 min) sessions at low intensity, without compromising the total training quality. It is not necessary to train every day in the heat, but no more than 2–3 days should elapse between exposures: it has been shown that exercising in the heat every third day for 30 days resulted in the same degree of acclimatization as exercising every day for 10 days (Fein *et al.*, 1975). It takes time to reverse the adaptations to heat; for subjects who are completely acclimatized, some of the improved responses are still present after as long as 21 days in a cool climate (Pichan *et al.*, 1985). Acclimatization at home means that the athlete can introduce the heat acclimatization sessions gradually while continuing with normal training, and is not trying to cope with the effects of heat, jet lag and a new environment at the same time.

A disadvantage of training in a hot room may be that the exercise inevitably depends on the facilities available and probably consists of cycle ergometer exercise, treadmill running, skipping or circuit training. From the point of view of acclimatization to the heat, the type of exercise is not important, but rather that a period of prolonged (60–100 min), moderately strenuous exercise is carried out in hot conditions. The intention is to raise body temperature and to stimulate sweating: these are the factors that promote adaptation. There is evidence that full acclimatization is most effectively achieved when the duration of exercise in the heat is about 100 min, and that there is no advantage in spending longer periods than this exposed to heat (Lind and Bass, 1963). After exercise in the heat, the athlete should aim to reduce body temperature rather quickly by seeking shade or an air-conditioned environment to cool down and hasten the recovery process. Intermittent exercise is likely to be as effective as continuous exercise: the total exposure time, including short breaks, should again be 100 min for the most effective adaptation. More recent evidence, however, suggests that exercise at higher intensities for shorter periods of time may be equally effective in bringing about beneficial adaptations, and that even 30 min per day at in intensity equal to about 75 per cent of maximum oxygen uptake (VO_{2max}) is as effective as 60 min at 50 per cent of VO_{2max} (Houmard *et al.*, 1990).

If acclimatization is carried out at a hot weather camp, information on local weather patterns is essential. In most countries, temperature will be highest near the middle of the day, with humidity being highest when the temperature is lower in the early morning and late afternoon. The acclimatization programme may have to be modified to take account of the prevailing conditions. The time-scale should be sufficient to allow for a few (at least 3–4, but perhaps as many as 5–10) days of reduced training: both total training volume and the amount of training at high intensity should be reduced, the extent of the reduction depending on the individual response. Because of the heat and the effects of travel, training for the first few days should be reduced to light recreational levels, if sufficient time is available, progressively increasing in volume and intensity as the athlete adapts. Normal training can then be re-established for a few days while the acclimatization process continues and before tapering for competition begins. The vital 'quality training' should continue, with enhanced periods of rest and recovery, over the final week before competition. Remember that recovery will be faster and more complete if it is possible to find a cool shady place for this. Again it must be stressed that every individual is different, and the extent and duration of the period of reduced training will vary between individuals: the coach must be alert to warning signs in those having difficulty in coping with the conditions. The whole process needs at least 10–14 days on average, but a longer or shorter period may be appropriate for some athletes.

The ideal may be a combination of both approaches, with an increasing level of heat exposure at home during the last 1–2 weeks before travelling (Montain *et al.*, 1996). This might be of particular benefit to those most at risk, i.e. those whose sport will result in the greatest exposure and those who have been found by experience to have difficulty in coping with the heat. It is strongly recommended that every opportunity to experience hot, humid weather conditions be taken, so that individuals who encounter problems can be identified and an effective strategy devised. Where a team travels together, it is especially important to remember that everyone will adapt at different rates and some individualization of training schedules will be necessary to take account of this.

The ideal temperature and humidity for the acclimatization process are not well established, and practicalities will have a large influence on the choice of venue. If the temperature is too hot, training will be reduced. A temperature of at least 32°C but not more than 35°C, with a relative humidity of at least 70 per cent, may be proposed. Somewhere in the same time zone as the competition is to be preferred. Attempts to take short cuts by compressing the whole process should not be undertaken lightly: the acclimatization process requires the athlete to be exposed to sufficient heat stress for the necessary adaptations to take place, but there is a real danger that taking the process too far or too quickly can result in acute heat injury.

Formulation of rehydration fluids

Maintaining hydration status is essential if exercise is to be performed in the heat. Provision of both water and carbohydrate can improve exercise performance and there is evidence that the effects are independent and additive (Below, 1995). The effects of ingestion of water and carbohydrate are summarized here before the issue of the most effective combination of these ergogenic components is considered.

An intake of exogenous carbohydrate during exercise can increase exercise capacity (measured as the time for which a fixed power output can be maintained) and this effect may be due to a sparing of the endogenous muscle glycogen stores (Hargreaves *et al.*, 1984), although this is by no means a consistent finding (Fielding *et al.*, 1985; Coyle *et al.*, 1986; Hargreaves and Briggs, 1988) and it seems likely that other mechanisms may be involved. Fatigue during prolonged exercise appears to be closely related to the depletion of the glycogen reserves in the exercising muscles, at least in cycling exercise when the ambient temperature is not high, so there is good reason for supposing that the provision of additional carbohydrate should delay the onset of fatigue in these conditions. Ingestion of large amounts of carbohydrate allows exercise to continue even when the muscle glycogen content has fallen almost to zero in well-trained cyclists (Coyle *et al.*, 1986), and it is commonly recommended that an intake of at least 30–60 g of carbohydrate per hour is necessary to achieve the greatest benefit (Coyle, 1992).

Several studies have shown that the ingestion of plain water can improve exercise performance in a variety of different situations, although others have not reported a significant difference between water and no-drink trials. It may be important to distinguish here between a statistically significant effect observed in the laboratory, which usually requires a difference between trials of something of the order of 5–10 per cent, and a difference in competition, where the margin between victory and defeat is often much smaller. The effects of water ingestion have been less thoroughly investigated than those of carbohydrate–electrolyte solutions: early studies in this area were reviewed by Maughan (1991). Barr *et al.* (1991) studied the responses of individuals to prolonged (6 h) low- intensity cycling exercise in the heat (30°C) when given water, a sodium chloride (25 mmol l^{-1}) solution or no drink during exercise. On the no-drink trial, exercise was terminated after a mean time of 4.5 h, although the exercise task was completed by seven of the eight subjects on the other two trials, clearly suggesting an improved exercise tolerance with water replacement. In another study of prolonged walking (5–6 h), Strydom *et al.* (1966) observed sweat losses of about 4.5 l: one group of subjects, whose fluid intake was restricted, had higher rectal temperatures than the other group who were allowed water *ad libitum*, but no measures of performance were made. In shorter duration exercise lasting 70–90 min, which is more relevant to the time-scale of most sports events, it has been reported that endurance time at a workload of 70 per cent of VO_{2max} was improved by ingestion of an isotonic glucose–electrolyte solution, but was not significantly improved by ingestion of solutions containing large amounts of CHO or by the ingestion of water (Maughan *et al.*, 1989). There was a small (6 min), not statistically significant ($P = 0.10$), increase in the mean time to exhaustion in the trial where water was given. This last finding of a possible benefit from ingestion of plain water during prolonged cycling, is supported by more recent results of the same authors which showed a significant improvement in exercise time (from 80.7 to 93.1 min) when water was consumed at a rate of 100 ml every 10 min during exercise (Maughan *et al.*, 1996). It is worth noting that in this latter study, ingestion of dilute glucose–electrolyte solutions was again more effective than water in improving performance. In a study by Robinson *et al.* (1995), administration of flavoured water in a volume of 1.5 l over a 60-min cycle ergometer exercise test resulted in a reduction in the total distance covered compared with a trial where no fluid was given. The reduced performance was ascribed to sensations of gastric discomfort, and the reluctance to drink such large volumes was clearly apparent as the intake volume was less than that prescribed. It seems clear that the subjects would not voluntarily have chosen to drink such large volumes and the effects of ingestion of a smaller, more acceptable, volume of water were not investigated in this study.

Below *et al.* (1995) have established in a well-controlled study that the effects of provision of carbohydrate and of water on performance of a high-intensity test which followed 50 min of cycling at an intensity of about 80 per cent of VO_{2max} are independent and additive. They found that when only a small volume (200 ml) of water was given during the initial 50-min cycling period, the mean time taken to complete the set task was 11.34 min. Ingestion of the same volume with the addition of 79 g of carbohydrate and ingestion of a large (1330 ml) volume of plain water both resulted in significant improvements in performance time, to 10.55 min and 10.51 min respectively. Ingestion of the same large fluid volume, but this time as a 6 per cent carbohydrate solution (which contained the same amount of carbohydrate as the small volume of the concentrated solution) was more effective than either of the treatments individually, and the mean exercise time on this trial was 9.93 min. Although the improved performance when a large fluid volume was ingested was associated with a reduced heart rate and core temperature during the prolonged exercise, the improvement associated with carbohydrate ingestion was not associated with this effect.

In spite of the apparent effectiveness of plain water in improving performance, Burgess *et al.* (1991) have reported that administration of a glucose–electrolyte solution with a low (1.8 per cent) carbohydrate content which provided only 13 g of CHO per hour is not effective in improving performance. More recent results, however, have suggested that ingestion of electrolyte-containing solutions with a low carbohydrate content (1.6 per cent) may be an effective way of improving exercise capacity in prolonged cycling (Maughan *et al.*, 1996). In this latter study, the dilute glucose solution was more effective than plain water, but there was no difference in endurance time between the 1.6 per cent glucose–electrolyte solution and a 3.6 per cent glucose–electrolyte solution (Figure 7.4).This discrepancy with regard to the effects of the administration of dilute carbohydrate–electrolyte solutions is surprising in view of the well-known effects of these solutions in maximizing the rate of rehydration that can be achieved by stimulation of intestinal water transport (Leiper and Maughan, 1988) and the negative effects of dehydration on exercise performance (Walsh *et al.*, 1994). It also conflicts with previous reports which show that provision of even small amounts of carbohydrate in the form of glucose–electrolyte solutions can result in a substantial improvement in exercise performance (Maughan *et al.*, 1989). Sweat losses during prolonged exercise will cause a reduction in circulating blood volume which may result in a decreased blood flow to the skin (Fortney *et al.*, 1984) and a reduced sweating rate (Sawka *et al.*, 1985), leading to an elevated core temperature (Gisolfi and Copping, 1974). Many studies have shown that fluid ingestion during a range of different exercise intensities and durations can attenuate the rise in body temperature which occurs, whether glucose–electrolyte drinks or plain water are taken, but there is no good evidence that an elevated core temperature is in itself the cause of fatigue in prolonged exercise.

The composition of drinks to be taken will be influenced by the relative importance of the need to supply fuel and water, and this in turn depends on the intensity and duration of the exercise task, on the ambient temperature and humidity, and on the physiological and biochemical characteristics of the individual athlete. Carbohydrate depletion will result in fatigue and a reduction in the exercise intensity which can be sustained, but is not normally a life-threatening condition. Disturbances in fluid balance and temperature regulation will also impair exercise performance, but have potentially more serious consequences and it may be, therefore, that the emphasis for the majority of participants in endurance events should be on proper maintenance of fluid and electrolyte balance by ingestion of dilute carbohydrate–electrolyte drinks.

Water overload and hyponatraemia

Even at rest, the thirst mechanism is normally insufficient to maintain water balance in the short term, although a long-term equilibrium clearly exists. When exercise and thermal stresses are added, voluntary fluid intakes are seldom sufficient to balance fluid losses, resulting in a progressive dehydration and an increased risk of heat illness in prolonged exercise when the ambient temperature is high. Wyndham and Strydom

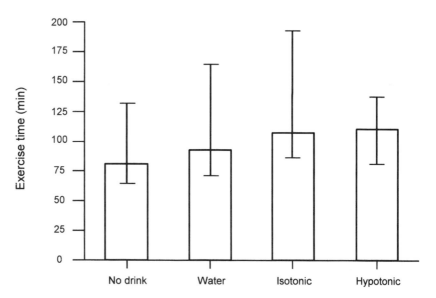

Figure 7.4. Exercise time to ingestion during a prolonged cycling test where subjects drank either no fluid, water or one of two dilute glucose–electrolyte solutions. See text for further details. (Data from Maughan *et al.*, 1996)

(1969) noted that marathon runners typically drink only about 100 ml h^{-1} and more recent evidence suggests that the intakes of serious runners are not much higher than this (Noakes, 1988). It seems that neither the physiological drive to drink nor the educational effort directed at these athletes is sufficient to maintain fluid balance. The advice often given to endurance athletes is that they should make a conscious effort to ensure a high fluid intake by drinking even when not thirsty and by following a strict fluid replacement regimen which prescribes fixed volumes at set intervals. It has also been recommended that drinks should contain low levels of glucose and electrolytes so as not to delay gastric emptying (American College of Sports Medicine, 1984). It is now recognized that the addition of electrolytes has relatively little effect on the rate of gastric emptying and the revised ACSM guidelines for fluid replacement (American College of Sports Medicine, 1996) support the addition of low levels of sodium. In accordance with these recommendations, most CHO–electrolyte drinks intended for consumption during prolonged exercise have been formulated to have a low electrolyte content, with sodium and chloride concentrations typically in the range of 10–20 mmol l^{-1}. While this might represent a reasonable strategy for providing substrates and water (although it can be argued that a higher sodium concentration might confer some benefits and that a higher carbohydrate content would increase substrate provision), these recommendations may not be appropriate in all circumstances.

Cases of collapse among runners at the end of long distance races are relatively rare, although they can be rather alarming when they do occur. Some of the major city marathons that have been held in recent years have attracted as many as 30 000 runners and in some of these there have been a significant number of casualties. This is perhaps unsurprising considering the poor preparation of the majority of participants. Problems are most often encountered in warm or hot weather and may be more frequent in marathon races taking place on a warm spring day when the participants have had little opportunity for heat acclimation. In most of these individuals, who typically collapse within a few minutes of completing the race, hypovolaemia resulting from pooling of blood in the legs is likely to be the cause. Hyperthermia associated with dehydration and hypernatraemia are normally observed, and the condition resolves relatively rapidly if the runner lies down with the feet raised. Oral or intravenous administration of fluids will accelerate the recovery process. It has, however, become clear that a small number of individuals at the end of very prolonged events may be suffering from hyponatraemia in conjunction with either hyperhydration or dehydration (see Maughan, 1994a, for a review of these studies).

All the cases of post-exercise hyponatraemia reported in the literature have been associated with ultramarathon or prolonged triathlon events. Most have occurred in events lasting in excess of 8 h and there are few reports of cases where the exercise duration is less than 4 h. These athletes may have encountered difficulties by adhering too closely to the inappropriate recommendations for fluid intake. Noakes *et al.* (1985) reported four cases of exercise-induced hyponatraemia; race times were between 7 and 10 h and post-race serum sodium concentrations were between 115 and 125 mmol l^{-1}, so that these individuals were clearly hyponatraemic. Estimated fluid intakes were between 6 and 12 l and consisted of water or drinks containing low levels of electrolytes; estimated total sodium chloride intake during the race was 20–40 mmol. These individuals were therefore adhering to the ACSM guidelines, which recommend an intake, at the upper end of the range, of about $1\,l\,h^{-1}$. It seems clear that the fluid requirements of the slower runner are much more variable than those of the elite competitor and, because of the lower exercise intensity and longer duration, it is possible to consume large volumes of fluid. In most big city marathons, plain water is the only fluid provided.

Reports of hyponatraemic collapse in ultramarathon runners are interesting and indicate that some supplementation with sodium chloride may be required in extremely prolonged events where large sweat losses can be expected and where it is possible to consume large volumes of fluid. This should not, however, divert attention away from the fact that electrolyte replacement during exercise is not a priority for most participants in most sporting events, although it is certainly helpful after the event to restore body water and electrolyte content. These occasional cases should also not be used as a reason to discourage the overwhelming majority of athletes from making every effort to increase their fluid intake.

Rehydration and recovery

In most sports, there is a need to recover as quickly and as completely as possibly after training or competition to begin preparation for the next event or training session. The importance of ingesting carbohydrate to replenish the muscle glycogen stores is now well recognized, but replacement of the water and electrolytes lost in sweat is equally important. The need for replacement will obviously depend on the volume of sweat lost and on its electrolyte content, but will also be influenced by the amount of time available before the next exercise bout. Rapid rehydration may also be important in events such as wrestling, boxing and weight lifting where competition is by weight category. It is common for competitors in these events to undergo acute thermal and exercise-induced dehydration to make weight, with weight losses of 10 per cent of body mass sometimes being achieved within a few days. The time interval between the weigh-in and competition may be as short as 3 h, although it may be longer, and is not sufficient for full recovery when significant amounts of weight have been lost, though some recovery is possible. The practice of acute dehydration to make weight has led to a number of fatalities, usually where exercise has been performed in a hot environment while wearing waterproof clothing to prevent the evaporation of sweat, and should be strongly discouraged, but it will persist and there is a need to maximize rehydration in the time available.

The ingestion of large volumes of fluids with a low sodium content has been reported to induce hyponatraemia during exercise of long duration. Ingestion of plain water or other drinks with a low electrolyte content in the post-exercise period also results in a rapid fall in the plasma sodium concentration and in plasma osmolality. These two variables are closely related and the falling plasma sodium level has the effect of reducing the subjective sensation of thirst, thus reducing the stimulus to drink, and of stimulating an increased urine output. The overall effect is to delay the rehydration process. Effective rehydration after exercise requires that both the water volume lost in sweat and the electrolytes lost are replaced. To allow for ongoing losses of urine during the recovery period, the volume ingested must be greater than the volume of sweat lost: this can be estimated from the loss of body mass, as 1 kg of mass loss is more or less 1 litre of water loss (Shirreffs *et al.*, 1996). Where an adequate volume is consumed during the recovery period, the fluid will not be retained unless the sodium content exceeds the sweat sodium loss, and urine production will be stimulated even when dehydration persists unless there is an adequate replacement of electrolytes (Maughan and Shirreffs, 1997). The subjective sensation of thirst is unlikely to ensure adequate rehydration and a conscious effort must be made to ensure volume replacement.

It is clear from the results of these studies that rehydration after exercise can only be achieved if the sodium lost in sweat is replaced as well as the water, and it might be suggested that rehydration drinks should have a sodium concentration similar to that of sweat (Figure 7.5). The sodium content of sweat varies widely, and no single formulation will meet this requirement for all individuals in all situations (Maughan, 1994a). The upper end of the normal range for sweat sodium concentration (80 mmol l^{-1}), however, is similar to the sodium concentration of many commercially produced oral rehydration solutions (ORS) intended for use in the treatment of diarrhoea-induced dehydration, and some of these are not unpalatable. The ORS recommended by the World Health Organisation for rehydration in cases of severe diarrhoea has a sodium content of 90 mmol l^{-1}, reflecting the high sodium losses which may occur in this condition. By contrast, the sodium content of most sports drinks is in the range of 10–25 mmol l^{-1} and is even lower in some cases. Most commonly consumed soft drinks contain virtually no sodium and these drinks are therefore unsuitable when the need for rehydration is crucial. The problem with high sodium concentrations is that this may exert a negative effect on taste, resulting in a reduced consumption. Where solid food containing electrolytes is ingested, additional salt may not be necessary, and the use of salt tablets is seldom required. Where the recovery time is short, however, and only liquid intake is possible, it is

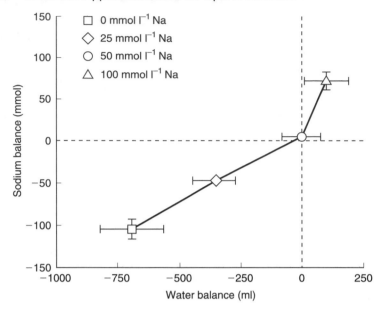

Figure 7.5. Restoration of water balance after exercise in relation to replacement of sodium. These measurements were made by dehydrating subjects by 2 per cent of body mass and requiring them to drink a volume of fluid containing sodium at different concentrations: whole body fluid and sodium balance were calculated 6 h into the recovery period. It is clear that positive fluid balance is not achieved unless sufficient sodium is ingested to allow restoration of sodium balance. (Redrawn from Maughan and Leiper, 1995)

important to ensure an adequate intake of electrolytes, especially sodium and also, to a lesser extent, potassium.

Practical implications for the athlete

Living in the heat

In many hot climates, living accommodation, as well as most indoor areas, will be air conditioned. It is not unusual for the temperature to be rather low, usually about 20°C, but sometimes as low as 12–15°C. Repeated changes from the heat outdoors to the cool indoor conditions seem to increase upper respiratory tract symptoms such as sore throat, cough and runny nose which may interfere with training. There are, however, advantages in having a cool place where recovery from training can take place: this may be a common-room or dining area rather than a bedroom. It is, however, wrong to think that there is an advantage in terms of acclimatization in switching the air-conditioning system off. A bedroom temperature of between 16 and 23°C is recommended. This is a wide range, which gives scope for individual preference. It should be noted, however, that disturbances of sleep have been shown to increase as the temperature of the room increases. When fluid losses are high, a water bottle by the bed allows drinks to be taken during the night with minimum inconvenience.

Monitoring of responses

Some degree of monitoring of individual responses to heat stress and of the rate and extent of adaptation is an essential part of preparation for hot weather competition. Training camps and any other hot weather training or competition opportunities should be used to collect information on individuals and on squads. Measurements made on individuals are also a crucial part of the education process in demonstrating the negative effects of dehydration and hyperthermia (increased body temperature), and the ways in which these effects can be minimized.

When exposed to the heat, athletes will generally become dehydrated despite the availability of fluids. Regular monitoring of body mass can give useful information on the athlete's hydration status, provided some precautions are taken to standardize the measurement conditions. These results, however, only have value if they can be compared with baseline measurements made in normal training conditions at home. Each athlete must know their own optimum body mass for training and competing, and must also know how much their body mass normally varies on a daily basis. Small variations (perhaps as much as 1–2 kg for some individuals) usually have no significance, but for those athletes whose mass is normally very constant, this can be an early warning sign. It is therefore crucial that the individual athlete knows what the normal range is. Body mass measurements should always be made at the same time of day, under the same conditions. Ideally, this will be done first thing in the morning, before breakfast or training, but after a visit to the toilet. If this is not possible, it may be done before training each day. Measurement of mass loss during training sessions should also be monitored, so that these measurements can be combined and compared with the normal daily pattern: 1 kg of mass loss represents approximately 1 litre of sweat loss, and should be replaced with 1.5 litres of fluid (Shirreffs *et al.*, 1996). A progressive decrease in body mass in Atlanta may be an indication of dehydration which is not being compensated for by an increased fluid intake. Alternatively, it may reflect a loss of appetite and decreased food intake, which is common in hot conditions. A decrease in mass may also be an early warning of overtraining. An increase in body mass is also possible, reflecting overeating resulting from the increased availability of high quality free food and increased leisure time. If large volumes of carbohydrate-containing drinks are consumed, these can contribute a large amount of energy to the athlete's diet; this is of particular concern to those in weight category sports.

Athletes should also be encouraged to keep, in their training diary, a record of subjective symptoms associated with travel, training and competition, to see what patterns emerge. This diary might record, as well as body mass, some information on urine output: the time of day urine is passed, an estimate of the volume (simply done with a measuring cylinder – and beaker if necessary), and the colour (by comparison with a colour chart). Urine colour is a sensitive and reliable measure of hydration status (Armstrong *et al.*, 1994). Other measures, such as urine osmolality, specific gravity or conductivity can also be helpful (Shirreffs and Maughan, 1998). This information gives an indication of hydration status, but the return of the normal pattern of urine output is a good index of the recovery from jet lag and the re-establishment of normal body rhythms. Again, this only has real value if the information collected in hot conditions can be compared with the normal pattern established over a period of at least a few weeks at home in normal training conditions immediately prior to departure. It is appreciated that this is not acceptable to everyone, but it is nonetheless vital that some sort of monitoring is carried out before and during visits to hot weather venues.

Team coaches and support staff have a responsibility to ensure that athletes appreciate the need to collect this information by explaining in advance its value. They must also keep an eye on the individual records and pay particular attention to anyone who appears to be having difficulty coping with training. Each athlete should try to encourage team mates to take extra fluids.

Warm-up

Contrary to popular belief, there is little, if any, evidence that warm-up prevents or reduces the risk of injury. Warming up before training or competition does, however, ensure adequate physiological and psychological preparation. In cool climates, the purpose of the warm-up is to elevate body temperature and increase blood flow to the muscles and associated soft tissues. In contrast, in hot climates, the body temperature should not be markedly increased during the warm-up due to the real possibility of reduced performance because of hyperthermia and dehydration. In explosive events this may be disregarded, but where exercise continues for more than perhaps 2 or 3 min, body temperature should not be markedly increased before exercise begins, and there may be real benefits of reducing the body temperature before events lasting more than about 30 min (Lee and Haymes, 1995; Booth *et al.*, 1997). The coach, athlete and physiotherapist need to look at modifications to the warm-up to ensure that the elevation of core temperature is limited without compromising the physiological and psychological preparation. It is absolutely essential that this is practised well in advance so that the athlete is comfortable with any changes made. Basic modifications must include warming up in the shade and drinking plenty of fluids, and the warm-up must be tailored to each individual's state of acclimation and sweating response. The modified warm-up will have to be practised and adjusted while at warm weather training camps, and perhaps also in heat chambers at home, so that the athlete becomes comfortable with any changes made. Practising the modified warm-up prior to training or competition while living in a cool climate may cause problems because of the need for an increased body temperature to produce the optimum physiological preparation.

Rehydration

Although athletes may be tempted to believe that the need for fluid replacement will decrease as they become adjusted to the heat, heat acclimatization will actually increase the requirement for fluid replacement because of the enhanced sweating response. So you not only have to drink more in the heat, but you have to drink even more as you become acclimatized and begin to sweat more. If dehydration is allowed to occur, the improved ability to tolerate heat which results from the acclimatization process will disappear completely (Sawka and Pandolf, 1990). There is no way of adapting to dehydration: attempting to do so is futile and dangerous.

Heat experience

As well as the physiological adaptations that occur in response to living and training in the heat, athletes gain valuable experience which allows them to develop coping strategies. The need for attention to fluid intake and for wearing the most appropriate clothing, and how to monitor fluid balance are not learned easily other than by experience. The most effective acclimatization programme for any individual can also be learned only by trial and error. Those individuals whose performance is most affected by heat can be identified and a strategy to meet their needs developed. Some athletes find great difficulty in hot, humid conditions and there may be implications for team selection. These aspects may be almost as important as the physiological adaptations that result.

Fluid replacement

Although the basic principles that govern fluid replacement strategies for athletes are well established, there are some real difficulties in putting these into practice. Athletes and their advisers want a prescription for the composition, amount and timing of fluid intake that will cover all situations. Even within a single event, however, the requirement will vary so much between individuals, depending on the physiological and biochemical characteristics of the individual as well as on the training load and on other factors such as taste preference, that such recommendations can only be made on an individual basis. When the possible effects of different climatic conditions and different training and competition schedules are added, the problems in making a simple recommendation are multiplied.

These difficulties are immediately apparent when any of the published guidelines for fluid intake during exercise are examined. Guidelines are generally formulated to include the needs of most individuals in most situations, with the result that the outer limits become so wide as to be at best meaningless and at worst positively harmful. The guidelines of the American College of Sports Medicine, published in their 1984 Position Statement on the prevention of heat illness in distance running, were more specific than an earlier (1975) version of these guidelines. The recommendation for marathon runners was for an intake of 100–200 ml every 2–3 km, giving a total intake of 1400–4200 ml at the extremes. Again, taking these extreme values, it is unlikely that the elite runners, who take only a little over 2 h to complete the distance, could tolerate a rate of intake of about 2 l h^{-1}, and equally unlikely that an intake of 300 ml h^{-1} would be adequate for the slowest competitors except perhaps when the ambient temperature was low. These same guidelines also recommended that the best fluid to drink during prolonged exercise is cool water. In view of the accumulated evidence presented above, this recommendation seems even less acceptable than it was in 1984. This has been recognized and the updated version of the guidelines (American College of Sports Medicine, 1996) are in accord with the current mainstream thinking: for events lasting more than 60 min, they favour the use of drinks containing 'proper amounts of carbohydrates and/or electrolytes'. The evolution of this series of ACSM position stands demonstrates the progress made in our understanding of this complex area.

Because of the difficulty in making specific recommendations that will meet the needs of all individuals in all situations, the only possible way forward is to formulate some general guidelines and to indicate how these should be modified in different circumstances. Assuming that athletes are willing and able to take fluids during training, the recommendations for fluid use in training will not be very different from those for competition, except in events of very short duration. The sprinter or pursuit cyclist, whose event lasts a few seconds or minutes, has no opportunity or need for fluid intake during competition, but should drink during training sessions which may stretch over 2 h or more. The body does not adapt to repeated bouts of dehydration: training in the dehydrated state will impair the quality of training and confers no advantage. The choice of the fluid to be used is again a decision for the individual. Water ingestion is better than fluid restriction, but dilute carbohydrate–electrolyte drinks will provide greater benefits than water alone. The optimum carbohydrate concentration in most situations will be in the range of about 2–8 per cent, and a variety of different carbohydrates, either alone or in combination, are effective. Glucose, sucrose, maltose and glucose oligomers are all likely to promote improved performance. Addition of small amounts of fructose to drinks containing other carbohydrates seems to be acceptable, but high concentrations of fructose alone are best avoided. Some sodium should probably be present, with the optimum concentration somewhere between 10 and 60 mmol l^{-1}, but there is also a strong argument that, in events of short duration, this may not be necessary. There is little evidence to suggest that small variations in the concentration of these components of ingested fluids will significantly alter their efficacy. There is not at present any evidence to support the addition of other components (potassium, magnesium, other minerals or vitamins) to drinks intended to promote or maintain hydration status. Palatability is, however, an important issue, and flavouring of drinks to promote consumption is crucial.

Individuals who begin exercise in a hypohydrated state will, in almost every exercise situation, but especially when there is an additional heat stress imposed by the environmental conditions, demonstrate a reduced exercise capacity. Full hydration prior to exercise is therefore essential, although it is not at present clear how beneficial attempts to over-hydrate might be. Evidence continues to accumulate that acute restoration of fluid losses after dehydration induced by exercise together with food and fluid restriction may not restore exercise capacity (Burge *et al.*, 1993). Where large sweat losses are incurred, it seems clear that more effective restoration is achieved by ingestion of solutions containing electrolytes, especially sodium, and there is good evidence that carbohydrate ingested at this time is also beneficial.

Restoration of fluid and electrolyte losses is a crucial part of the recovery process. Athletes should be encouraged to record body mass changes during training as an estimate of sweat losses. Full replacement requires an intake of water in excess of the sweat loss and also requires that electrolyte losses are replaced. Where no solid food is taken, these electrolytes must be present in the drinks consumed.

References

American College of Sports Medicine (1975). Position statement on prevention of heat injuries during distance running. *Med. Sci. Sports*, **7**, vii–ix.

American College of Sports Medicine (1984). Position stand on prevention of thermal injuries during distance running. *Med. Sci. Sports Exerc.*, **16**, ix–xiv.

Armstrong, L.E., Costill, D.L. and Fink, W.J. (1985). Influence of diuretic-induced dehydration on competitive running performance. *Med. Sci. Sports Exerc.*, **17**, 456–461.

Armstrong, L.E., Maresh, C.M., Castellani, J.W., Bergeron, M.F., Kenefick, R.W., LaGasse, K.E. and Riebe, D. (1994). Urinary indices of hydration status. *Int. J. Sport Nutr.*, **4**, 265–279.

Astrand, I. (1960). Aerobic work capacity in men and women. *Acta Physiol. Scand.*, **49** (Suppl. 169), 64–73.

Barr, S.I., Costill, D.L. and Fink, W.J. (1991). Fluid replacement during prolonged exercise: effects of water, saline or no fluid. *Med. Sci. Sports Exerc.*, **23**, 811–817.

Below,P.R., Mora-Rodriguez, R., Gonzalez-Alonso, J. and Coyle, E.F. (1995). Fluid and car- bohydrate ingestion independently improve performance during 1 h of intense exercise. *Med. Sci. Sports Exerc.*, **27**, 200–210.

Booth, J., Marino, F. and Ward, J.J. (1997). Improved running performance in hot humid conditions following whole body precooling. *Med. Sci. Sports Exerc.*, **29**, 943–949.

Brengelmann, G.L. (1983). Circulatory adjustments to exercise and heat stress. *Ann. Rev. Physiol.*, **45**, 191–212.

Brown, N.J., Stephenson, L.A., Lister, G. and Nadel, E.R. (1982). Relative anaerobiosis during heavy exercise in the heat. *Fed. Proc.*, **41**, 1677.

Burgess, W.A., Davis, J.M., Bartoli, W.P. and Woods, J.A. (1991). Failure of low dose carbo- hydrate feeding to attenuate glycoregulatory hormone responses and improve endurance performance. *Int. J. Sports Nutr.*, **1**, 338–352.

Coyle, E.F., Coggan, A.R., Hemmert, M.K. and Ivy, J.L. (1986). Muscle glycogen utilisation during prolonged strenuous exercise when fed carbohydrate. *J. Appl. Physiol.*, **61**, 165–172.

Dawson, B. (1994). Exercise training in sweat clothing in cool conditions to improve heat tolerance. *Sports Med.*, **17**, 233–244.

Febbraio, M., Parkin, J.A., Baldwin, J., Zhao, S. and Carey, M.F. (1996). Metabolic indices of fatigue in prolonged exercise at different ambient temperatures. *J. Sports Sci.*, **14**, 361.

Fein, L.W., Haymes, E.M. and Buskirk, E.R. (1975). Effects of daily and intermittent exposure on heat acclimation of women. *Int. J. Biometeorol.* **19**, 41–52.

Fielding, R.A., Costill, D.L., Fink, W.J., King, D.S., Hargreaves, M. and Kovaleski, M.E. (1985). Effect of carbohydrate feeding frequencies on muscle glycogen use during exercise. *Med. Sci. Sports Exerc.*, **17**, 472–476.

Fortney, S.M., Wenger, C.B., Bove, J.R. and Nadel, E.R. (1984). Effect of hyperosmolality on control of blood flow and sweating. *J. Appl. Physiol.* **57**, 1688–1695.

Galloway, S.D.R. and Maughan, R.J. (1997). Effects of ambient temperature on the capacity to perform prolonged cycle exercise in man. *Med. Sci. Sports Exerc.*, **29**, 1240–1249.

Gisolfi, C.V. and Copping, J.R. (1974). Thermal effects of prolonged treadmill exercise in the heat. *Med. Sci. Sports Exerc.*, **6**, 108–113.

Gonzalez, R.R. (1988). Biophysics of heat transfer and clothing considerations. In *Human Performance Physiology and Environmental Medicine at Terrestrial Extremes* (K.B. Pandolf, M.N. Sawka and R.R. Gonzalez, eds), pp. 45– 95. Benchmark.

Hargreaves, M. (1994). Carbohydrates and exercise. In *Foods, Nutrition and Sports Performance* (C. Williams and J.T. Devlin, eds), pp. 19–33. Spon.

Hargreaves, M. and Briggs, C.A. (1988). Effect of carbohydrate ingestion on exercise meta- bolism. *J. Appl. Physiol.*, **65**, 1553–1555.

Hargreaves, M., Costill, D.L., Coggan, A., Fink, W.J. and Nishibata, I. (1984). Effect of car- bohydrate feedings on muscle glycogen utilisation and exercise performance. *Med. Sci. Sports Exerc.*, **16**, 219–222.

Houmard, J.A., Costill, D.L., Davis, J.A., Mitchell, J.B., Pascoe, D.D. and Robergs, R.A. (1990). The influence of exercise intensity on heat acclimation in trained subjects. *Med. Sci. Sports Exerc.*, **22**, 615–620.

Lamb, D.R. (1984). *Physiology of Exercise*. MacMillan.

Lee, D.T. and Haymes, E.M. (1995). Exercise duration and thermoregulatory responses after whole body precooling. *J. Appl. Physiol.*, **79**, 1971–1976.

Leiper, J.B. and Maughan, R.J. (1988). Experimental models for the investigation of water and solute uptake in man: implications for oral rehydration solutions. *Drugs*, **36** (Suppl. 4), 65– 79.

Leithead, C.S. and Lind, A.R. (1964). *Heat Stress and Heat Disorders*. Cassell.

Lind, A.R. and Bass, D.E. (1963). Optimal exposure time for development of heat acclimation. *Fed. Proc.*, **22**, 704–708.

Maughan, R.J. (1991). Effects of CHO–electrolyte solution on prolonged exercise. In *Perspectives in Exercise Science and Sports Medicine* (D.R. Lamb and M.H. Williams, eds), pp. 35–85. Benchmark Press.

Maughan, R.J. (1994a). Fluid and electrolyte loss and replacement in exercise. In *Oxford Textbook of Sports Medicine* (Harries, Williams, Stanish and Micheli, eds), pp. 82–93. Oxford University Press.

Maughan, R.J. (1994b). Physiology and nutrition for middle distance and long distance running. In *Perspectives in Exercise Science and Sports Medicine. Volume 7: Physiology and Nutrition in Competitive Sport* (Lamb, Knuttgen and Murray, eds), pp. 329–371. Cooper.

Maughan, R.J. and Leiper, J.B. (1995). Effects of sodium content of ingested fluids on post-exercise rehydration in man. *Eur. J. Appl. Physiol.*, **71**, 311–319.

Maughan, R.J. and Shirreffs, S.M. (1997). Recovery from prolonged exercise: restoration of water and electrolyte balance. *J. Sports Sci.*, **15**, 297–303.

Maughan, R.J., Fenn, C.E. and Leiper, J.B. (1989). Effects of fluid, electrolyte and substrate ingestion on endurance capacity. *Eur. J. Appl. Physiol.*, **58**, 481–486.

Maughan, R.J., Bethell, L. and Leiper, J.B. (1996). Effects of ingested fluids on homeostasis and exercise performance in man. *Exp. Physiol.*, **81**, 847–859.

Montain, S.J., Maughan, R.J. and Sawka, M.N. (1996). Heat acclimatization strategies for the 1996 Summer Olympics. *Athletic Ther.Today*, **1**, 42–46.

Nadel, E.R. (1988). Temperature regulation and prolonged exercise. In *Perspectives in Exercise Science and Sports Medicine. Volume 1: Prolonged Exercise* (D.R. Lamb and R. Murray, eds), pp. 125–152. Benchmark.

Neilsen, B (1996). Olympics in Atlanta: a fight against physics. *Med. Sci. Sports Ex.* **28**, 665–668.

Nielsen, B., Kubica, R., Bonnesen, A., Rasmussen, I.B., Stoklosa, J. and Wilk, B. (1982). Physical work capacity after dehydration and hyperthermia. *Scand. J. Sports Sci.*, **3**, 2–10.

Nielsen, B., Hales, J.R.S., Christensen, N.J., Warberg, J. and Saltin, B. (1993). Human circulatory and thermoregulatory adaptation with heat acclimation and exercise in a hot, dry environment. *J. Physiol.*, **460**, 467–485.

Nielsen, M. (1938). Die Regulation der Korpertemperatur bei muskelarbeit. *Skand. Arch. Physiol.*, **79**, 193–230.

Noakes, T.D. (1988). Why marathon runners collapse. *S. Af. Med. J.*, **73**, 569–571.

Pichan, G., Sridharan, K., Swamy, Y.V., Joseph, S. and Gautam, R.K. (1985). Physiological acclimatization to heat after a spell of cold conditioning in tropical subjects. *Aviat. Space Environ. Med.*, **56**, 436–440.

Piwonka, R.W. and Robinson, S. (1967). Acclimatization of highly trained men to work in severe heat. *J. Appl. Physiol.*, **22**, 9–12.

Rehrer, N.J. and Burke, L.M. (1996). Sweat losses during various sports. *Aust. J. Nutr. Diet.*, **53**, S13–S16.

Robinson, T.A., Hawley, J.A., Palmer, G.S., Wilson, G.R., Gray, D.A., Noakes, T.D. and Dennis, S.C. (1995). Water ingestion does not improve 1-h cycling performance in moderate ambient temperatures. *Eur. J. Appl. Physiol.*, **71**, 153–160.

Rowell, L.B. (1983). Cardiovascular aspects of human thermoregulation. *Circ. Res.*, **52**, 367–379.

Rowell, L.B. (1986). *Human Circulation*. Oxford University Press.

Santee, W.R. and Gonzalez, R.R. (1988). Characteristics of the thermal environment. In *Human Performance Physiology and Environmental Medicine at Terrestrial Extremes* (K.B. Pandolf, M.N. Sawka and R.R. Gonzalez, eds), pp. 1–43. Cooper, Carmel.

Sawka, M.N. and Pandolf, K.B. (1990). Effects of body water loss on physiological function and exercise performance. In *Perspectives in Exercise Science and Sports Medicine*, Vol. 3 (C.V. Gisolfi and D.R. Lamb, eds), pp. 1–38. Benchmark.

Sawka, M.N., Andrew, A.J., Francesconi, R.P., Muza, S.R. and Pandolf, K.B. (1985). Thermoregulatory and blood responses during exercise at graded hypohydration levels. *J. Appl. Physiol.*, **59**, 1394–1401.

Sawka, M.N., Young, A.J., Latzka, W.A., Neufer, P.D., Quigley, M.D. and Pandolf, K.B. (1992). Human tolerance to heat strain during exercise: influence of hydration. *J. Appl. Physiol.*, **73**, 368–375.

Shirreffs, S.M. and Maughan, R.J. (1998). Urine osmolality and conductivity as markers of hydration status. *Med. Sci. Sports Exerc.*, **30**, 1598–1602.

Shirreffs, S.M., Taylor, A.J., Leiper, J.B. and Maughan, R.J. (1996). Post-exercise rehydration in man: effects of volume consumed and sodium content of ingested fluids. *Med. Sci. Sports Exerc.*, **28**, 1260–1271.

Walsh, R.M., Noakes, T.D., Hawley, J.A. and Dennis, S.C. (1994). Impaired high-intensity cycling performance time at low levels of dehydration. *Int. J. Sports Med.*, **15**, 392–398.

Wenger, C.B. (1988). Human heat acclimatisation. In *Human Performance Physiology and Environmental Medicine at Terrestrial Extremes* (K.B. Pandolf, M.N. Sawka and R.R. Gonzalez, eds), pp. 153–197. Benchmark.

Wyndham, C.H. and Strydom, N.B. (1969). The danger of an inadequate water intake during marathon running. *S. Afr. Med. J.*, **43**, 893–896.

Further reading

Bar-Or, O. (1989). Temperature regulation during exercise in children and adolescents. In *Perspectives in Exercise Science and Sports Medicine. Volume 2: Youth, Exercise and Sport* (C.V. Gisolfi and D.R. Lamb, eds), pp. 335–362. Benchmark.

Maughan, R.J. (1994). Physiology and nutrition for middle distance and long distance running. In *Perspectives in Exercise Science and Sports Medicine. Volume 7: Physiology and Nutrition for Competitive Sport* (D.R. Lamb, H.G. Knuttgen and R. Murray, eds), pp. 329–372. Cooper.

Nadel, E.R. (1980). Circulatory and thermal regulations during exercise. *Fed. Proc.*, **39**, 1491–1497.

Saltin, B. and Costill, D.L. (1988). Fluid and electrolyte balance during prolonged exercise. In *Exercise, Nutrition, and Metabolism* (E.S. Horton and R.L. Terjung, eds), pp. 150–158. Macmillan.

8

Immunology

Michael Gleeson and Nicolette C. Bishop

Interest in the acute and chronic effects of exercise on immune function in recent years has been prompted by an increasing scientific body of evidence which suggests that athletes involved in prolonged strenuous training are more susceptible to communicable opportunistic infections than their sedentary counterparts. Although increased incidence of infection in athletes may be partly attributable to increased exposure and facilitated pathogen transmission, the literature generally supports the idea of immunological dysfunction in athletes. This chapter gives a brief summary of the structure and function of the immune system and discusses which specific components of the immune system are affected by exercise, the time-course of such effects and the possible mechanisms by which exercise and heavy training cause an alteration in immune function. Many scientists believe that the effect of intense exercise on immune function may be similar to that of other forms of stress that are known to suppress immune function such as surgical trauma, physical and thermal injury, sepsis and extreme emotional distress. Exercise can be viewed as a very useful model of stress, since its duration and intensity can be accurately controlled and reproduced in the laboratory. For practical purposes, research into the effects of exercise on immune function may elucidate with what frequency and intensity athletes should train to provide the necessary physiological adaptations to increase performance while avoiding the detrimental effects of exercise on immune function and hence susceptibility to infection

Altered susceptibility to infection in athletes

Anecdotal reports of increased incidence of infection in athletes training hard are legion. Several epidemiological reports suggest that athletes training for endurance events such as the marathon are at increased risk of upper respiratory tract infection (URTI) and some recent reviews of this information are available (Nieman, 1994a,b, 1996). Additional risk factors for URTI appear to include ultradistance events, the 1–2 week period following marathon-type race events and engaging in prolonged exercise during the winter months (Nieman, 1996). Most epidemiological studies have used questionnaires to assess incidence of symptoms of supposed URTI in athletes and non-athletes. Unfortunately, this approach leaves such studies open to the criticism that the reporting of respiratory symptoms was increased by increased body awareness, respiratory muscle fatigue or inhalation of air pollutants in regularly exercising individuals rather than by a specific infection of the upper respiratory tract. Furthermore, if the reported incidence of respiratory symptoms is compared with anticipated infection rates for the general population, there may be a response bias. In the study by Nieman *et al.* (1990), only 46.9 per cent of questionnaires were returned, and the respondents may have been mainly those who developed symptoms.

Other confounding factors that could give rise to an increased incidence of infection in athletes other than through an exercise-induced depression of immune function include exposure to contaminated air or water, increased lung ventilation and breathing through the mouth as well as the nose, a reduction of tracheal ciliary or mucosal secretory activity by the inhalation of cold air, modified diet, physical contact and skin abrasions and psychological stress.

Normal immune function

Components of the immune system

The immune system protects against, recognizes, attacks and destroys elements which are foreign to the body (Brenner *et al.*, 1994). This statement succinctly defines the functions of this homeostatic system, which, nevertheless, are far more complex than the above remark initially indicates. It involves the precise co-ordination of many different cell types and molecular messengers and yet, like any other homeostatic system, the immune system is composed of redundant mechanisms to ensure that essential processes are carried out. The immune system is particularly important in defending the body against pathogenic (disease-causing) micro-organisms including bacteria, protozoa, viruses and fungi.

The immune system can be divided into two broad functions: innate (natural or non-specific) and adaptive (acquired or specific) immunity which work together synergistically. The attempt of an infectious agent to enter the body immediately activates the innate system. This first line of defence (Table 8.1) comprises three general mechanisms with the common goal of restricting micro-organism entry into the body: (1) physical/structural barriers (skin, epithelial linings, mucosal secretions); (2) chemical barriers (pH of bodily fluids and soluble factors); and (3) phagocytic cells (e.g. neutrophils, monocytes/macrophages) and other non-specific killer cells (e.g. natural killer (NK) lymphocytes). Failure of the innate system and the resulting infection activates the adaptive system, which

Table 8.1.   Innate (non-specific) first line of defence mechanisms

Skin	• Tough barrier. • Secretions on surface lower pH and suppress pathogenic bacterial division. Natural bacteria, adapted to conditions, contribute to secretions.
Membranes and secretions	• Lysozyme in sweat attacks cell walls of many bacteria. • Acid in stomach. • Hairs, mucus and cilia in respiratory tract. • Saliva contains IgA, lysozyme and α-amylase which have antibacterial properties. • Low pH of urine.
Phagocytes	• Macrophages (from monocytes in blood) and neutrophils: ingest (phagocytose) and destroy foreign material.
NK cells	• Natural killer (NK) cells, a non-specific lymphocyte, attack membranes of virus-infected cells and tumour cells, causing lysis.
Inflammation	• Injury to cells triggers inflammatory response. Small blood vessels near injury site dilate and leak more leading to classical signs of redness, warmth and swelling. • Leukocytes leave blood and enter damaged tissue. • Clotting proteins enter interstitial fluid and help seal off infected area. • Chemicals released from injured cells, including histamine, prostaglandins and various peptides, initiate inflammation. Some chemicals dilate blood vessels, others increase capillary permeability, attract and activate leukocytes, signal the bone marrow to release more neutrophils and cause pain.
Pyrogens	• Chemicals released from damaged tissues and activated leukocytes (e.g. interleukin-1) or invading micro-organisms (lipopolysaccharides). Cause fever by resetting of hypothalamic thermostat. Mild to moderate fever stimulates phagocytosis and inhibits bacterial growth. High fever is dangerous.

Table 8.1.   (Continued)

Antimicrobial proteins	• Interferons are proteins released from virus-infected cells that cause other cells to resist virus infection by inhibiting virus replication inside them. Some interferons mobilize NK cells, others activate macrophages and stimulate the specific immune response.
	• Complement proteins circulate as inactive form in blood: activated by onset of immune response and can increase histamine release, coat invading organisms, attract and activate phagocytic cells and form membrane attack complex causing lysis of bacteria.
Acute phase proteins	• Made in the liver, secreted into the blood.
	• Encourage leukocyte migration to sites of injury and infection. Activate complement and stimulate phagocytosis.

aids recovery from infection. The adaptive immune system responds with a proliferation of cells which either attack the invader directly or produce specific defensive proteins, i.e. antibodies (also known as immunoglobulins, Ig), which help to counter the pathogen in various ways. This is helped greatly by receptors on the cell surface of T and B lymphocytes that recognize the antigen (foreign substance – usually the proteins located on the surface of the bacteria or virus), engendering specificity and 'memory' that enable the immune system to mount an augmented response when the host is reinfected by the same pathogen (Cannon, 1993).

The components of the immune system comprise cellular and soluble elements (Table 8.2). The immune cells have diverse functions despite their common origin: the haemipoietic stem cell of the bone marrow. Leukocytes (white blood cells, WBC) consist of the granulocytes (60–70 per cent of circulating leukocytes), monocytes (10–15 per cent) and lymphocytes (20–25 per cent). Various subsets of the latter can be identified by the use of monoclonal antibodies to identify cell surface markers (clusters of differentiation, CD). The characteristics of the various leukocytes and lymphocyte subsets are summarized in Tables 8.3 and 8.4, respectively.

Soluble factors of the immune system act in several ways: (1) to activate leukocytes; (2) as neutralizers (killers) of foreign agents; and (3) as regulators of the immune system (Mackinnon, 1992). Such factors include the cytokines. These polypeptide messenger substances stimulate the growth, differentiation and functional development of leukocytes via specific receptor sites on either secretory cells (autocrine function) or immediately adjacent leukocytes (paracrine function) (Shephard *et al.*, 1994). The actions of cytokines are not confined to the immune system; they also

Table 8.2.   Main components of the immune system

Innate components	Adaptive components
Cellular: Natural killer cells (CD16+, CD56+) Phagocytes (neutrophils, eosinophils, basophils, monocytes, macrophages)	**Cellular:** T lymphocytes (CD3+, CD4+, CD8+) B lymphocytes (CD19+, CD20+, CD22+)
Soluble: Acute phase proteins Complement Lysozyme Cytokines (interleukins (IL), interferons (IFN), colony-stimulating factor (CSF), tumour necrosis factors (TNF)) Cytokine receptor antagonists	**Soluble:** Immunoglobulins (IgA, IgD, IgE, IgG, IgM)

influence the neuroendocrine system, an action of importance to this review. Other soluble factors include complement, lysozyme and the specific antibodies secreted from B lymphocytes. The actions of the innate non-specific soluble factors relevant to this review are summarized in Table 8.5.

Origins and tissue locations of cells of the immune system

All blood cells originate in the bone marrow from common stem cells. The latter are capable of differentiating into erythrocytes, neutrophils, monocytes (precursors of tissue macrophages), lymphocytes, eosinophils and basophils. Initially, all lymphocytes are alike. After circulating in the blood as immature lymphocytes, they continue their maturation either in the thymus, a gland in the upper chest, where they become T lymphocytes, or in the bone marrow where they become B lymphocytes. As they mature, the lymphocytes develop immunocompetence: each cell becomes competent at recognizing one particular antigen and mounting an immune response against that antigen alone. During the development of immunocompetence, specific receptor proteins (similar to antibodies) are synthesized and appear on the surface of the lymphocyte. Each cell has receptors that can bind to only one kind of antigen. The T and B cell populations include hundreds of thousands of subpopulations, each made up of cells bearing unique antigen receptors on their surfaces. Each lymphocyte becomes rigidly programmed to recognize and respond to a specific antigen before encountering it and the immune system is prepared for an almost unlimited variety of potential infections. Thus, the versatility of the immune system is not due to flexible cells that change their antigenic targets on demand; rather it depends on the presence of an enormous diversity of lymphocytes with different receptor specificities.

Table 8.3.   A summary of the characteristics of leukocytes

Leukocyte	Main characteristics
Neutrophil	• 55–70% of leukocytes • Phagocytose foreign substances including whole bacteria • Phagocytose antigen–antibody complexes • Display little or no capacity to recharge their killing mechanisms once activated; limited lifespan ($\sim$ 2 days) and half-life in circulation ($\sim$ 9 h)
Eosinophil	• 2–5% of granulocytes • Phagocytose parasites • Triggered by IgG to release toxic lysosomal products
Basophil	• 0–2% of granulocytes • Produce chemotactic factors • Tissue equivalent is the mast cell, which releases an eosinophil chemotactic factor and histamine; important in allergic reactions
Monocytes/ Macrophages	• 10–15% of leukocytes • Egress into tissues (e.g. liver, spleen) and differentiate into the mature form: the macrophage • Phagocytose foreign material enabling antigen presentation • Secrete immunomodulatory cytokines • Retain their capacity to divide after leaving the bone marrow
Lymphocytes	• 20–25% of leukocytes • Activate other lymphocyte subsets • Produce lymphokines • Recognize antigens • Produce antibodies (immunoglobulins) • Exhibit memory • Exhibit cytoxicity

Circulating immunocompetent lymphocytes concentrate in lymph nodes, arranged along an extensive network of lymph vessels, and the spleen, through which passes most of the circulating blood. Most pathogens getting through the outer defences appear in lymph fluid, since lymph vessels drain nearly all the body's tissues, returning lymph to the circulation. Lymphocytes located in the lymph nodes are strategically located to remove antigens before they reach the blood. Lymph nodes contain large numbers of macrophages, which ingest pathogens swept into the lymph nodes by the flow of lymph fluid. Macrophages play a key role in activating lymphocytes. As macrophages and lymphocytes resist invasion, lymph nodes may swell; a common sign of infection.

Table 8.4.   Lymphocyte functions and characteristics

Lymphocyte subset	Main function and characteristic
T cells (CD3+): T-H (CD4+)	• 60–75% of lymphocytes • 60–70% of T cells • 'Helper' cells • Recognize antigen to co-ordinate the acquired response • Secrete cytokines that stimulate T and B cell proliferation and differentiation
T-C/T-S (CD8+)	• 30–40% of T cells • T-S ('suppressor') cells involved in the regulation of proliferation of B cells and other T cells • T-S cells may be important in 'switching off' the immune response • T-C ('cytotoxic') cells kill a variety of targets, including some tumour cells and virus-infected cells • Exhibit memory
B cells (CD19+, CD20+, CD22+)	• 5–15% of lymphocytes • Produce and secrete immunoglobulins (Ig) • Exhibit memory
Natural killer (NK) cells (CD16+, CD56+)	• 10–20% of lymphocytes • Large, granular lymphocytes • Express spontaneous cytolytic activity against a variety of tumour cells and virus-infected cells • MHC-independent • Do not express the CD3 cell-surface antigen • Triggered by IgG • Control foreign materials until the antigen-specific (adaptive) immune system responds

General mechanism of the immune response

The introduction of an infectious agent to the body initiates an inflammatory response which augments that of the immune system. Acute inflammation increases the perfusion of the infected area, and this – coupled with augmented vascular permeability – facilitates the entry of leukocytes and plasma proteins into the infected tissue. The immune response itself varies according to the nature of the infectious agent (parasitic, bacterial, fungal, viral) but a general response pattern is evident (Figure 8.1). The phagocytosis (ingestion) of the invading micro-organism by a macrophage initiates a chain of events. Lysosomal digestive enzymes and oxidizing agents (e.g. hydrogen peroxide and superoxide radicals) are released into the intracellular vacuole containing the foreign material within the macrophage. The foreign proteins (antigens) normally found on the micro-organism's surface are processed by the macrophage and incorporated into its own cell surface. The antigens can now be presented

Table 8.5.   Producers and actions of the major innate soluble factors

Soluble factor	Producer(s) and immune actions
Cytokines: IL-1	• Produced mainly from activated macrophages • IL-1α tends to remain cell associated • IL-1β acts as a soluble mediator • Stimulates IL-2 production from CD3+ and CD4+ cells • Increases IL-1 and IL-2 receptor expression • Increases B cell proliferation • Increases TNF-α, IL-6 and CSF levels • Stimulates secretion of prostaglandins • Appear to be endogenous pyrogens
IL-2	• Produced mainly by CD4+ cells • Stimulates T and B cell proliferation and expression of IL-2 receptors on their surfaces • Stimulates release of IFN • Stimulates NK cell proliferation and killing
IL-6	• Produced by activated T-H cells, fibroblasts and macrophages • Stimulates the differentiation of B cells, inflammation and the acute phase response
TNF-α	• Produced from monocytes, T, B and NK cells • Enhances tumour cell killing and antiviral activity
Acute phase proteins (APP)	• Made in the liver, secreted into the blood • Encourage cell migration to sites of injury and infection • Activate complement • Stimulate phagocytosis
Complement proteins	• Found in the serum • Consist of 20 or more proteins • Stimulate phagocytosis, antigen presentation and neutralization of infected cells • The 'amplifier' of the immune response

to the other cellular immune components. T-helper lymphocytes (CD4+ expressing cells) co-ordinate the response via cytokine release to activate other immune cells. Stimulation of mature B lymphocytes results in their proliferation and differentiation into immunoglobulin-secreting plasma cells. Immunoglobulins or antibodies are important to antigen recognition and memory of earlier exposure to specific antigens (Mackinnon, 1992).

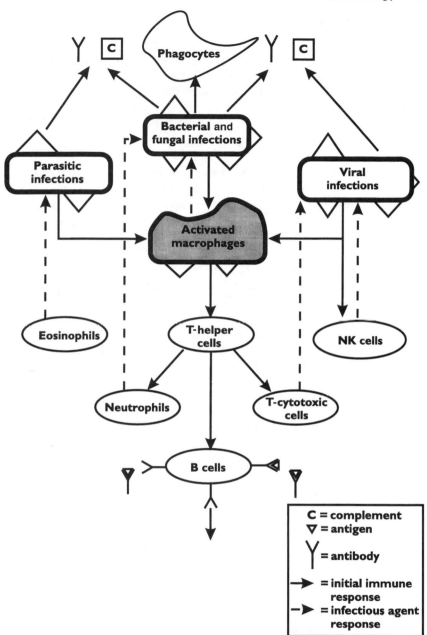

Figure 8.1. The general scheme of the immune response to various pathogens. The key player is the macrophage which ingests foreign material and presents antigens on its cell surface which then activates T and B lymphocytes specific for the antigen. Infectious agents also activate non-specific (innate) host defence mechanisms including complement, phagocytic cells (e.g. neutrophils) and natural killer cells

Clonal selection and immunological memory

An antigen entering the body selectively activates only a tiny fraction of the quiescent lymphocytes, which then grow and divide to form a clone of identical effector cells. This selective activation is called clonal selection. Each antigen (usually a foreign protein or lipopolysaccharide) may carry several antigenic determinants, each activating a different clone, and an invading bacterium will carry a number of antigens. So a particular species of bacterium invading the body will activate a number of clones of lymphocytes.

The first encounter with any antigen causes the primary immune response to that antigen. There is a lag period of several days before clones of lymphocytes selected by the antigen can multiply and differentiate to become effector B and T cells. From B cells it takes several days for specific antibodies to appear in the blood. During the lag period, pathogenic organisms may gain entry to the body and multiply in sufficient numbers to cause symptoms of illness.

A second exposure to the same antigen (even years later) produces a much more rapid, stronger and longer lasting secondary response. This depends on memory cells, which are produced at the same time as effector cells during the primary response. Effector cells usually only last for a few days, but memory cells may last for decades. When there is a second exposure to an antigen, they rapidly multiply and differentiate to give large numbers of effector cells and large quantities of antibodies dedicated to attacking the antigen.

The ability of the immune system to distinguish self from non-self depends largely on a group of protein markers known as the major histocompatibility complex (MHC). These markers are present on the surface of every cell and are slightly different in each individual.

Cellular immune response

Many pathogens, including all viruses, are parasites that can only reproduce within host body cells. The cellular immune response fights pathogens that have already entered cells. Activated T lymphocytes include memory cells, and T-cytotoxic (killer) cells, which attack infected host cells or foreign cells. There are also helper and suppressor T cells, very important in mobilizing and regulating the whole immune response. When T-helper cells bind to specific antigenic determinants displayed with MHC proteins on the cell surface of macrophages, the macrophage is stimulated to release a cytokine called interleukin-1 (IL-1), which stimulates the T cells to grow and divide. The activated T cells release another cytokine, interleukin-2 (IL-2), which further stimulates proliferation and growth of T-helper and T-cytotoxic cells. IL-2 and other cytokines from T-helper cells also stimulate B cells to respond to specific antigens by differentiating to antibody forming plasma cells. T-cytotoxic cells recognize and attach to cells which have on their surface appropriate antigenic determinants coupled with MHC complex. T-cytotoxic cells then release perforin, a protein which causes break up of the cell membrane so that the infected host cell breaks up (lyses). The fragments are ingested and digested by phagocytes.

Humoral (fluid) immune response

B lymphocytes are also coated with receptors which are specific for particular antigenic determinants. Most antigens activate B cells only when the B cells are stimulated by cytokines from T-helper cells: they are T cell dependent antigens. Some antigens are T cell independent; they usually have a repetitive structure, and bind with several receptors on the B cell surface at once, a process called capping. The antigen is taken into the cell and activates it. Exposure to an antigen causes appropriate clones of B cells to proliferate and differentiate into memory cells and plasma cells. The latter are the effector cells of humoral immunity and are capable of secreting large amounts of antibody during their brief life of 4–5 days. The antibodies circulate in the blood and lymph, binding to antigen and contributing to the destruction of the organism bearing it. Antibodies are all proteins, belonging to a class of proteins called immunoglobulins (Ig). Each antibody molecule has the ability to (a) bind to a specific antigen and (b) assist with the antigen's destruction. Every antibody has separate regions for each of these two functions. The regions that bind the antigen differ from molecule to molecule and are called variable regions. Only a few humoral effector mechanisms exist to destroy antigens, so only a few kinds of regions are involved; these are called constant regions. An antibody molecule consists of two pairs of polypeptide chains – two short, identical light (L) chains, and two longer, identical heavy (H) chains. The chains are joined together to form a Y-shaped molecule. The variable regions of H and L chains are located at the ends of the arms of the Y, where they form the antigen binding sites. Thus on each antibody molecule there are two antigen binding sites, one at each tip of the antibody's two arms. The rest of the antibody molecule, consisting of the constant regions of the H and L chains, determines the antibody's effector function. There are five types of constant region and hence five major classes of antibody, called IgM, IgG, IgA, IgD and IgE. Their different roles in the immune response are described in Table 8.6. Remember that within each class there will be a multitude of subpopulations of antibodies, each specific for a particular antigen.

Antibodies do not have the power to destroy antigen-bearing invaders directly. Instead, they effectively tag foreign molecules and cells for destruction by various effector mechanisms. Each mechanism is triggered by the selective binding of antigens to antibodies to form antigen–antibody complexes. The antibodies may simply block the potential toxic actions of some antigens (a process called neutralization) or they may

Table 8.6.   Properties of the five classes of immunoglobulins

Class	Mean adult serum level ($g\ l^{-1}$)	Serum half-life (days)	Function
IgM	1.0	5	• Complement fixation • Early immune response • Stimulation of ingestion by macrophages
IgG	12.0	25	• Complement fixation • Placental transfer • Stimulation of ingestion by macrophages
IgA	1.8	6	• Localized protection in external secretions, e.g. saliva
IgD	0.03	3	• Function unknown
IgE	0.0003	2	• Stimulation of mast cells • Parasite expulsion

cause clumping together of antigens or foreign cells (agglutination) which can then be ingested by phagocytes. Precipitation is a similar mechanism, in which soluble antigen molecules are cross-linked to form inactive and immobile precipitates that are captured by phagocytes. Antibody–antigen complexes on the surfaces of invading micro-organisms usually cause complement activation. Once activated, complement proteins attack the membrane of the invader, or by coating the surface of foreign material make it attractive to phagocytes (a process known as opsonization).

This brief overview of the immune system has been given in order to facilitate the following discussion of the acute and chronic effects of exercise on immunity. In parts it has been greatly simplified and the complexity of the immune system and its precise co-ordinated responses should not be underestimated. For further details, the interested reader is recommended to consult the excellent textbooks of Roitt (1994) and Kuby (1997).

Exercise and the immune response

It would be easy to write a whole book on this subject alone, such is the large amount of literature available due to renewed interest in this area in recent years. However, this has been reviewed at length elsewhere (see, for example, Hoffman-Goetz, 1996; Mackinnon, 1992; Nieman, 1997; Pedersen and Bruunsgaard, 1995; Shephard *et al.*, 1991, 1994) and as such this discussion will only scrape the surface of what is one of the 'hot topics' in immunology at present.

Acute effects of exercise on immune function

Methodological problems

The reported response of various components of the immune system to exercise is transient and quite variable, depending upon the type of exercise, the immunological methodology used, the intensity of effort relative to the fitness of the individual and the timing of the observations (Shephard *et al.*, 1991). Effects disappear usually within 6 h post-exercise (Nieman, 1994b). Many findings are method-dependent; blood analyses are time-consuming and so some investigators collect few blood samples. Delaying taking samples by 30 min post-exercise may lead to quite different results and all blood measures will be affected by haemoconcentration. Responses may also be influenced by natural circadian variations in circulating lymphocyte numbers and plasma hormone (e.g. cortisol) concentrations (Figure 8.2), yet many studies do not include non-exercising time controls in their protocols. Overall and differential white blood cell counts can also be modified by changes in blood volume, margination and demargination of cells, modification of leukocyte/endothelial interactions, sympathetic and parasympathetic neural activity and cell redistribution with the release of granulocytes from bone marrow (Shephard *et*

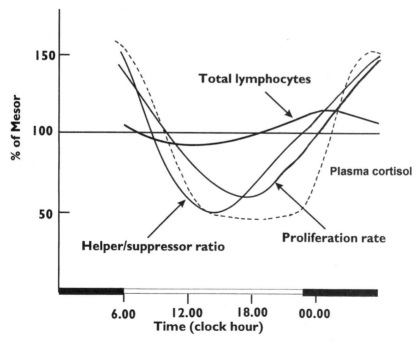

Figure 8.2. Circadian variations in the plasma cortisol concentration, total circulating lymphocyte count, ratio of T-helper to T-suppressor cells and *in vitro* lymphocyte proliferation response to mitogens. (Adapted from Cannon, 1993)

al., 1991). Thus, changes in populations of cells may be responsible for some apparent changes in leukocyte functions.

Numerous studies report effects of exercise on functions of isolated leukocytes when these cells are stimulated *in vitro* by added antigens or mitogens. However, it is difficult to extrapolate from the *ex vivo* stimulated response of isolated cells to predict how these same cells would respond in the far more complex *in vivo* environment. In addition to the presence of antigens, leukocyte function is also influenced by endogenous chemicals including hormones, neurotransmitters and cytokines, and the plasma concentration of these may change during exercise. The pH and temperature of the blood also change during exercise, but these factors are often ignored in experiments on isolated cell types. Thus, separating cells from their *in vivo* environment is somewhat artificial and to a large degree excludes the effects of exercise-induced chemical changes in the blood that will undoubtedly modify leukocyte function. The closest one can get to the *in vivo* condition is by performing measurements on whole blood, in which the proximity between the leukocytes and the extracellular milieu is retained.

Finally, only 0.2 per cent of the total leukocyte mass is circulating at any moment (Cannon, 1993); the remainder is in lymphoid tissue, the bone marrow and other tissues. It may thus be more important to assess the status of leukocytes in the skin, mucosa and lymph nodes rather than in the blood. Nevertheless, there is sufficient reliable data with which to establish the immunological response to acute exercise.

Increases in circulating numbers of leukocytes during exercise

Leukocytosis (an increase in the number of circulating leukocytes) is one of the most striking and consistent changes observed during exercise (Mackinnon, 1992). Acute exercise provokes an increase in peripheral leukocyte count, the magnitude of which is proportional to exercise intensity and duration, and inversely proportional to fitness level (Mackinnon, 1992; Shephard and Shek, 1994). The time it takes for the leukocyte count to return to normal after exercise is also dependent on the exercise intensity and duration. After very intense (> 100 per cent $\dot{V}O_{2max}$) brief (< 10 min) exercise the leukocyte count may continue to rise for up to 15 min into recovery (Gleeson *et al.*, 1995a). After less strenuous exercise of up to 1 h duration the blood leukocyte count immediately falls on cessation of exercise and usually takes 10–60 min to return to basal levels.

An acute bout of high-intensity exercise (> 70 per cent $\dot{V}O_{2max}$) of less than 1 h duration is associated with a biphasic perturbation of the circulating leukocyte count (McCarthy and Dale, 1988; Nieman, 1994b). Immediately post-exercise, total leukocytes are increased by around 50–100 per cent compared with rest, represented evenly by lymphocytes and neutrophils, accompanied by a smaller increase in monocytes. Within 1 h of recovery, lymphocytopenia occurs (Figure 8.3) with a greater decrease

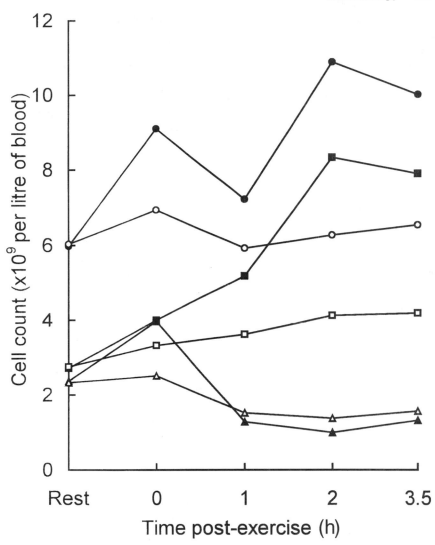

Figure 8.3. Changes in the circulating counts of total leukocytes (circles), neutrophils (squares) and lymphocytes (triangles) after 45 minutes of exercise and high intensity (closed symbols) or moderate intensity (open symbols). Note the larger rise in neutrophils and greater fall in lymphocytes following the higher intensity exercise. (adapted from Nieman *et al.*, 1994)

in lymphocyte number after high- as opposed to moderate-intensity exercise of the same duration (Nieman *et al.*, 1994). Levels remain low for 3–6 h (Nieman, 1994b). Eosinophil count is decreased (Nieman *et al.*, 1994; Shinkai *et al.*, 1993) but basophils remain fairly constant (Nieman *et al.*, 1994). The sustained leukocytosis at this time is due to a pronounced neutrophilia (Gleeson, 1994; Nieman *et al.*, 1994; Pedersen and Bruunsgaard, 1995) which appears to be due to release of neutrophils from the bone marrow as a result of the delayed effects of the steroid hormone cortisol. The actions of this hormone are also responsible for the fall in the lymphocyte count during very prolonged exercise and during recovery.

At least for exercise lasting less than 1 h, most of these extra leukocytes do not enter the circulation from the bone marrow, but rather are released from the marginated pool of leukocytes that are normally adhered to the vascular endothelium at rest. The sizes of the marginated and circulating pools of leukocytes are approximately equal at rest, so complete demargination could potentially double the circulating leukocyte count. The mechanism of demargination during exercise probably involves both the mechanical effects of increased blood flow rate, physically moving cells into the circulating stream, and the effects of adrenaline which decreases the adherence of leukocytes to the endothelium via interaction with β receptors on both cell types (Figure 8.4). There is also an influx of lymphocytes from lymphatic vessels and release of some leukocytes from temporary storage sites in the liver and spleen sinusoids. Another possible source is from recruitment of previously unperfused capillaries in muscle and the lungs. The movement of leukocytes away from the walls of the lung capillaries could contribute to the increased incidence of respiratory infections in athletes. Remember that during physical activity, exposure of the lung tissue to airborne pathogens is increased due to the increased rate and depth of breathing during exercise. Hence, a rise in the circulating leukocyte count cannot simply be interpreted as an improvement in immune defence. Indeed, the first response to injury or infection involves inflammation of the damaged tissue and movement of leukocytes from the blood through capillary walls into the tissue. The first leukocytes to enter the infected tissue will be the ones that are already adhered to the local vascular endothelium. Demargination of leukocytes due to exercise could only be expected to delay this process, perhaps allowing invading organisms time to establish a colony of proliferating cells!

Acute exercise and phagocytic cell function

There is some convincing evidence that macrophages and neutrophils become activated during exercise and several authors have reported increased levels of granular enzymes (e.g. elastase and myeloperoxidase) indicative of neutrophil degranulation (Dufaux and Order, 1989; Blannin *et al.*, 1996b). Phagocytic activity is also generally reported to be higher

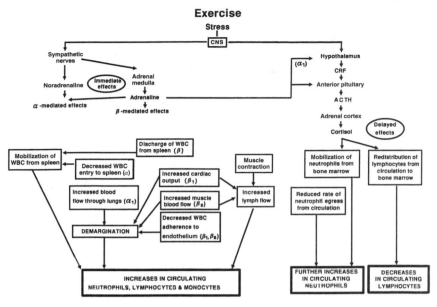

Figure 8.4. Mechanisms contributing to the immediate and delayed leukocytosis of exercise. The catecholamines are largely responsible for the increase in the circulating leukocyte count during the early stages of exercise. Cortisol appears to be involved in the secondary rise in neutrophils that occurs in the later stages of prolonged exercise or during recovery from short-term high intensity exercise

immediately after bouts of moderate-intensity exercise, and these effects are thought to be mediated by increased concentrations of growth hormone and/or activated complement fragments during exercise. However, for several hours after exercise the ability of neutrophils to respond to bacterial stimulation seems attenuated. This may be a manifestation of a reduced responsiveness following neutrophil activation or may represent an altered neutrophil population, with less mature cells having entered the circulation from the bone marrow (Pyne, 1994). Such effects may be compensated for by the increased circulating numbers of neutrophils which can last for several hours after exercise has stopped (Figure 8.3).

Acute exercise and lymphocyte subsets

Of the three major lymphocyte subpopulations (T, B and NK cells), NK cells are by far the most responsive to exercise (Nieman, 1994b). The extent of such changes depends on the intensity of effort; high-intensity activity leads to the rapid recruitment of large numbers of NK cells from the peripheral lymphoid tissue to the circulation (Shephard *et al.*, 1994). Nieman *et al.* (1993) demonstrated a 50 per cent increase in NK cell number after 45 min of treadmill exercise at 80 per cent $\dot{V}O_{2max}$ compared with a 36 per cent decrease at 50 per cent $\dot{V}O_{2max}$. The NK cell cytotoxic activity (NKCA) of blood is a measure of the 'killing' capacity of NK cells and increased 40 per cent immediately post-exercise, probably due to NK cell recruitment. In the 2 h post-exercise, the blood NKCA decreased by 33 per cent (Figure 8.5). These results are consistent with other findings (Shephard *et al.*, 1994). The NKCA expressed per NK cell increased significantly (by 61 per cent) after high-intensity exercise. However, this included NK cells expressing both CD16+ (NK cell specific) and CD56+ (common to NK and T-cytotoxic cells) antigens. T-cytotoxic cells increase following maximal exercise (Shephard and Shek, 1994) and thus may account for this result.

Exercise-induced changes in interleukin and interferon concentration may alter the surface properties of NK cells, and thus their lytic properties

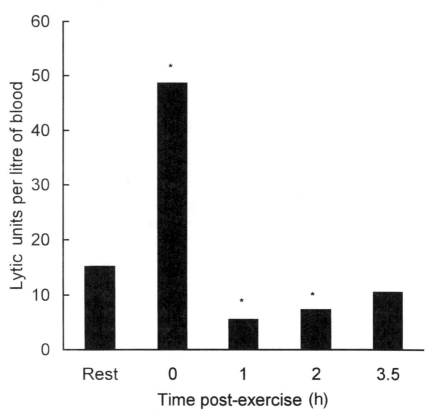

Figure 8.5. Natural killer cell cytotoxic activity (NKCA) of the blood compartment: response to high intensity exercise. The asterisks indicate significant differences from the resting state. Note the rise in NKCA immediately post-exercise and the sustained fall in NKCA during the recovery period. (From Nieman *et al.*, 1993)

(Shephard and Shek, 1994). Exhaustive exercise produces less favourable results. Shinkai *et al.* (1993) demonstrated a temporary decrease in CD16+ cells (which exert NK activity) after a triathlon, supporting the previous findings of Shek *et al.* (1992), who found a decrease in both NK cell number and activity after a single 90–120 min bout of exercise at 65 per cent $\dot{V}O_{2max}$ which persisted for over 1 week.

Exercise is associated with a transient redistribution of lymphocytes and alterations in the CD4+:CD8+ or T-H:T-S/C ratio (T-helper:T-suppressor/cytotoxic cell ratio) (Frisna *et al.*, 1994). This ratio has a critical influence upon susceptibility to infection and values below 1.5 are believed to be associated with impaired immunity (Shephard and Shek, 1994). In the acquired immune deficiency syndrome (AIDS), T-helper cells are attacked by the human immunodeficiency virus, rendering the sufferer extremely susceptible to a wide range of opportunistic infections. After exercise, Berk *et al.* (1986) found no significant difference in total T cell number but found the T-H:T-S/C ratio decreased from 1.94 to 1.36, due to a 30 per cent decrease in T-helper cell numbers.

In late recovery and continuing for the 24 h after exercise the T-H:T-S/C ratio is elevated mainly because of a reduction in T-suppressor cells (Shephard and Shek, 1994). Exercise also seems to increase the numbers of T-cytotoxic cells (Shephard and Shek, 1994). In general there is a small decrease in B cell proportion after 30 min of vigorous treadmill exercise (Shephard and Shek, 1994). Tvede *et al.* (1989) found that the B cell suppression induced by 1 h of high-intensity cycling lasted for at least 2 h post-exercise because of an inhibitory effect of prostaglandins secreted from activated monocytes.

Acute maximal exercise can lead to an apparent reduction in the mitogen-stimulated lymphocyte proliferative response (e.g. Nieman *et al.*, 1994; Fry *et al.*, 1992b; Lewicki *et al.*, 1987), but Fry *et al.* (1992b) commented that this decrease may be the result of an increase in the proportion of NK cells rather than a down-regulation of B cell function.

Acute exercise and soluble factors

A 24.4 per cent decrease in salivary IgA level concentration was reported to occur immediately following exhaustive treadmill exercise, which remained depressed (16.9 per cent) 1 h later (McDowell *et al.*, 1992). Schouten *et al.* (1988), however, found the opposite to be true in young, healthy habitual exercisers and others (e.g. Blannin *et al.*, 1998) have not observed any change in salivary IgA after repeated bouts of high-intensity exercise. Since increased sympathetic drive during exercise increases total protein secretory rates into saliva independent of salivary flow rate, Cannon (1996) has argued that there is no simple way to interpret changes in the concentration of a single salivary protein.

Acute maximal and submaximal exercise is further associated with a transient increase in serum Ig levels (Nieman and Nehlsen-Cannarella,

1991), but this is likely to be due to a decrease in plasma volume (i.e. haemoconcentration) (Nieman and Nehlsen-Cannarella, 1991) and/or increased lymph flow (Nieman, 1994b).

Of the cytokines it appears that only IL-2 is adversely affected by exercise. Its production and levels are decreased both during and 24 h after acute exercise (Mackinnon, 1992). IL-1, IL-6 and TNF-α all appear to be elevated after prolonged running (Sprenger et al., 1992). Pedersen and Bruunsgaard (1995) hypothesized that high-intensity eccentric exercise causes a more pronounced increase in the muscle and plasma levels of cytokines involved in acute inflammatory responses (IL-1, TNF-α and IL-6). These are possibly derived from macrophages, endothelial cells and fibroblasts in the muscle and may play an important role in the recruitment and activation of NK cells. Short-term exercise results in the activation of the complement proteins C3 and C4 (Smith et al., 1990), probably to aid repair of damaged tissues.

Chronic exercise and the immune response

Chronic adaptations to exercise have been generally measured via cross-sectional comparisons of the immune systems of athletes and non-athletes (e.g. Lewicki et al., 1987; Nieman and Nehlsen-Cannarella, 1991; Blannin et al., 1996a). Several studies (reviewed by Mackinnon, 1992) suggest that well trained athletes exhibit lower resting leukocyte numbers, but this has been disputed by Lewicki et al. (1987), amongst others, who found similar leukocyte counts in trained and untrained men. Any differences may be dependent on the training load, duration of training and the selection of appropriate controls. Blannin et al. (1996a) found significantly lower total leukocyte, neutrophil and lymphocyte counts in cyclists who had been training regularly for over 10 years compared with age- and weight-matched sedentary controls. The expansion of the plasma volume in response to endurance training is probably at least partly responsible for the lower circulating leukocyte counts in such athletes.

The decrease in bactericidal neutrophil activity after acute exercise (Hack et al., 1992), the reduction in lymphocyte proliferation responsiveness following prolonged acute exercise (MacNeil et al., 1991), and resting serum Ig levels (Nieman and Nehlsen-Cannarella, 1991), have all been shown to be similar in trained persons and sedentary controls. In contrast, it appears that serum complement (Smith et al., 1990) and salivary IgA levels (Thorp and Barnes, 1990) are lower in athletes than non-athletes. During periods of high-intensity training, neutrophil function has been reported to be lower in athletes compared with less active controls (Hack et al., 1994; Pyne, 1994; Blannin et al., 1996a). Some athletes also exhibit abnormally low neutrophil counts. Since acute bouts of prolonged or high-intensity exercise are associated with a marked release of neutrophils from the bone marrow, it may be that repeated bouts of exercise could deplete the bone marrow of its store of ready-to-release neutrophils. The normal marrow contains a 3-day reserve of neutrophils available for rapid release as needed. This store may be severely depleted in athletes engaged in regular heavy exercise; the normal time period for production of new granulocytes from stem cells is 5–10 days. Even this might be prolonged if the athlete's diet is deficient in protein or certain vitamins. A reduced resting neutrophil count and/or impaired function would make the individual particularly susceptible to bacterial infections (Pyne, 1994).

Exhaustively (or over-) trained athletes demonstrate a whole range of immune dysfunctions (e.g. depressed lymphocyte, macrophage and neutrophil functions) which have been discussed at length elsewhere (e.g. Rowbottom et al., 1995, 1996). Such effects have been variously attributed to chronic elevation of glucocorticoid hormones, micronutrient deficiencies and abnormally low plasma levels of glutamine.

The relationship between exercise and susceptibility to infection has been modelled in the form of a 'J' curve (Nieman, 1994b). This model suggests that, while engaging in moderate activity may enhance immune function above sedentary levels, excessive amounts of prolonged high-intensity exercise induce detrimental effects on immune function. However, although the literature provides evidence in support of the

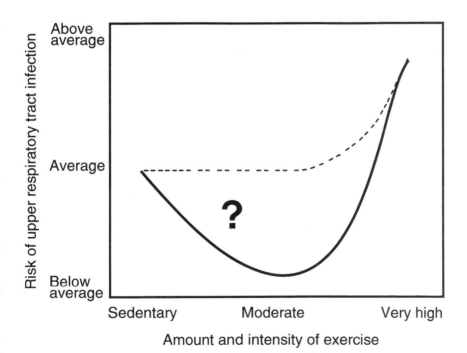

Figure 8.6. Model of the relationship between varying amounts of exercise and the incidence of upper respiratory tract infection. The dashed line indicates the present authors' interpretation of the literature. (Adapted from Nieman, 1994b)

latter point, little evidence is available to suggest any difference in immune function between sedentary and moderately active persons. Thus, it may be more realistic to 'flatten' out the portion of the curve representing this part of the relationship

According to Pedersen and Bruunsgard (1995), the immune system is only suppressed following exercise of one hour's duration or more. While this is somewhat of an oversimplification, because exercise intensity is not taken into account, it follows that prolonged, frequent, high-intensity bouts of activity potentiate the immunosuppressive effect. It is not training *per se* that is the great risk; rather, it is the increased training regimen that many athletes adopt in order to push themselves to what they believe is their best, which compromises immune function.

Environmental and psychological factors

Environmental and psychological as well as physiological factors can compound the negative influence that heavy exertion has on the immune system. Associated competitive and environmental stressors modify the immune response, (Shephard and Shek, 1994) and appear to augment the suppressive endocrine response to prolonged exercise. Indeed plasma levels of the stress hormones are influenced by psychological and environmental stressors (Khansari *et al.*, 1990; Cannon, 1993). Such factors can thus be considered as potential causes of immunosuppression in athletes.

Facilitated pathogen transmission

The very involvement in a sporting activity may predispose the individual to infection, although not always because of suppressed immune function. According to Cannon (1993), abrasive interpersonal exchanges in contact sports, crowded locker rooms and shared drinking containers all enhance transmission of infectious micro-organisms. Hanley (1976) found that retention of water in the ear canal leading to swimmer's ear (external otitis) was prevalent in both water polo and swimming teams of that year's USA Olympic squad. Furthermore, the commonest cause of diarrhoea was overeating and the consumption of unusual amounts of fruit, and not gastrointestinal infection.

Cannon (1993) commented that facilitated transmission could readily account for many infectious episodes and has questioned whether it is really necessary to infer some underlying exercise-induced immunosuppression as a cause of these events. The findings of Linde (1987) certainly could be interpreted either as the result of facilitated pathogen transmission or exercise-induced immunosuppression. The incidence of upper respiratory tract infection (URTI) was compared over a year in trained orienteers, a sport in which individuals run alone, outdoors, and non-athletic controls and shown to be 50 per cent higher in the former. It could be that athletes do not have suitable rest periods after an infectious episode, reducing the ability of the body to fight disease and increasing the risk of complicating infections. Athletes training for outdoor sports, such as orienteering, in areas such as Scandinavia are exposed to cold and wet weather which is considered to predispose them to URTI (Linde, 1987). Cold temperature may affect respiratory mucous and cilia function as well as IgA secretion in the mucosal fluids. Housh *et al.* (1991) demonstrated that salivary IgA secretion was unaffected by 30 min of treadmill running at ambient temperatures of 6, 19 and 34°C, but these were not as low as those temperatures experienced by Linde's (1987) orienteers during the Scandinavian winter, and levels of IgA secretion in the mucosal fluids of the respiratory tract were not measured. Furthermore, the exercise bout used by Housh *et al.* (1991) was not of sufficient duration for any significant immunosuppressive response as, according to Pedersen and Bruunsgaard (1995), immunosuppressive effects are only evident following exercise of 1 h duration or more. A seasonal distribution of URTI was evident in Linde's (1987) controls; low in summer, high in winter. It was much more evenly spread in the orienteers, possibly indicating a suppressed innate immune system.

However, Linde (1987) suggested that as the majority of training camps are in the summer, the communal living conditions would have been optimal for pathogen transmission. Conversely, it could be argued that the increased training load experienced by the orienteers at these camps led to suppressed immune function. Linde (1987) did not measure any immune function variables; hence, the actual cause of the increased episodes of URTI could not be established. It is likely that all of the conditions contributed in some way.

Psychological stress

Psychological stress is thought to influence immune function through autonomic nerves innervating lymphoid tissue and by hormone-mediated alteration of immune cell functions (Cohen *et al.*, 1991). Chronic psychological stress also appears to lower salivary IgA levels, evidenced by a transient decrease in the levels of salivary IgA in students under academic examination stress (Jemmott *et al.*, 1983). Psychological stress may also modify immune responses through the adoption of coping behaviours, e.g. increased alcohol consumption, or smoking (Cohen *et al.*, 1991). The literature concerning the relationship between psychological stress and immunosuppression is inconsistent, largely due to the numerous variables that need to be controlled. However, Cohen *et al.* (1991) carried out a well controlled study (including controls for education, shared housing and personality differences) in which subjects were intentionally exposed to one of five respiratory viruses via nasal drops. The results indicated that psychological stress is associated with an increased risk of infection independent of the possibility of transmission, the strain of administered virus, and of an exercise index that included frequency of running, walking, jogging, swimming, aerobic exercise and housework.

Environmental pollutants

The poor air quality of inner cities may have important implications for immunocompetence in city marathon runners. Few studies have concentrated on this area yet many of the epidemiological studies concerning URTI incidence following acute bouts of prolonged strenuous exercise have focused on athletes competing in such events (e.g. Nieman, 1990). Furthermore, the increased lung ventilation rate associated with exercise facilitates an increased exposure of the exercising individual to airborne pollutants and pathogens. Animal and human studies have shown that NO_2 has minimal effects on immune function, but high levels of SO_2 may adversely affect leukocyte numbers in the bronchial lavage fluid of humans (Cannon, 1993). A combined inhalation of high levels of ozone (O_3) and *Streptococcus pyogenes* led to a two-fold increase in mortality in exercising mice compared with their non-exercising counterparts (Illing *et al.*, 1980). However, it must be taken into consideration that demargination of leukocytes from the pulmonary capillary bed during exercise may effectively remove the first line of defence against airborne pathogens, rendering the athlete more susceptible to infection.

The personal and surrounding environment of the athlete appear to be 'external causes' (as opposed to any biochemical/hormonal/nutritional ones) of immunosuppression in athletes. However, the role of facilitated pathogen transmission must not be overlooked. The psychological stress associated with personal achievement, parental or peer pressure, and the financial consequences of success, coupled with the physiological stress of exercise itself, presents a very real risk to the proper functioning of the athlete's immune system.

Temperature

Rises in body temperature during strenuous exercise or during prolonged exercise in a hot environment may have an effect on immune function. Increasing the body temperature of humans to 39.5°C by immersion in a hot water-bath caused immune alterations that resembled the changes in response to exercise, but without much change in plasma catecholamine concentrations (Kappel *et al.*, 1991). As mentioned previously, exercising in the cold may impair immune defence of the upper respiratory tract via a reduction in salivary IgA secretion, mucosal secretions and ciliary function caused by the inhalation of cold air (Mackinnon, 1992).

Hormonal influences

In response to exercise above an intensity of about 60 per cent of $\dot{V}O_{2max}$, the blood concentrations of a number of stress hormones, including the catecholamines, cortisol, growth hormone and β-endorphin, increase (Hoffman-Goetz and Pedersen, 1994). These hormones are capable of modifying leukocyte numbers and functions (Cupps and Fauci, 1982; Khansari *et al.*, 1990) and a brief description of their specific effects follows.

Catecholamines

In response to exercise, discharge from the sympathetic splanchic nerves innervating the adrenal medulla results in the release of adrenaline and noradrenaline into the plasma. The main source of noradrenaline in the plasma, however, is from leakage from sympathetic nerve endings.

Sympathetic nerve endings which densely innervate the lymphoid tissues have β_2-adrenergic receptors (Murray *et al.*, 1992). Acute *in vivo* exposure to catecholamines via exercise-induced release and by catecholamine infusion elevates β_2-adrenergic receptor density in circulating lymphocytes, which appears to be mediated by the β-adrenergic agonist, adrenaline, rather than the α_1-, β_1-selective agent, noradrenaline (Maisel *et al.*, 1990; Van Tits *et al.*, 1990). This increase is due to a redistribution of circulating cell subsets that differ in their β_2-adrenergic receptor number (Maisel *et al.*, 1990). Adrenaline decreases cell adhesion to vascular endothelium, thus increasing the demargination of cells. Freshly released splenic lymphocytes appear to carry more β_2-adrenergic receptors than those found in the circulation (Van Tits *et al.*, 1990).

Lymphocyte proliferation is dependent on IL-2 receptor expression. Exercise-induced impairment of these two immune responses may be directly related to large increases in circulating adrenaline (Murray *et al.*, 1992). Indeed β-agonists *in vivo* demonstrate an inhibition of *de novo* expression of IL-2 receptors, down-regulation of previously expressed IL-2 receptor subpopulations on mature T cells and impairment of IL-2 production (Murray *et al.*, 1992). Furthermore, the ability of exogenously administered isoproterenol (a β-adrenergic agonist) to decrease lymphocyte mitogen responsiveness *in vitro* has been documented (Van Tits *et al.*, 1990). Increases in receptor sensitivity via exercise-induced increases in β_2-receptor density render lymphocytes more susceptible to the inhibiting effects of catecholamines on proliferative responses.

The widely observed reduction in T-H:T-S/C ratio may also be catecholamine mediated. Van Tits *et al.* (1990) demonstrated 41 per cent and 107 per cent increases in plasma levels of T-helper and T-suppressor/ cytotoxic subsets, respectively. A subsequent decrease in the T-H:T-S/C ratio from 1.7 to 0.5 after isoproterenol infusion mimicked exercise-induced changes. Tonesson *et al.* (1987) demonstrated adrenaline-mediated leukocytosis, lymphocytosis and neutrophilia following 1 h of continuous intravenous adrenaline infusion.

NK cells have the greatest density of β_2-receptors among the various subsets (Murray *et al.*, 1992). Maisel *et al.* (1990) observed a 35 per cent increase in receptor density following dynamic exercise. Intravenous infusion of adrenaline resulted in circulating numbers of NK cells identical to those obtained following 1 h of cycling at 75 per cent $\dot{V}O_{2max}$ (Kappel *et al.*, 1991). The NK cell concentration 2 h after adrenaline infusion also mimicked that seen after exercise. Furthermore, NKCA was similar under both conditions and the authors concluded that increased plasma adrenaline concentration during physical stress causes a redistribution in mononuclear cell subpopulations that results in altered function of NK cells.

Glucocorticoids

Exercise is a potent stimulus for adrenocorticotrophic hormone (ACTH) secretion, which in turn stimulates adrenal production of the steroid hormone, cortisol (Galbo, 1983). ACTH has been found to regulate the functions of most of the major types of leukocytes (Blalock, 1989). It augments B cell proliferation, yet suppresses the synthesis of both Ig and IFN-γ and mediates macrophage activation. This latter action may be as part of a feedback mechanism: exercise elevates IL-1 production from activated macrophages. This cytokine stimulates the release of cortisol releasing factor (CRF) from the hypothalamus which in turn stimulates ACTH secretion from the anterior pituitary. As a result, cortisol is released from the adrenal cortex. The inhibitory effect of cortisol on macrophage activity subsequently decreases the production of IL-1, thus restoring IL-1 levels to those prior to exercise.

A critical exercise intensity of 60 per cent $\dot{V}O_{2max}$ stimulates cortisol release during short-term exercise and the plasma cortisol concentration is highest following near maximal intensity exercise. Levels may remain elevated for over 2 h (Nieman, 1994b). During more prolonged exercise, the plasma cortisol concentration rises progressively and observations from our laboratory indicate that it may attain higher levels after 3 h at 55 per cent $\dot{V}O_{2max}$ compared with fatiguing exercise at 80 per cent $\dot{V}O_{2max}$ lasting about 40 min.

The secondary (delayed) leukocytosis which occurs following brief high-intensity exercise is predominantly due to a cortisol-stimulated release of leukocytes (mainly neutrophils) from the bone marrow. As exercise continues, cortisol stimulation of the bone marrow induces a strong and sustained neutrophilia (Nieman, 1994b). Moreover, cortisol inhibits the entry of lymphocytes into the circulation and facilitates their egress from the blood into other lymphoid tissues (Shephard and Shek, 1994). Whereas adrenaline causes rapid yet transient lymphocytosis, longer-lasting cortisol dominates events during recovery, causing a marked and prolonged lymphocytopenia and neutrophilia (Nieman, 1994b) and elevating the T-H:T-S/C ratio via a cortisol-induced reduction in the number of T-S/C cells (Shephard and Shek, 1994). This may be to compensate for the suppression of NKCA and neutrophil bactericidal activity at this time, which correlate negatively with serum cortisol levels. Adrenaline and cortisol exert opposite effects on NKCA (Kappel *et al.*, 1991); the immediate increase in NKCA post-exercise is adrenaline-mediated, whereas the post-exercise suppression is cortisol-mediated. NKCA has been shown to be depressed 24–48 h after administration of long-acting glucocorticoids (Gatti *et al.*, 1987; Tonnesen *et al.*, 1987). That is not to say that cortisol is the sole mediator of NKCA suppression; the action of prostaglandins released from macrophages and neutrophils has also been implicated (Pedersen *et al.*, 1988, 1990; Kappel *et al.*, 1991).

Growth hormone

The plasma concentration of growth hormone (GH) increases (with a delay which is short-lasting and inversely related to intensity) in proportion to the work rate and is initiated at intensities as low as 30–40 per cent $\dot{V}O_{2max}$. The response may be diminished at higher intensities or at exhaustion (Howlett, 1987). Kappel *et al.* (1993) observed that infusion of GH in physiological concentrations characteristic of exercise had no effect on mononuclear cell subsets, NKCA, cytokine production or lymphocyte function but did induce a significant increase in neutrophil concentration. GH is also an activator of neutrophil phagocytosis and may influence the proliferation of T lymphocytes and their differentiation into effector cells (Blalock, 1989).

β-Endorphin

The release of the endogenous peptide β-endorphin from the anterior pituitary is enhanced at high exercise intensities (80 per cent $\dot{V}O_{2max}$). Furthermore, the increase in levels occurs rapidly (30–60 s) and lasts for up to 2 h. β-Endorphin binds to monocytes, lymphocytes and granulocytes and, *in vitro*, appears to have variable effects on NK cells (Hoffman-Goetz and Pedersen, 1994). The *in vivo* administration of the opioid antagonist naloxone in young women inhibited the characteristic post-exercise rise in NKCA following a maximal cycle ergometer test, although the percentage of lymphocytes bearing the NK cell surface marker CD16+ did not change (Fiatarone *et al.*, 1988). These authors suggested a major role for the opioid system in NK cell modulation during physiological stress. β-Endorphin is also thought to stimulate chemotaxis and phagocytosis in macrophages.

Prostaglandins

The suppression of NKCA that is evident 1–2 h after prolonged exercise has been previously ascribed to numerical shifts in NK cells as, when adjusted per-NK cell, a 61 per cent increase is evident (Nieman *et al.*, 1993). However, the number of NK cells included cells expressing both the CD16+ (NK cell specific) and CD56+ marker (common to NK and T-cytotoxic cells). T-cytotoxic cells increase following maximal exercise (Shephard and Shek, 1994), and thus may account for this result. A number of previous reports implicate the role of prostaglandins (PGs) released from monocytes and neutrophils (Pedersen *et al.*, 1988, 1990; Kappel *et al.*, 1991) in down-regulating NKCA. Prostaglandins, though technically not hormones, are often considered to be (Willmore and Costill, 1994). Several PGs (PGE$_1$, PGE$_2$, PGA and PGA$_2$) are known NKCA inhibitors (Mackinnon, 1992) and PGE$_2$ production by monocytes significantly increases after acute exercise (Pedersen *et al.*, 1990). The pattern of NKCA following 60 min of cycle exercise at 80 per cent $\dot{V}O_{2max}$ and the corresponding findings that (a) the proportion of CD16+ cells was normal when NKCA was suppressed, (b) indomethacin, an inhibitor of PG synthesis, fully restored NKCA *in vitro* and (c) there was a two-fold increase in monocyte (CD20+) proportions 2 h after exercise, strongly indicated an inhibitory role of monocyte-derived PG after heavy exertion (Pedersen *et al.*, 1988).

Prostaglandins have been implicated as suppressors of T cell proliferation (Gordon *et al.*, 1979; Kunkel, 1986). The exogenous addition of interleukin-2 (IL-2) to macrophage cultures caused an increase in PGE$_2$ levels, whereas the addition of prostacyclin (PGI$_2$) or PGE$_2$ resulted in a dose-dependent suppression of macrophage IL-2 production (Kunkel *et al.*, 1986). Prostaglandins thus act as self-induced inhibitors of IL-2 production, which results in inhibition of the lymphocyte proliferative response. As such the decreased IL-2 production post-exercise could be attributable to the inhibitory effects of the increased levels of PG. It has been hypothesized that the administration of indomethacin by athletes would counter such prostaglandin-influenced immunosuppression (Shephard and Shek, 1994).

Exercise induces a cascade of co-ordinated hormonal responses that influence the behaviour of immune cells (Hoffman-Goetz and Pedersen, 1994). The exercise-induced increases in the plasma levels of adrenaline, cortisol, β-endorphin and prostaglandins impart immunosuppressive effects on the immune system, which could account for much of the depressed immune functions observed in athletes. Many other hormones, such as prolactin and dihydroxyadrostenedione-sulphate (DHEA-S) (Blalock, 1989) also appear to be immunomodulatory, but as yet no work has elucidated any connection between these and exercise-induced immunosuppression.

Nutritional factors

Dietary habits

The diet of the athlete appears to be a further potential cause of immuno-suppression, yet few papers have concentrated on this theme. Many athletes try to control their body weight by restriction of dietary energy intake in order to gain a competitive edge. Alarmingly, it has been demonstrated that a loss of just 2 kg over a 2 week period adversely affects the defence mechanisms of even healthy athletes (Kono et al., 1988). Macrophage phagocytic function decreased after reduction of the dietary energy intake, suggesting that human immune function is influenced by changes in both physical activity and nutritional status. Although in this study the lymphocyte proliferative response remained unchanged, this may have been due to the minor degree of malnutrition employed. According to Kono et al. (1988), further dietary energy restriction may 'affect other cellular functions, leading to extensive dysfunction of the immune system'.

The daily protein requirement is approximately doubled in athletes compared with the sedentary population. An intake of less than 1.6 g of protein per kg body mass per day is likely to be associated with a negative nitrogen balance in athletes who are training hard, particularly endurance athletes (Lemon, 1992). Protein deficiency has been long associated with impaired immune function (Roitt, 1994). In the quest to restore muscle and liver glycogen, athletes have been encouraged to consume large amounts of carbohydrate ($8–10$ g kg^{-1} body mass day^{-1} is currently recommended: Hawley, 1995). If this is done to the neglect of protein intake then this could have dire consequences for immune function. A recent study indicated that supplementing overtained athletes' diets with an additional $20–30$ g protein day^{-1} for a period of 3 weeks, restored depressed plasma glutamine levels to normal and enabled a return to increased training in 60 per cent of athletes given the supplement (Kingsbury et al., 1998). Unfortunately, the authors did not measure any associated changes in immune function during this period.

Polyunsaturated fatty acids (PUFA) inhibit the lymphocyte proliferative response in vitro probably via inhibition of IL-2 secretion (Calder and Newsholme, 1992), indicating that T cell activation and the immune response may be modulated by dietary PUFA intake. No athletic study has been done as yet and the relevance of this to the dietary habits of top class athletes is questionable; nevertheless IL-2 production is suppressed by exercise and a high PUFA diet could potentiate this.

Trace elements

Cross-sectional studies of athletes and non-athletes indicate that long-term physical training may lead to a chonic depression of plasma iron and zinc (Cannon and Kluger, 1983). Zinc deficiency results in decreased macrophage ingestion and phagocytosis, whereas iron is needed by NK cells, neutrophils and lymphocytes for optimal function (Chandra, 1990). Depression of plasma levels of these trace elements appears to be via the action of endogenous cytokines released from monocytes and macrophages and the subsequent release of iron and zinc chelating proteins from activated neutrophils. These cytokines include IL-1α, IL-1β and TNF-α (Cannon *et al.*, 1989), all of which are elevated following exercise (Mackinnon, 1992). Elevated concentrations of IL-1β have been found in muscle tissue 5 days after prolonged eccentric muscular exercise (Cannon *et al.*, 1989). Dietary supplements of iron and zinc could hypothetically ensure that sufficient levels are maintained to reduce the risk of compromised immune function.

Vitamins

The oxygen free-radical formation that accompanies the dramatic increase in oxidative metabolism during exercise could potentially inhibit immune responses (Cannon, 1993). Reactive oxygen species (ROS) have also been implicated in exercise-induced muscle damage (Duthie *et al.*, 1996). An up to 10-fold increase in oxygen utilization occurs during prolonged exhaustive exercise (Robertson *et al.*, 1991), enhancing superoxide radical (O_2^-) leakage from the mitochondria into the cytosol (Duthie *et al.*, 1996). These ROS may inhibit leukocyte chemotaxis (Peters *et al.*, 1993). Sustained endurance training appears to be associated with an adaptive up-regulation of the antioxidant defence system which nevertheless can be further improved by the dietary intake of antioxidant vitamins and trace element cofactors of antioxidant enzymes (Robertson *et al.*, 1991) such as selenium (a cofactor of glutathione peroxide) and manganese (a cofactor of superoxide dismutase) (Mertz, 1981). However, such adaptations may be insufficient to protect individuals who train extensively and such individuals should consider increasing their intakes of nutritional antioxidants such as vitamins C and E (Duthie *et al.*, 1996).

Vitamin C

Findings of Peters *et al.* (1993) support the suggestion of Duthie *et al.* (1996). Using a double-blind placebo research design, it was determined that a daily supplementation of 600 mg of vitamin C reduced the incidence of symptoms of URTI (68 per cent compared with 33 per cent in age- and sex-matched control runners) after participation in a 90 km ultramarathon. The authors suggested that because heavy exertion enhances the production of ROS, vitamin C, with its antioxidant properties, is required in greater quantities. Gleeson *et al.* (1987) demonstrated an increase in lymphocyte ascorbic acid (vitamin C) concentration directly after a 21 km race, probably due to uptake from the plasma. The plasma ascorbic acid concentration dipped 20 per cent below pre-exercise levels 24 h after the race, and remained low for the next 2 days. Increased vitamin C is present in sweat and urine following prolonged exercise and there may be an increased turnover of this vitamin during exercise (Peters *et al.*, 1993). The findings outlined above indicate that the vitamin C requirements of athletes are increased by prolonged, heavy exertion, rendering athletes more susceptible to vitamin C deficiency and the subsequent detrimental effects on immune function.

Vitamin E

Animal studies have shown an increased oxidation of vitamin E during exercise and a resulting possible reduction in antioxidant protection (Quintanilha and Packer, 1983). Cannon *et al.* (1991) highlighted a further role of vitamin E in minimizing the immunosuppressive effects suffered by athletes. Dietary vitamin E stimulates mononuclear cell production of IL-1β via its influence on the arachidonic acid metabolic pathways (Cannon *et al.*, 1991). Cytokine production is further facilitated by a vitamin E-influenced inhibition of PGE_2 production, as shown by Meydani *et al.* (1990). Severe vitamin E deficiency results in impaired cell-mediated immunity and decreased antibody synthesis (Chandra, 1990).

Other vitamins

Chandra (1990) highlights two other vitamins essential for immunocompetence: vitamins A and B_6. Decreases in the lymphocyte proliferative response to mitogens and antigen-specific antibody production result from vitamin A deficiency and, although isolated vitamin B_6 deficiency is rare in humans, the profound effects on immune function seen in animals include impaired cell-mediated immunity and reduced T lymphocyte cytotoxicity. Vitamin B_{12} and folic acid are essential for the normal production of red and white blood cells in the bone marrow.

It has been shown that the poor nutritional status of some athletes may predispose them to immunosuppression. A well-balanced diet and appropriate supplementation of minerals and vitamins appear to reduce this risk. Nevertheless, the dangers of oversupplementation should be highlighted; many micronutrients given in quantities beyond a certain threshold will in fact reduce immune responses (Chandra, 1990).

Glutamine

Exercise-induced immunosuppression may be attributable to a lack of lymphocyte and monocyte energy supply, of which there are two major sources: glucose and glutamine (Hoffman-Goetz and Pedersen, 1994).

Glutamine is the most abundant free amino acid in human muscle and plasma and is utilized at very high rates by leukocyte to provide energy and optimal conditions for nucleotide biosynthesis. Indeed, glutamine is considered important, if not essential, to lymphocytes and other rapidly dividing cells including the gut mucosa and bone marrow stem cells. It is also required for optimal macrophage phagocytic activity. The normal plasma glutamine concentration in overnight-fasted healthy adult humans is 450–750 μmol l^{-1}. Glutamine homeostasis depends on an equilibrium between its synthesis and utilization. This is placed under stress in various catabolic states including surgical trauma, infection and prolonged exercise (Rowbottom *et al.*, 1996). At such times, glutamine reserves in skeletal muscle are depleted, the plasma glutamine concentration falls and this may contribute to immunosuppression.

Parry-Billings *et al.* (1992) demonstrated a 16 per cent decrease in plasma glutamine in runners following a marathon, whereas levels remain unchanged or increase after short-term high-intensity exercise. Sewell *et al.* (1994) observed a rise in the plasma glutamine concentration (662 μmol l^{-1} compared with 757 μmol l^{-1}) following exhaustive treadmill exercise lasting 2–3 min. This could be wholly accounted for by haemoconcentration.

The acute effects of exercise on plasma glutamine level may be cumulative since overload training has been shown to result in low plasma glutamine levels (< 450 μmol l^{-1}), requiring long periods of recovery (Rowbottom *et al.*, 1996). Furthermore, athletes suffering from the overtraining syndrome have demonstrated lower resting levels of plasma glutamine, compared with active healthy controls (Kingsbury *et al.*, 1998; Parry-Billings *et al.*, 1992). Therefore, muscle activity directly affects glutamine availability to the leukocytes, thus influencing immune function.

In vitro experiments suggest that falls in glutamine concentration below 600 μmol l^{-1} in the incubation medium are associated with reduced RNA synthesis, IL-2 production, immunoglobulin synthesis and proliferative responses to mitogens in lymphocytes and a decreased rate of phagocytosis in macrophages (Parry-Billings *et al.*,1992). However, some caution must be exercised when interpreting these results as the methodology involved incubation of the isolated cells with specific concentrations of glutamine at the start of the experiment. It is likely that these concentrations will have fallen over the 24–48 h required to obtain significant lymphocyte proliferative and other responses, due to utilization of glutamine by the lymphocytes as an energy source or in the biosynthesis of nucleotides. The concentration of glutamine in the cultures was neither monitored during the experiments nor at the end. It is, therefore, possible that glutamine levels dropped below physiological concentrations or decreased to zero, an occurrence which does not happen in the body, rendering the results invalid; the experiments may have become effectively a measure of glutamine utilization. However, physiological concentrations of glutamine have been shown to increase the proliferative response of the cytokine-activated killer cell activity of blood mononuclear cells isolated from normal healthy subjects (Rohde *et al.*, 1995).

Literature concerning the time-course of recovery of the depressed glutamine levels after exercise is sparse, but Rowbottom *et al.* (1996) observed depressed plasma levels for at least 8 h following high-intensity exercise. However, these workers used a 'unique' bioassay method, using a strain of *Escherichia coli* that is dependent on glutamine for replication, and which appears to give glutamine values that are double the plasma concentrations found by standard enzymatic spectrophotometric techniques. A bioassay method may not be valid for studies investigating changes in plasma glutamine concentration during and after exercise, as other factors may change in the blood plasma during exercise that could influence the growth of bacteria in culture.

Exogenous provision of glutamine may be beneficial by preventing impairment of immune function. Castell *et al.* (1996) reported a lower incidence of URTI in athletes given glutamine supplementation after very prolonged running compared with placebo-treated control runners. The decrease in plasma glutamine levels in runners following a marathon was attenuated following supplementation with branched chain amino acids (BCAA) (Parry-Billings *et al.*, 1992). Natural enhancement of glutamine and BCAA levels via dietary manipulation (additional protein) would avoid supplementation and there is some new evidence that this can restore depressed plasma glutamine levels in overtrained athletes (Kingsbury *et al.*, 1998).

Carbohydrate ingestion during exercise

Since the ingestion of carbohydrate during prolonged exercise is known to attenuate the rise in plasma catecholamines and cortisol, it seems likely that this practice could minimize the immune dysfunction associated with heavy exertion. A recent double-blind placebo-controlled study has demonstrated that the consumption of carbohydrate during 2.5 h of running (77 per cent $\dot{V}O_{2max}$) blunts the rise in IL-6 and reduces trafficking of most leukocytes and lymphocyte subsets (Nehlsen-Cannarella *et al.*, 1997).

Further research is required to determine whether the effects of carbohydrate ingestion on immune cell concentrations and function will lower the risk of URTI following competitive endurance events.

Summary

Immunosuppression in athletes involved in heavy training cannot be assigned to a specific source; it is undoubtedly a multifactoral occurrence. Heavy prolonged exertion places significant stress on the immune system.

This is associated with numerous hormonal and biochemical changes, many of which have detrimental effects on immune function. Furthermore, environmental factors, such as pollutants, psychological stress and improper nutrition, can compound the negative influence of heavy exertion on immunocompetence. Training and competitive surroundings may also increase the athlete's exposure to pathogens and provide optimal conditions for pathogen transmission.

Although it is impossible to counter the effects of all of the causes which contribute to exercise-induced immunosuppression, it has been shown to be possible to minimize the effects of many factors. Athletes can help themselves by eating a well-balanced diet which includes adequate protein and carbohydrate, supplemented by certain micronutrients such as vitamin C and zinc, reducing other life stresses, maintaining good oral and skin hygiene, obtaining adequate rest, and spacing prolonged training sessions and competition as far apart as possible.

References

Berk, L.S., Ton, S.A., Nieman, D.C. and Eby, E.C. (1986). The suppressive effect of stress from acute exhaustive exercise on T–lymphocyte helper/suppressor ratio in athletes and non–athletes. *Med. Sci. Sports Exerc.*, **18**, 706.

Blalock, J.E. (1989). A molecular basis for bidirectional communication between the immune and endocrine systems. *Physiol. Rev.*, **69**, 1–32.

Blannin, A.K., Chatwin, L.J., Cave, R. and Gleeson, M. (1996a). Effects of submaximal cycling and long term endurance training on neutrophil phagocytic activity in middle aged men. *Brit. J. Sports Med.*, **30**, 125–129.

Blannin, A.K., Gleeson, M., Brooks, S. and Cave, R. (1996b). Acute effect of exercise on human neutrophil degranulation. *J. Physiol.*, **495**, 140P.

Blannin, A.K., Robson, P.J., Walsh, N.P., Clark, A.M., Cook, L. and Gleeson, M. (1998). No change occurs in saliva immuno-globulin A concentration after intermittent high intensity exercise despite increases in total protein concentration and α-amylase activity. *J. Sports Sci.*, **16**, 37.

Brenner, I.K.M., Shek, P.N. and Shephard, R.J. (1994). Infection in athletes. *Sports Med.*, **17**, 86–107.

Calder, P.C. and Newsholme, E.A. (1992). Polyunsaturated fatty acids suppress human peripheral lymphocyte proliferation and interleukin-2 production. *Clinical Sci.*, **82**, 695–700.

Cannon, J.G. (1993). Exercise and resistance to infection. *J. Appl. Physiol.*, **74**, 973–981.

Cannon, J.G. (1996). Exercise and the acute phase response. In *Exercise and Immune Function* (L. Hoffman-Goetz, ed.), pp. 39–54. CRC Press.

Cannon, J.G., Fielding, R.A., Fiatarone, M.A. *et al.* (1989). Increased interleukin-1β in human skeletal muscle after exercise. *Am. J. Physiol.*, **257**, R451–R455.

Cannon, J.G. and Kluger, J.J. (1983). Endogenous pyrogen activity in human plasma after exercise. *Science*, **220**, 617–619.

Cannon, J.G., Meydani, S.N., Fielding, R.A. *et al.* (1991). Acute phase response in exercise. II. Association between vitamin E, cytokines, and muscle proteolysis. *Am. J. Physiol.*, **260**, R1235–R1240.

Castell, L.M., Poortmans, J.R. and Newsholme, E.A. (1996). Does glutamine have a role in reducing infections in athletes? *Eur. J. Appl. Physiol.*, **73**, 488–490.

Chandra, R.K. (1990). Nutrition and immunity: lessons from the past and a new insights into the future. *Am. J. Clin. Nutrition*, **53**, 1087–1101.

Cohen, S., Tyrrell., D.A. and Smith A.P. (1991). Psychological stress and susceptibility to the common cold. *New Eng. J. Med.*, **325**, 606–612.

Cupps, T.R. and Fauci, A.S. (1982). Corticosteroid-mediated immunoregulation in man. *Immunol. Rev.*, **65**, 133–155.

Dufaux, B. and Order, U. (1989). Plasma elastase-α1-antitrypsin, neopterin, tumor necrosis factor, and soluble interleukin-2 receptor after prolonged exercise. *Int. J. Sports Med.*, **10**, 434–438.

Duthie, G.G., Jenkinson, A.M., Morrice, P.C. and Arthur, J.R. (1996). Antioxidant adaptations to exercise. In *Biochemistry of Exercise IX* (R.J. Maughan and S.M. Shirreffs, eds). Human Kinetics.

Fehr, H.G., Lötzerich, H. and Michna, H. (1989). Human macrophage function and physical exercise: phagocytic and histochemical studies. *Eur. J. Appl. Physiol.*, **58**, 613–617.

Fiatarone, M.A., Morley, J.E., Bloom, E.T. *et al.* (1988). Endogenous opioids and the exercise-induced augmentation of natural killer cell activity. *J. Lab. Clinical Med.*, **112**, 544–552.

Fry, R.W., Morton, A.R., Crawford, G.P.M. and Keast, D. (1992a). Cell numbers and *in vitro* responses of leucocytes and lymphocyte subpopulations following maximal exercise and interval training sessions of different intensities. *Eur. J. Appl. Physiol.*, **64**, 218–227.

Fry, R.W., Morton, A.R. and Keast, D. (1992b). Acute intensive interval training and T-lymphocyte function. *Med. Sci. Sports Exer.*, **24**, 339–345.

Galbo, H. (1983). *Hormonal and Metabolic Adaptation to Exercise*. Thieme-Stratton.

Gatti, G., Cavallo, R., Sartori, M.L. *et al.* (1987). Inhibition by cortisol of human natural killer (NK) cell activity. *J. Steroid Biochem.*, **26**, 49–58.

Gleeson, M. (1994). Exercise and immune function. *Physiological Soc. Mag.*, **15**, 8–9.

Gleeson, M., Robertson, J.D. and Maughan, R.J. (1987). Influence of exercise on ascorbic acid status in man. *Clin. Sci.*, **73**, 501–505.

Gleeson, M., Blannin, A.K., Sewell, D.A. and Cave, R. (1995a). Short-term changes in the blood leucocyte and platelet count following different durations of high-intensity running. *J. Sports Sci.*, **13**, 115–123.

Gleeson, M., Blannin, A.K., Zhu, B. *et al.* (1995b). Cardiorespiratory, hormonal and haematological responses to submaximal cycling performed 2 days after eccentric or concentric exercise bouts *J. Sports Sci.*, **13**, 471–479.

Gordon, D., Hendersen, D.C. and Westwick, J. (1979). Effect of prostaglandins E_2 and I_2 on human lymphocyte transformation in the presence and absence of inhibitors of prostaglandin synthesis. *Brit. J. Pharmacol.*, **67**,17–22.

Hack, V., Strobel, G., Rau, J.P. and Weicker, H. (1992). The effect of maximal exercise on the activity of neutrophil granulocytes in highly trained athletes in a moderate training period. *Eur. J. Appl. Physiol.*, **65**, 520–524.

Hack, V., Strobel, G., Weiss, M. and Weicker, H. (1994). PMN cell counts and phagocytic activity of highly trained athletes depend on training period. *J. Appl. Physiol.*, **77**, 1731–1735.

Hanley, D.F. (1976). Medical care of the US Olympic team. *J. Am. Medical Assoc.*, **236**,146–147.

Hawley, J.A., Dennis, S.C., Lindsay, F.H. and Noakes, T.D. (1995). Nutritional practices of athletes: Are they sub-optimal? *J. Sports Sci.*, **13** (Special Issue), S75–S81.

Heath, G.W., Macera, C.A. and Nieman, D.C. (1992). Exercise and URTI: is there a relationship? *Sports Med.*, **14**, 353–365.

Heath, G.W., Ford, E.S., Craven, T.E. *et al.* (1991). Exercise and the incidence of upper respiratory tract infections *Med. Sci. Sports Exerc.*, **23**, 152–157.

Hoffman-Goetz, L. (ed.) (1996). *Exercise and Immune Function*. CRC Press. Raton.

Hoffman-Goetz, L. and Pedersen, B.K. (1994). Exercise and the immune system: a model of the stress response? *Immunol. Today*, **15**, 382–387.

Housh, T.J., Johnson, G.O., Housh D.J. *et al.* (1991). The effect of exercise at various temperatures on salivary levels of immunoglobulin A. *Int. J. Sports Med.*, **12**, 498–500.

Howlett, T.A. (1987). Hormonal responses to exercise and training: A short review. *Clinical Endocrinol.*, **26**, 723–742.

Illing, J.W., Miller, F.J. and Gardner, D.E. (1980). Decreased resistance to infection in exercised mice exposed to NO_2 and O_3. *J. Toxicol. Environment. Health*, **6**, 843–851.

Jemmot, J.B., Borysenko, M., Chapman, R. *et al.* (1983). Academic stress, power motivation, and decrease in secretion rate of salivary secretory immunoglobulin A. *Lancet*, 1400–1402.

Kappel, M., Tvede, N., Galbo H. *et al.* (1991). Evidence that the effect of physical activity on natural killer cell activity is mediated by epinephrine. *J. Appl. Physiol.*, **70**, 2530–2534.

Khansari, D.N., Murgo, A.J. and Faith, R.E. (1990). Effects of stress on the immune system. *Immunol. Today*, **11**, 170–175.

Kingsbury, K.J., Kay, L. and Hjelm, M. (1998). Contrasting plasma amino acid patterns in elite athletes: association with fatigue and infection. *Brit. J. Sports Med.*, **32**, 25–33.

Kono, I., Matsuda, H.K.M., Haga, S. *et al.* (1988). Weight reduction in athletes may adversely affect the phagocytic function of monocytes. *Physician Sports Med.*, **16**, 56–65.

Kuby, J. (1997). *Immunology*, 3rd Edn. W.H. Freeman at Macmillan Press.

Kunkel, S.L., Chensue, S.W. and Phan S.M. (1986). Prostaglandins as endogenous mediators of interleukin-1 production. *J. Immunol.*, **136**, 186–193.

Lemon, P.W.R. (1992). Effect of exercise on protein requirements. In *Foods, Nutrition and Sports Performance* (C. Williams and J. Devlin, eds), pp. 65–86. E. and F.N. Spon.

Lewicki, R., Tchorzewski, H., Denys, A. *et al.* (1987). Effect of physical exercise on some parameters of immunity in conditioned sportsmen. *Int. J. Sports Med.*, **8**, 309–314.

Linde, F. (1987). Running and URTI. *Scand. J. Sport Sci.*, **9**, 21–23.

Mackinnon, L.T. (1992). *Exercise and Immunology*. Human Kinetics.

MacNeil, B., Hoffman-Goetz, L., Kendall, A. *et al.* (1991). Lymphocyte proliferative responses after exercise in men: fitness, intensity, duration and effects. *J. Appl. Physiol.*, **70**,175–179.

Maisel, S.A., Harris, T., Rearden, C.A. and Michel, M.C. (1990). β-Adrenergic receptors in lymphocyte subsets after exercise. *Circulation*, **82**, 2003.

McDowell, S.L., Hughes, R.A., Hughes, R.J. *et al.* (1992). The effect of exhaustive exercise on salivary immunoglobulin A. *J. Sports Med. Phys. Fitness*, **32**, 412–415.

Mertz, W. (1981). The essential trace elements. *Science*, **213**, 1332–1338.

Meydani, S.N., Barklund, M.P., Liu, S. *et al.* (1990). Vitamin E supplementation enhances cell-mediated immunity in healthy elderly subjects. *Am. J. Clin. Nutrition*, **52**, 557–563.

Murray, D.K., Irwin, M., Rearden, A. *et al.* (1992). Sympathetic and immune interactions during dynamic exercise: Mediation via a $β_2$-adrenergic-dependent mechanism. *Circulation*, **86**, 203–213.

Nehlsen-Cannarella, S.L., Fagoaga, O.R., Nieman, D.C. *et al.* (1997). Carbohydrate and the cytokine response to 2.5 h of running. *J. Appl. Physiol.*, **82**(5), 1662–1667.

Nieman, D.C. (1994a). Exercise, infection and immunity. *Int. J. Sports Med.*, **15**, S131–S141.

Nieman, D.C. (1994b). Exercise, upper respiratory tract infection, and the immune system. *Med. Sci. Sports Exerc.*, **26**, 128–139.

Nieman, D.C. (1996). Prolonged aerobic exercise, immune response and risk of infection. In *Exercise and Immune Function* (L. Hoffman-Goetz, ed.) pp. 143–161. CRC Press.

Nieman, D.C. (1997). Immune response to heavy exertion. *J. Appl. Physiol.*, **82**(5), 1385–1394.

Nieman, D.C, Johansen L.M, and Lee, J.W. (1990). Infectious episodes in runners before and after the Los Angeles Marathon. *J. Sports Med. Phys. Fitness*, **30**, 316–328.

Nieman, D.C., Miller, A.R., Henson, D.A. *et al.* (1994). Effect of high- versus moderate-intensity exercise on lymphocyte subpopulations and proliferative response. *Int. J. Sports Med.*, **15**, 199–206.

Nieman, D.C., Miller, A.R., Henson, D.A. *et al.* (1993). Effects of high- versus moderate-intensity exercise on natural killer cell activity. *Med. Sci. Sports Exerc.*, **25**, 1126–1134.

Nieman, D.C. and Nehlsen-Cannarella, S.L. (1991). The effects of acute and chronic exercise on immunoglobulins. *Sports Med.*, **11**, 183–201.

Parry-Billings, M., Budgett, R., Koutedakis, Y. *et al.* (1992). Plasma amino acid concentrations in the overtraining syndrome: possible effects on the immune system. *Med. Sci. Sports Exerc.*, **24**, 1353–1358.

Pedersen, B.K. and Bruunsgaard, H. (1995). How physical exercise influences the establishment of infections. *Sports Med.*, **19**, 393–400.

Pedersen, B.K., Tvede, N., Klarlund, K. *et al.* (1990). Indomethacin *in vitro* and *in vivo* abolishes post-exercise suppression of natural killer cell activity in peripheral blood. *Int J. Sports Med.*, **11**, 127–131.

Pedersen, B.K., Tvede, N., Hansen, F.R. *et al.* (1988). Modulation of natural killer cell activity in peripheral blood by physical exercise. *Scand. J. Immunol.*, **27**, 673–678.

Peters, E.M. and Bateman, E.D. (1983). Ultramarathon running and URTI: an epidemiological survey. *S. Afr. Med. J.*, **64**, 582–584.

Peters, E.M., Goetzsche, J.M., Grobbelaar, B. and Noakes, T.D. (1993). Vitamin C supplementation reduces the incidence of post-race symptoms of URTI in ultramarathon runners. *Am. J. Clin. Nutrition*, **53**, 170–174.

Pyne, D.B. (1994). Regulation of neutrophil function during exercise. *Sports Med.*, **17**, 245–258.

Quintanhila, A.T. and Packer, L. (1983). Vitamin E, physical exercise and tissue oxidative damage. In *Biology of Vitamin E*, pp. 56–69. Pitman.

Robertson, J.D., Maughan, R.J., Duthie, G.G. and Morrice, P.C. (1991). Increased blood antioxidant systems of runners in response to training load. *Clin. Sci.*, **80**, 611–618.

Rohde, T., Ullum, H., Rasmussen, J.P. *et al.* (1995). Effects of glutamine on the immune system: influence of muscular exercise and HIV infection. *J. Appl. Physiol.*, **79**, 146–150.

Roitt, I. (1994). *Essential Immunology*, 8th Edn. Blackwell Science.

Rowbottom, D.G., Keast, D., Goodman, C. *et al.* (1995). The haematological, biochemical and immunological profile of athletes suffering from the overtraining syndrome. *Eur. J. Appl. Physiol.*, **70**, 502–509.

Rowbottom, D.G., Keast, D. and Morton, A.R. (1996). The emerging role of glutamine as an indicator of exercise stress and overtraining. *Sports Med.*, **21**, 80–97.

Schouten, W.J., Verschuur, R. and Kemper, H.C.G. (1988). Habitual physical activity, strenuous exercise, and salivary immunoglobulin A levels in young adults: The Amsterdam Growth and Health Study. *Int. J. Sports Med.*, **9**, 289–293.

Sevier, T.L. (1995) Common infectious diseases in athletes. *Sports Med. Arthros. Rev.*, **3**, 107–121.

Sewell, D.A., Gleeson, M. and Blannin, A.K. (1994). Hyperammonaemia in relation to high-intensity exercise duration in man. *Eur. J. Appl. Physiol.*, **69**, 350–354.

Shek, P.N., Sabiston, B.H., Vidal, D. *et al.* (1992). Immunological changes induced by exhaustive exercise in conditioned athletes. *Proc. The Int. Congr. Immunol.*, **8**, 706.

Shephard, R.J., Rhind, S. and Shek, P.N. (1994). Exercise and the immune system. *Sports Med.*, **18**, 340–369.

Shephard, R.J. and Shek, P.N. (1994). Potential impact of physical activity and sport on the immune system – a brief review. *Br. J. Sports Med.*, **28**, 247–255.

Shephard, R.J., Verde, T.J., Thomas, S.G. and Shek, P.N. (1991). Physical activity and the immune system. *Can. J. Sports Sci.*, **16**, 169–185.

Shinkai, S., Yurokawa, Y., Hino, S. *et al.* (1993). Triathlon competition induced a transient immunosuppressive change in the peripheral blood of athletes. *J. Sports Med. Phys. Fitness*, **33**, 70–78.

Smith, J.K., Chi, D.S., Krish, G. *et al.* (1990). Effect of exercise on complement activity. *Ann. Allergy*, **65**, 304–310.

Sprenger, H., Jacobs, C., Nain, M. *et al.* (1992). Enhanced release of cytokines, interleukin-2 receptors and neopterin after long distance running. *Clin. Immunol. Immunopathol.*, **62**, 188–195.

Tharp, G.D. and Barnes, M.W. (1990). Reduction in saliva immunoglobulin levels by swim training. *Eur. J. Appl. Physiol.*, **60**, 61–64.

Tønnesden, E., Christensen, N.J. and Brinkløv, M.M. (1987). Natural killer cell activity during cortisol and adrenaline infusion in healthy volunteers. *Eur. J. Clin. Investigation*, **17**, 497–503.

Tvede, N., Heilmann, C., Halkjaer Kristensen, J. and Pedersen, B.K. (1989). Mechanisms of B-lymphocyte suppression induced by acute physical exercise. *J. Clin. Lab. Immunol.*, **30**, 169–173.

Van Tits, L.J., Michel, M.C., Grosse-Wilde, H. and Happel, M. (1990). Catecholamines increase lymphocyte β_2-adrenergic receptors via a β_2-adrenergic, spleen-dependent process. *Am. J. Physiol.*, **258**, E191–E202.

Wilmore, J.H. and Costill, D.L. (1994). *Physiology of Sport and Exercise*, pp. 133–139. Human Kinetics.

9

Psychological outcomes of physical activity

William P. Morgan

Better to hunt in the fields for health unbought
Than fee the Doctor for a nauseous draught.
The wise for the cure on exercise depend.
Dryden, circa 1675

It has been estimated that nearly one half of those individuals who are treated for affective disorders are seen by primary care physicians, and depression is one of the most common problems seen in primary care settings (Muñoz *et al.*, 1994). Given the cost and time associated with traditional psychotherapy, as well as the cost and potential side- or after-effects of medications used in the treatment of mental disorders, it is understandable that inexpensive, low-risk interventions such as physical activity have become popular. There is evidence, for example, that many primary care physicians prescribe physical activity in the treatment of mental health problems such as anxiety and depression (Morgan, 1997). However, the enthusiasm with which workers in behavioural medicine and health psychology have employed exercise interventions has not always been matched by a compelling research basis.

The therapeutic efficacy of exercise in both the prevention and treatment of various physical and mental disorders has been addressed in a comprehensive manner. The Proceedings of the Second International Consensus Symposium on Physical Activity held in Toronto, Canada during May of 1992, contains 70 chapters, and much of the material deals with the influence of physical activity on physical or mental health (Bouchard *et al.*, 1994). This encyclopaedic volume includes consensus statements based on state-of-the-art views formulated by a panel of international authorities. The conditions and circumstances under which acute and chronic physical activity can be effective in the prevention of both physical and mental disorders is spelled out, as well as its efficacy in treatment once an illness occurs. It is clear from the material summarized in this volume that an association exists between vigorous physical activity on the one hand and positive mental health on the other. However, it is also apparent that causal linkages remain to be demonstrated in many cases. This is important, since there is evidence that physical fitness, as well as involvement in vigorous physical activity, is governed to a significant degree by genetic influences (Bouchard, 1988). Furthermore, much of the literature in the area of exercise and mental health has been characterized by numerous methodological problems (Morgan, 1997b). Finally, with few exceptions, most authors who have reviewed this research literature have done so in an uncritical manner, and research design issues of a fundamental nature have been largely ignored.

There has also been a tendency to think of exercise in a generic context, and there has been little attention paid to important considerations such as the type (i.e. mode), intensity, duration and frequency of physical activity. In other words, exercise 'dosage' has not been considered in a systematic or comprehensive manner. There has also been an implicit assumption that 'if a little exercise is good, a lot of exercise will be better'. As a consequence there has been a tendency to ignore problems such as exercise addiction and dependence (Morgan, 1979b), compulsive exercise (Polivy, 1994) and the recognized problems associated with overtraining (Morgan *et al.*, 1987; O'Connor, 1997; Morgan *et al.*, 1988; O'Connor *et al.*, 1991). It is important that the 'dark side' of physical activity be considered when using this intervention in both prevention and treatment settings.

A brief summary of earlier reviews is presented in this chapter, and this is followed by a discussion of selected methodological issues which must be considered when evaluating the efficacy of exercise. Most of the published research involving exercise and mental health has been concerned with the anxiolytic and antidepressant effects of exercise, and these topics will be considered as well. Any intervention that is sufficiently potent to result in anxiolytic and/or antidepressant effects would presumably be capable of producing undesirable effects if used inappropriately, and exercise is no exception in this regard. Therefore, the dark side of exercise is considered as well, and the chapter concludes with some modest suggestions regarding future directions.

Overview of previous reviews

The first comprehensive review dealing with the influence of physical activity on mental health appeared in a chapter by Layman (1960) entitled 'Physical activity as a psychiatric adjunct'. This chapter was published in a volume edited by Johnson (1960): *Science and Medicine of Exercise and Sports*. Layman (1960) pointed out in this chapter that physical recreation was employed in psychiatric rehabilitation for many years, but it was used for its 'diversional' value prior to 1940. It was not until after the Second World War that exercise therapy actually gained acceptance as an adjunct to psychiatric treatment. While physical activity may be promoted today as an innovative or unique method of treating psychopathology, this somatic therapy has been used in the treatment of various mental health problems for at least the past 60 years. Actually, physical activity was used in this manner for many centuries, but formal programmes of exercise therapy grew and flourished during the two decades following the Second World War.

There have also been some significant changes in the ways in which exercise therapy is typically employed today compared with earlier applications. Layman (1960) pointed out, for example, that the use of physical activity in the treatment of psychiatric patients was based on an understanding of the individual patient's needs, as well as '...a knowledge of the psychodynamics of different kinds of exercise' (p. 703). There is no reference to exercise prescriptions being based upon 'target heart rates', 'per cent of VO_2max' and so on in this review. Indeed, it appears that exercise prescriptions were developed on the basis of a given activity's potential for: (1) improving self-confidence; (2) facilitating self-expression; (3) gratifying narcissistic needs; (4) enhancing communication skills; (5) developing socialized attitudes and habits; (6) improving the patient's reality orientation; or (7) reducing tension. In other words, an attempt was made to first determine the patient's needs and then to select a physical activity that had the potential for meeting these needs. Furthermore, during this period of time, the development of exercise prescriptions and the planning of activities was the responsibility of the physiatrist and psychiatrist. Physical education, recreational and/or corrective therapists were responsible for carrying out the exercise prescriptions. These 'activity' therapists were also expected to note the patient's behaviour patterns and verbalizations, and patient logs were then given to the psychotherapist for use in planning and evaluating the ongoing psychotherapy.

It should also be noted that most hospitals employed 'total push' or 'milieu' therapy in efforts to rehabilitate psychiatric patients. These programmes included various 'adjunctive' therapies such as psychotherapy, drug therapy, physical activity therapy, shock therapy, occupational therapy and physical therapy. It was virtually impossible to discern the effect of a specific therapy since these interventions were employed as 'adjuncts' in these 'total push' efforts. These interventions were not based upon research trials that had demonstrated efficacy in most cases, and it was not possible to argue that physical activity led to a patient's improvement since gains might have been due to one of the other treatments being employed. In other words, the value of physical activity in the treatment of psychopathology was based largely on subjective data and anecdotal evidence until recent years. Layman (1960) emphasized in this comprehensive review that a need existed for more '...experimentation on the effects of different kinds of exercise on the psychiatric patient, and for more studies utilizing adequate controls' (p. 704). Exercise scientists have accepted this challenge, and the subsequent research and reviews suggest that we now have some research evidence supporting the efficacy of physical activity in the treatment of certain mental health problems. A cursory overview of these subsequent reviews follows.

Most of the articles and chapters dealing with the influence of physical activity on mental health published prior to 1970 dealt with psychiatric samples and, furthermore, a large number of the patients included in these studies were diagnosed as schizophrenics. These patient samples were sometimes contrasted with convenience samples composed of non-hospitalized 'normals' for comparison purposes. Finally, very few of these early studies actually employed longitudinal research designs in an effort to quantify the effects of physical activity. Rather, intact sample groups were typically administered tests of physical fitness, and the relationship between psychopathology and physical fitness was studied at a cross-sectional level (Layman, 1960; Morgan, 1969a; Rice *et al.*, 1961). This design strategy is problematic since it is recognized that both psychopathology (Holden, 1984) and physical fitness (Bouchard, 1988) possess substantial genetic components.

Despite the fact that cross-sectional studies often lack internal as well as external validity, this method possesses a number of advantages. Should previously active and sedentary samples fail to differ on physical fitness or another target criterion (such as psychopathology), for example, there would not be a strong basis for conducting more complex and expensive longitudinal studies. In other words, cross-sectional data supporting this relationship might be thought of as 'necessary' evidence, and this type of information can be useful in formulating hypotheses and designing longitudinal studies.

The initial review by Layman (1960) was updated by Morgan (1969a), and this summary revealed that an inverse relationship exists between physical fitness on the one hand and psychopathology on the other. That is, the greater the degree of psychopathology, the lower the level of physical fitness. This seemed to be the case regardless of how investigators defined physical fitness, and this relationship was also independent of how pathology was operationalized. In other words, the relationship existed whether fitness was defined as muscular strength, muscular endurance or cardiovascular fitness. Also, in a comprehensive report, Cureton (1963) summarized the findings of research conducted in the Physical Fitness Research Laboratory at the University of Illinois over a 10-year period. Cureton (1963) reported that these studies taken collectively revealed that personality deterioration was correlated with the following physical factors: (1) accumulation of body fat; (2) loss of muscular strength; (3) slowing of reaction time; (4) reduced ventilatory capacity; and (5) reduced physical working capacity.

The nature of the relationship between physical fitness and psychopathology may be far more complex than implied by Cureton (1963), Layman (1960) and Morgan (1969) in these early reviews. It is possible, for example, that depressed patients may not differ from non-depressed patients or normals on standard measures of muscular strength and endurance, but rather, they simply lack the motivation necessary to perform at a higher level. It is also possible that low levels of physical fitness seen in psychiatric patients may reflect genetic influences rather than past activity patterns. Most of the psychiatric patients evaluated in the earlier studies had been hospitalized for many years, and it could be argued that low fitness levels observed in these samples were due to prolonged hospitalization. This possibility was addressed by Rice *et al.* (1961) who compared the physical fitness of 62 recently hospitalized schizophrenics and 59 patients who had been hospitalized for a prolonged period of time. Physical fitness was measured with the Rogers Physical Fitness Index (PFI) and, while both groups scored below normal on the PFI, these samples did not differ from each other. This led Rice *et al.* (1961) to interpret these results as indicative of a direct relationship between schizophrenia and below-normal physical fitness, regardless of length of hospitalization.

In a related study using the PFI, Hodgdon and Reimer (1960) also demonstrated that schizophrenic patients scored below normal on physical fitness. However, one of the patients in this study had a score of 140 on the PFI, and this falls significantly above the average score of 100 for the general population. This patient was reported to be tense, mute and nervous at the time of testing, and the investigators tested the individual three times in order to be confident that an error had not been made in the assessment of physical fitness. This patient's exceptional fitness performance was replicated with repeated testing. It was necessary for this patient to be transferred to a maximum security unit because of aggressive and hostile behaviour. It is of considerable interest that this patient's PFI score dropped substantially as his psychiatric status improved. It has been known for many years in the field of exercise science that maximal physical efforts are usually governed by inhibitory mechanisms. This is thought to be beneficial since true maximal efforts might lead to injury (e.g. fractures, dislocations, strains), and it is also known that maximal physical performance can be enhanced in normal individuals where disinhibition of inhibitory mechanisms takes place. Under certain conditions, for example, it is possible to enhance physical performance above customary or baseline levels with the use of hypnosis (Morgan, 1993). It has also been shown that disinhibition of inhibitory mechanisms can be provoked with certain drugs (e.g. amphetamine), placebo ingestion and loud noises, as well as hypnosis (Ikai and Steinhaus, 1961). It would be reasonable to hypothesize that measured levels of physical fitness might undulate as a patient with bipolar depression cycled between manic and depressed states. Indeed, it would be surprising if this was not the case since psychomotor retardation and fatigue are common symptoms of depression.

The author's initial review (Morgan, 1969a) has been updated and expanded periodically to include new research directions and findings over the past 20 years. These reviews (Morgan, 1974, 1977, 1981, 1982, 1984, 1985, 1994b; Morgan and O'Connor, 1987, 1989; Morgan *et al.*, 1990) have each confirmed that physically active individuals are consistently found to score lower on self-report measures of mood than do sedentary individuals. These reviews have also suggested that adoption of exercise programmes by previously sedentary individuals is usually *associated* with an improvement in affective states. There does not appear to be any evidence supporting the view that this improvement in affect is *caused* by the exercise, but a number of hypothesized mechanisms seem to be tenable (Morgan, 1985, 1994b, 1997a). Furthermore, these reviews suggest that improved mood states in previously sedentary individuals are most likely to occur in those individuals with moderate levels of mood disturbance prior to adoption of a regular programme of physical activity (Morgan and Goldston, 1987). There is an absence of compelling research evidence that individuals scoring within the normal range on a self-report measure of depression, for example, experience a decrease in depression following the adoption of a physical activity programme. There are a few studies that suggest that 'normals can become more normal' following the adoption of an exercise programme, but these investigations have been characterized by serious methodological deficiencies (Hughes, 1984; Morgan, 1997b).

These more recent reviews are also in agreement with epidemiological reports by Ross and Hayes (1988) and Stephens (1988) indicating that individuals who regularly exercise are characterized by decreased symptoms of depression. In addition, the above cited reviews are also in general agreement with narrative reviews by other authors such as Martinsen (1990), Raglin (1990) and Taylor *et al.* (1985). It is believed by some investigators that quantitative reviews that rely on meta-analysis are more effective than narrative reviews of the type summarized in this section, but others have proposed that meta-analysis has a number of shortcomings (Dishman, 1994). While these diverse views cannot be addressed here, a more reasoned position would seem to be that meta-analysis is not inherently good or bad. At any rate, it is noteworthy that the two most recent meta-analyses dealing with the psychological effects of physical activity are in essential agreement with the narrative reviews mentioned above. The first involved a comprehensive meta-analysis performed by McDonald and Hodgdon (1991) that dealt with the psychological effects of aerobic fitness training. A subsequent review by Landers and Petruzzello (1994) actually focused on previous narrative reviews, as well as reviews based on meta-analysis, that dealt with the influence of physical activity on anxiety. The conclusions reached by these authors are in general agreement with the earlier narrative reviews. That is, irrespective of the methodology employed, reviewers have reported that physical activity is *associated* with desirable psychological states and traits. The issue of *causality* (Morgan and Goldston, 1987) remains to be addressed, and the mechanisms underlying the relationship have not been elucidated. However, there has been encouraging work involving animal models (primarily rat models) suggesting that physical activity may have a direct effect on brain chemistry. There is evidence that acute and chronic physical activity may influence brain levels of dopamine (Meeusen, 1996), endorphin (Hoffmann, 1997), norepinephrine (Dishman, 1997) and serotonin (Chaouloff, 1997).

There are several exceptions to the generalizations presented here regarding the association between physical activity and mental health, and these papers need to be considered in order to have a balanced overview. Following a review of the same literature examined by other authors, it was concluded by Hughes (1984) that little evidence exists to support the view that aerobic exercise has an antidepressant effect. Various methodological criteria were employed in order for a study to be included in this analysis, and only 12 of the 1100 published articles were judged as acceptable by Hughes (1984). The remaining studies were regarded as suffering from various methodological problems such as (1) absence of randomization, (2) small sample size, (3) inadequate psychological measures, (4) experimenter expectancy effects, and so on. It could also be argued that the psychological effect of physical activity must be quite potent since it is apparent despite the report by Hughes (1984) that 99 percent of the published studies are characterized by methodological problems. In other words, to observe a significant reduction in depression following an aerobic exercise programme even though sample size is small and experimental error is high (i.e. low statistical power) argues in favour of an antidepressant effect rather than against the effect.

The minority view expressed by Hughes (1984) was supported in a subsequent paper by Simons *et al.* (1985). These authors also pointed out that early research dealing with the antidepressant effect of exercise suffered from '...conceptual confusion and methodological problems' (p. 553). However, these reviewers also pointed out that more recent research in this area '...provides grounds for cautious optimism regarding the potential therapeutic effects of exercise' (p. 553). The caution urged by these authors seems warranted given the later review by Weinstein and Meyers (1988) who stated that it was not possible to draw '...definitive conclusions regarding the antidepressant properties of running' (p. 288). Due to the conceptual and methodological shortcomings of published research in this area, Weinstein and Meyers (1988) concluded that '...there is little clear evidence to support running as a strategy for modifying depression' (p. 296). These authors recommended that improved methodology was needed in this area, and this recommendation served to reinforce the earlier position advanced by Layman (1960) almost three decades earlier. The issue of methodology will be addressed in a later section of this chapter and it has also been addressed elsewhere (McDonald and Hodgdon, 1991; Morgan, 1981, 1985, 1994b, 1997b; Morgan *et al.*, 1990).

The common theme in the reviews by Hughes (1984), Simons *et al.* (1985) and Weinstein and Meyers (1988) involves the conceptual and methodological problems involving research dealing with the psycholo-

gical effects of physical activity. Due in part to the lack of agreement which existed at this point in time, the National Institute of Mental Health (NIMH) convened a consensus panel in 1985 for the purpose of attempting to summarize what was known at the time regarding the influence of physical activity on mental health. The proceedings of this workshop were subsequently published in an edited volume entitled *Exercise and Mental Health* (Morgan and Goldston, 1987), and this panel reached the following conclusions
(p. 156):

1. Physical fitness is positively *associated with* mental health and well-being.
2. Exercise is *associated with* the reduction of stress emotions such as state anxiety.
3. Anxiety and depression are common symptoms of failure to cope with mental stress, and exercise has been *associated with* a decreased level of mild to moderate depression and anxiety.
4. Long-term exercise is usually *associated with* reductions in traits such as neuroticism and anxiety.
5. Severe depression usually requires professional treatment which may include medication, electroconvulsive therapy and/or psychotherapy, with exercise as an adjunct.
6. Appropriate exercise results in reductions in various stress indices such as neuromuscular tension, resting heart rate and some stress hormones.
7. Current clinical opinion holds that exercise has beneficial emotional effects across all ages and in both sexes.
8. Physically healthy people who require psychotropic medication may safely exercise when exercise and medications are titrated under close medical supervision.

It should be noted that a reservation appears in the first four consensus statements and the panel did not wish to state or imply that a *causal link* existed. Therefore, the term 'associated with' is used in each case. Indeed, the panellists felt that the issue of *causality* should play a prominent role in the development of future research agendas (Morgan and Goldston, 1987).

A number of experimental investigations and reviews have been published since these consensus statements were formulated over 10 years ago. Despite the fact that a few isolated studies are not in agreement with these views, the consensus statements continue to possess currency. Reviewers sometimes point out that one of the few randomized trials using both control and exercise groups is the study by Stern and Cleary (1982), and these investigators failed to observe an antidepressant effect following 24 months of exercise. However, this study suffers from a number of serious methodological problems (Morgan, 1994b). The individuals studied by Stern and Cleary (1982), for example, were not depressed at the outset and, therefore, it is unclear why the investigators (or reviewers) would be surprised that an antidepressant effect was not observed. However, there has been a tendency for reviewers to ignore the matter of external validity when attempting to understand the published literature in this area. This problem has previously been discussed in detail (Morgan, 1997b; Morgan *et al.*, 1990). Reviewers have tended to make the assumption that research involving non-depressed samples, for example, can be generalized to depressed psychiatric patients and vice versa. This assumption, however, violates a number of fundamental principles that have been well established by generalizability theorists, as well as the basic assumptions underlying most inferential statistical models. This, and related methodological problems, will be considered in the following section. At any rate, it is clear that individuals with mild to moderate depression experience a reduction in depression following chronic physical activity (Greist *et al.*, 1979; Martinsen, 1987a,b; Martinsen, 1990; Martinsen *et al.*, 1985; Martinsen and Morgan, 1997).

Methodological issues

Much of the research dealing with physical activity and mental health has been characterized by various methodological problems. Indeed, many of these studies have 'fatal flaws' in terms of methodology and experimental design. This overall problem has been dealt with in earlier reviews (Layman, 1960; Morgan, 1981), as well as in a recent monograph by McDonald and Hodgdon (1991) and in several review articles and chapters by Morgan (1985, 1994b, 1997b) and Morgan *et al.* (1990). Therefore, the important issue of methodology will not be examined in detail in this chapter, but a few of the more significant issues will be discussed.

It has been recognized for many years that the perceived efficacy of a given intervention can be influenced by various behavioural artifacts (Morgan, 1997). It is also commonly accepted that experiments should be designed in an effort to control or minimize the impact of effects due to various behavioural artifacts when attempting to quantify the impact of a given treatment. Investigators with an interest in the efficacy of a new drug commonly employ a double-blind placebo trial in order to eliminate and/or quantify changes due to the Halo, Hawthorne and Rosenthal effects. In addition, efforts are usually made to control for factors such as demand characteristics, pre-test sensitization effects, bias due to a lack of randomization, and response distortion. Computation of optimal sample size is normally performed as well, since it is known that an inadequate number of subjects can suggest that no effect is present when, in fact, there is an effect. Conversely, a sample size that is too large can suggest that an effect is present when, in fact, the observed change is trivial.

An investigation that is frequently cited to support the view that exercise has an antidepressant effect is a paper by Stern and Cleary (1981). These investigators observed a 'statistically significant' reduction in depression from a mean score of 22.1 to 21.3 on the MMPI depression scale. The reason this trivial effect was found to be statistically significant was because of the sample size. There were 784 male participants in this study. Furthermore, these individuals had each experienced a documented myocardial infarction (MI) within the past 3 years. This study illustrates another major problem with the literature in this area. Reviewers have tended to ignore the fact that these results cannot be generalized to (1) females, (2) healthy males or females, or (3) depressed inpatients or outpatients. In other words, the study lacks *external validity* where one is interested in generalizing beyond non-depressed, post-MI males.

Another classic illustration of problems involving external validity involves a paper by Jankowski *et al.* (1976). This paper is often cited as evidence that exercise is superior or equivalent to psychotherapy and drug therapy. The frequent suggestion that this study provides evidence that exercise can reduce depression in adult females and males, normal or depressed, is inappropriate since the study dealt with adolescent males engaged in outpatient or inpatient therapy! Furthermore, a review of the original paper reveals that it has numerous design problems (e.g. lack of randomization, raters not blinded, no statistical analyses, invalid rating scales, fitness measures not defined) and there is *no evidence* that exercise was equivalent or superior to the other therapies. A more detailed analysis appears in a review by Morgan (1994b). This summary emphasizes the importance of distinguishing between sound evidence and the evangelical zeal that often exists in the exercise/mental health literature.

Some authors who have written about the mental health benefits of exercise have admitted that design factors can be a problem, but they have argued that a meta-analysis, or simply combining a large number of studies in a narrative review, can overcome these shortcomings. This may be true in the case of *random error*, but it is more likely that there has been considerable *systematic error* in many of these studies. In responding to self-report questionnaires designed to measure variables such as anxiety, depression or self-esteem, for example, it is likely that participants in exercise intervention studies have been more likely to 'fake good' than they have been to 'fake bad'. The influence of expectancy effects and demand characteristics is effectively illustrated in the seminal paper by Desharnais *et al.* (1993). These investigators randomly assigned volunteers to an expectancy group and a control group. The participants in both groups trained aerobically for 10 weeks, and both groups experienced a significant improvement in maximal aerobic power. Both groups were assessed on self-esteem at the outset, during training and following the experiment. The only difference was that subjects in the 'expectancy' group were led to believe that they would experience positive psychological changes. The hypothesis was confirmed, and this study emphasizes that investigators must consider expectancy effects when designing exercise trials. It is noteworthy that very few investigators have commented on the possibility that observed effects may have been due to expectancy, and the use of response distortion measures (i.e. lie scales) has been largely ignored in this area of inquiry.

Exercise prescription

There are many considerations that must be made when developing an exercise prescription, and there has been a great deal written about this topic. The most comprehensive treatment of this subject to date is contained in the edited volume by Bouchard *et al.* (1994). Excellent introductions to the overall nature of exercise prescription appear in chapters by Haskell (1987, 1994), and the earlier chapter by Layman (1960) is particularly valuable where one is concerned with psychological outcomes. Layman (1960) appears to have been the first author to emphasize activity selection on the basis of patient needs. The most recent discussions of exercise 'dose' ignore the personalization of exercise on the basis of patient needs, and there continues to be a fixation on group effects at fixed intensities of the same physical activity (Rejeski, 1994). There is little reason to believe that exercise prescriptions of this type would be effective. Layman (1960), on the other hand, not only discusses the patient's personalized needs, but the development of exercise prescriptions on the basis of a physical activity's psychodynamic potential is also emphasized in this review. The chapter by Layman (1960) has currency today and, despite the passage of time, it continues to be instructive.

There are some very basic considerations that one should make in developing an exercise prescription, and it is likely that problems associated with exercise adherence (Dishman, 1987a,b; Dishman and Sallis, 1994; Morgan, 1977) are due in large measure to inappropriate prescriptions. The exercise **mode** (e.g. walking, running, swimming) is obviously one of the most important considerations, followed by the **intensity** (e.g. light, moderate, heavy), **duration** (e.g. time per session) and **frequency** (e.g. times per day/week). It is well documented that these are very important considerations where one is concerned principally with physiological outcomes. However, there is a lack of compelling research evidence regarding the optimal mode, intensity, duration and frequency of exercise where one is concerned primarily with psychological outcomes. Furthermore, there is published research indicating that groups of individuals fail to experience psychological changes even though significant gains in muscular strength, muscular endurance and /or aerobic power occur. Conversely, there is also evidence that reductions in anxiety and depression, as well as improved self-esteem, can take place even though gains in physical fitness do not occur (Morgan, 1994b, 1997b). There is simply an absence of hard data suggesting that the exercise prescription must lead to improved physical fitness in order for psychological improvement to occur. It has been hypothesized (Bahrke and Morgan, 1978; Morgan, 1985; Raglin and Morgan, 1987, 1997) that improved affect following exercise may be due to the distraction (i.e. 'time out') from the cares and worries of the day rather than the exercise *per se*. It is possible that muscle tissue undergoes cellular adaptation, and there may even be neurochemical changes that take place in the CNS (Chauloff, 1997; Dishman, 1997; Hoffmann, 1997) despite the failure to observe changes in various physiological parameters commonly employed by exercise scientists. In other words, the distraction hypothesis should not be viewed as 'psychological' since it may reflect significant 'physiological' changes at a local or central level. At any rate, the distraction hypothesis continues to be tenable, and efforts to support or refute this hypothesis should not be approached from a psychological or physiological perspective alone. It has been recognized for some time that psychobiological inquiry is the most efficacious approach in exercise and sport science (Morgan, 1973), and this position has recently been reinforced in a comprehensive review by Dishman (1994). Since we do not know how much exercise an individual needs in order to derive positive psychological effects, it would seem prudent to recommend lower exercise volumes when developing prescriptions. It is also important that the individual's psychological needs be considered when prescribing exercise (Layman, 1960), and this parameter has simply not been included in contemporary proposals (Rejeski, 1994).

Anxiolytic effects

The possibility of using physical activity as a means of reducing anxiety has been discussed for a number of years (Morgan, 1968, 1971), and it is known that many primary care physicians routinely prescribe exercise for this purpose (Morgan and Goldston, 1987). However, the view that vigorous physical activity is actually contraindicated for anxiety neurotics has become institutionalized within the field of psychiatry (Lader, 1985), and this misconception is based largely on the report by Pitts and McClure (1967). The basis for this belief is the report that anxiety and panic attacks occur in patients diagnosed as anxiety neurotics as a consequence of excess lactate production (Pitts and McClure, 1967). However, there is compelling evidence refuting the lactate hypothesis of exercise-induced anxiety (Grosz and Farmer, 1969; Martinsen *et al.*, 1998; Morgan, 1973, 1979; Raglin, 1997).

Most of the earlier research involving the tension-reducing properties of physical activity was concerned with the influence of *acute* physical activity on *state anxiety* (Bahrke and Morgan, 1978). However, the participants in the NIMH Workshop on Exercise concluded that *chronic* physical activity was also effective in reducing *trait anxiety* (Morgan and

Goldston, 1987). A subsequent review dealing with the exercise/anxiety literature contains a summary of 159 studies (Landers and Petruzello, 1994), and Raglin (1997) has presented a comprehensive update of this literature. The conclusions reached by these authors confirm and extend the earlier reports by the NIMH consensus panel (Morgan and Goldston, 1987).

One of the first experimental investigations dealing with the anxiolytic effect of acute physical activity was performed by Bahrke and Morgan (1978), who randomly assigned 75 adult males to: (1) an exercise condition ($n = 25$) that consisted of walking on a motor-driven treadmill for 20 min at 70 percent of maximum; (2) 20 min of non-cultic meditation ($n = 25$); or (3) quiet rest ($n = 25$). The participants in the last group sat quietly in a sound-filtered room for 20 min. It was observed that all three groups experienced significant reductions in state anxiety as measured by the State–Trait Anxiety Inventory (STAI) (Spielberger *et al.*, 1983). These findings have been replicated and extended to include physically challenged college students (Brown *et al.*, 1993). The results fit with theoretical expectations for the exercise and meditation conditions, but the anxiolytic effect noted for quiet rest was not anticipated. Incidentally, the magnitude of the anxiolytic effect was comparable for the three conditions. Does exercise reduce anxiety? Does meditation reduce anxiety? Or is it the distraction from the cares and worries of the day afforded by exercise and meditation that results in the anxiolytic effect? These questions remain to be answered, as does the question of whether or not these interventions have differential chronic effects.

In an effort to quantify the length of time the anxiolytic effect persists following acute physical activity, Raglin and Morgan (1987) evaluated state anxiety and blood pressure before, immediately following and every 30 min for 3 h following exercise and quiet rest. It was found that both conditions resulted in reduced anxiety and blood pressure within minutes following the cessation of treatment. However, the improvement following exercise persisted for 2 h, whereas the effect only lasted for 30 min following quiet rest. Whether or not these two conditions would differ in outcome if compared following a chronic intervention is not known. At any rate, it appears that the anxiolytic effect of exercise persists for about 2 h, and this finding was confirmed in the subsequent summary by Landers and Petruzello (1994) which included additional studies. A comprehensive update of research dealing with the anxiolytic effect of physical activity by Raglin (1997) extends these earlier reviews to include more recent work dealing with resistance exercise.

Antidepressant effects

There is an emerging body of literature suggesting that physical activity is effective in the prevention and management of depression (Morgan,

1994b). The earliest research on this relationship was of a cross-sectional nature, and this work revealed that depression was inversely correlated with measures of physical fitness such as muscular endurance (Morgan, 1968) and physical working capacity as measured by the PWC150 test (Morgan, 1969). This research also demonstrated that depressed psychiatric patients scored below published norms on physical working capacity (Morgan, 1970a). Furthermore, it was observed that muscular strength and endurance at the time of admission to a psychiatric facility was significantly correlated with length of hospitalization (Morgan, 1970b). That is, patients with higher scores on tests of muscular strength and endurance experienced shorter hospital stays than did patients scoring lower on these tests. This cross-sectional research was initially followed by two intervention studies (Morgan et al., 1970, 1971) which served to emphasize the importance of investigating the antidepressant effects of exercise at both acute and chronic levels. Most of the subsequent research on this problem has been focused on the latter, and a brief review of this literature follows.

The first intervention study dealing with the antidepressant effect of physical activity consisted of a quasi-experimental design, and the results have been described in papers by Morgan et al. (1970) and Roberts and Morgan (1971). The participants in this study consisted of 140 healthy adult males ranging in age from 22 to 62 years (mean = 39 years, SD = 9). These individuals exercised two to three times per week at approximately 85 per cent of predicted maximal heart rate. It was found that gains in physical working capacity as measured by standard treadmill and bicycle ergometer tests varied as a function of exercise mode and frequency, but all of the exercise groups had greater gains than the non-exercise control group (Roberts and Morgan, 1971). Depression was assessed before and following the intervention with the Self-Rating Depression Scale (SDS) (Zung, 1965). None of the exercise groups, irrespective of the fitness gains, experienced a reduction in depression, nor did the exercise groups differ from the control group before or following the 6-week intervention.

The mean depression scores for each of the groups in this study fell within the normal range on the SDS and, therefore, a reduction in depression should not have been expected. Also, there are now quite a few studies demonstrating that normal, non-depressed individuals do not experience a reduction in depression following the adoption of exercise programmes (Morgan, 1994b). Indeed, if such changes were noted, one would suspect that behavioural artefacts (e.g. demand characteristics, response distortion) were probably responsible for the changes. However, there is one additional finding from this study that warrants attention. Eleven of the participants scored above 53 on the SDS and Zung (1965) has reported that scores in this range reflect depression of clinical significance. This subgroup actually experienced a significant reduction in depression, and the antidepressant effect was independent of the mode and frequency of exercise. In other words, an antidepressant effect took place in these moderately depressed individuals with 6 weeks of aerobic exercise. These findings were replicated and extended to include the efficacy of exercise compared with traditional psychotherapy by Greist *et al.* (1979), and this study will be reviewed here since it served as the impetus for much of the research that followed in the next decade.

The study by Greist *et al.* (1979) represented a significant advance in several respects. First of all, the participants were outpatients who were diagnosed as possessing mild to moderate depression. Second, rather than comparing exercise with an untreated control group, exercise effects were compared with traditional therapy. The patients were assigned to exercise therapy (i.e. running), time-limited psychotherapy or time-unlimited psychotherapy. In other words, rather than comparing exercise with nothing (i.e. a control group), the antidepressant effect of exercise was contrasted with the effect observed for two forms of psychotherapy. It was found that exercise resulted in a significant improvement, and the antidepressant effect observed for exercise was comparable to that found for time-limited psychotherapy and superior to that noted for time-unlimited psychotherapy. Furthermore, the exercise group remained non-depressed at the 12-month follow-up, while approximately half of the patients in the psychotherapy groups were depressed at follow-up.

The report by Greist *et al.* (1979) was replicated by Martinsen *et al.* (1985) with psychiatric inpatients. The work by Martinsen and his associates has been significant for a number of reasons. First, it has been shown that inpatients suffering from unipolar depression experience a decrease in depression when treated with exercise (Martinsen, 1987a, 1990). Second, it has been reported by Martinsen (1987b) that patients receiving antidepressant medications can exercise providing the exercise and medication are titrated under the supervision of a physician. An overview of the interaction of exercise and drug prescriptions has recently been presented by Martinsen and Stanghelle (1997). Third, while groups of patients suffering from unipolar depression experience a reduction in depression with exercise, there are important individual differences. Martinsen (1987a) has reported that aerobic exercise is of great help for some patients, but '... others experience no antidepressant effect at all' (p. 99). Finally, Martinsen (1987a) has made the important point that our understanding about the mechanisms underlying the antidepressant effect of exercise is unsatisfactory. There have been additional investigations demonstrating that exercise is associated with an antidepressant effect in individuals suffering from unipolar depression in the mild to moderate range, and these studies have been summarized by a number of authors (Martinsen, 1990; Martinsen and Morgan, 1997; McDonald and Hodgdon, 1991; Morgan, 1994; Morgan and Goldston, 1987; North *et al.*, 1990; O'Connor *et al.*, 1993).

Most of the research dealing with the antidepressant effects of exercise has been based upon chronic physical activity lasting for periods of 6 weeks or longer. There has been a limited amount of research involving the acute effects of a single episode of exercise on depression. Since it is well documented that transient reductions in anxiety occur following acute bouts of exercise, it is also possible that temporary reductions in depression occur following acute physical activity. Indeed, this might explain why many authors have reported that participants in exercise studies report that they experience improved mood states following involvement in chronic exercise, but these reports are often not associated with psychological changes as measured by standardized depression scales.

In an attempt to evaluate the acute effect of a single bout of exercise on depression Morgan *et al.* (1971) randomly assigned 120 adult males to exercise bouts designed to produce heart rate responses of 150, 160, 170 or 180 beats per minute. These individuals were randomly assigned to a treadmill or bicycle ergometer for the exercise session, and a post-test-only randomized groups design was employed in order to eliminate pre-test sensitization effects. All participants completed the Depression Adjective Check List (DACL) following the exercise, and results on this measure of depression were compared with published norms (Lubin, 1967). The post-exercise depression scores were lower than published norms for both exercise modes and all exercise intensities. The effect sizes for these interventions are summarized in Table 9.1, and these calculations were performed using the standard deviation reported for the published norms. The findings of this study suggest that acute physical activity of the type employed is associated with levels of depression that fall below published norms for non-depressed individuals. This study was not designed in such a way that causality can be inferred, nor does it permit speculation concerning the mechanisms involved. Also, if the observed levels of depression were due to the actual exercise, the effect was probably transitory since non-depressed individuals do not experience reduced depression following chronic physical activity (Martinsen and Morgan, 1997; Morgan, 1994b).

Table 9.1. Effect sizes for depression (DACL) following bicycle ergometer and treadmill exercise performed at selected intensities (adapted from Morgan *et al.*, 1971)

	Exercise heart rate in beats per minute (bpm)			
	150 bpm	160 bpm	170 bpm	180 bpm
Bicycle ergometer group (*n* = 60)	0.14	0.15	0.63	0.69
Treadmill group (*n* = 60)	0.60	0.85	0.48	0.69

The influence of acute physical activity on depression has not been studied systematically during the two decades that have passed since the publication of the above study. However, this question was addressed recently by Nelson and Morgan (1994), who evaluated the effect of 20 min of acute physical activity performed at 40, 60 and 80 per cent of predicted maximal heart rate on depression in six depressed and six non-depressed women referred from a college counselling service. The Beck Depression Inventory (BDI) was employed for the purpose of determining the presence or absence of depression, and the level of depression before and following exercise was quantified with the depression scale of the Profile of Mood States (POMS). Physical working capacity was assessed on the first day of the study, and the exercise intensities were presented in randomized order on three separate days. The depressed group experienced a significant reduction in depression following exercise at each intensity, but there was no difference in the antidepressant effect across intensities. Also, the non-depressed group did not experience a decrease in depression following exercise at any intensity. This study revealed that the antidepressant effect of exercise was transitory and that the baseline level of depression returned within 24–48 h of the acute exercise bout. Since the acute effect was noted for each exercise intensity, it would appear that an exercise prescription based on an intensity of 40 per cent of predicted maximum may be sufficient. This research needs to be replicated, and it is also necessary that the chronic effect of selected intensities be investigated as well. It is also possible that an exercise intensity based upon the individual's 'preferred exertion' (Morgan, 1994a, 1997b) will ultimately prove to possess the greatest efficacy, and this issue needs to be explored in future research.

The dark side of exercise

The potential psychological advantages of exercise are now well documented. The anxiolytic and antidepressant effects of physical activity have been discussed in this chapter, and there are additional benefits associated with regular exercise. There is empirical evidence and a theoretical rationale in support of the view that physical activity can influence self-esteem, but this topic has not been addressed in this chapter. Summaries of the research literature dealing with physical activity, physical fitness and self-esteem are available (Sonstroem, 1984, 1997; Sonstroem and Morgan, 1989). It is clear that physical activity leads to improved physical fitness, and this improved physical status is associated with enhanced estimation of physical ability. This enhanced perception of physical ability is in turn associated with an improvement in self-esteem. These positive psychological changes are well documented in the exercise literature, but little has been written about the potential negative consequences of exercise. Overtraining and exercise addiction represent two related problems that have been recognized in sports medicine for many years, and these problems will be discussed briefly. While both of these problems involve excessive exercise, the latter tends to be self-imposed whereas the former is usually governed in part or whole by another person (such as a coach).

Exercise addiction

The problem of exercise addiction or dependence has been recognized for a number of years (Morgan, 1979b). While there is an absence of epidemiological research dealing with the incidence of this syndrome, it is clear that compulsive exercise leading to self-destructive behaviour is a significant problem for a subset of regular exercisers (Polivy, 1994). The symptoms of exercise addiction resemble those of other major addictions, and individuals who are exercise dependent have been reported to experience withdrawal symptoms if deprived of exercise (Morgan, 1979b; Polivy, 1994). In a recent report by Mondin *et al.* (1996), for example, it was shown that habitual exercisers experience mood disturbance within 48 h of exercise deprivation. Indeed, it was proposed by De Coverley Veale (1987) that exercise dependence be included in DSM-IV on the grounds that the symptoms of this syndrome resemble the criteria for dependence or addiction. This problem will not be addressed in detail here, but anyone contemplating the use of exercise therapy should be aware of the potential for abuse when employing this intervention with compulsive individuals. A comprehensive discussion of this problem has been presented by Polivy (1994).

Overtraining

The problem of overtraining has been recognized in the field of sports medicine for many years. The syndrome that results from overtraining has been labelled staleness and it is characterized by a number of distress markers. Some of the more common symptoms are: anxiety, depression, chronic fatigue, increased effort sense, muscle soreness, elevated creatine kinase, elevated cortisol with decreased testosterone, elevated plasma catecholamines, elevated blood pressure, increased resting and exercise pulse, insomnia, loss of appetite, weight loss, inability to maintain regular exercise programmes and decreased performance (O'Connor, 1997). In other words, many of the positive changes associated with adoption of a physical activity programme are reversed with overtraining. Overtraining is frequently provoked by an athlete's coach, but the athlete can be, and often is, a willing participant. Also, this problem is not restricted to competitive athletes in the traditional sense. Overtraining can be one of the signs of exercise addiction, and this can occur in individuals who initially become involved in an exercise programme for health reasons.

It has been well documented that healthy young men and women experience significant increases in anxiety and depression when exercise becomes excessive (Morgan *et al.*, 1987, 1988; O'Connor, 1997; O'Connor *et al.*, 1991). Furthermore, this effect is thought to be *causal* for three reasons. First, other college students maintain baseline levels of anxiety and depression during the same period of time (Morgan *et al.*, 1988). In other words, the effect is not due to the psycho-social stressors inherent in the college environment. Second, the nature of the mood disturbance can be described as a dose–response function, and the stepwise increase in stress markers can be predictably and reliably reversed by reducing the training volume (Morgan *et al.*, 1988). In other words, systematic titration of exercise volume produces predictable mood disturbance and/or improved mood in a law-like fashion. Third, there are physiological changes that accompany overtraining (e.g. hypercortisolism), and hence the staleness syndrome possesses biological plausibility (O'Connor, 1997). Finally, it is wrong to think of this problem as reflecting psychological or physiological problems alone since a psycho-biological explanation has been shown to be the most efficacious (Morgan *et al.*, 1988).

Future directions

The research reviewed in this chapter demonstrates that physical activity is effective in reducing anxiety and depression. This applies to both acute and chronic activity, but the evidence is less compelling for the anti-depressant effect of acute exercise. While the anxiolytic effects of exercise have been shown to occur in individuals with elevated anxiety as well as those scoring in the normal range, antidepressant effects of exercise are most likely to occur in individuals with mild to moderate elevations in depression (Martinsen and Morgan, 1997). Despite these positive psycho-logical changes that are known to accompany physical activity, paradox-ical effects occur with overtraining.

There are a number of future directions that must be taken in order for research and application to advance in this area. First, it is imperative that rigorous research design and methodology be employed in future work. Second, there is a need to focus research efforts on the elucidation of mechanisms underlying the antidepressant and anxiolytic effects of exercise. Third, there is a need to study exercise prescription from a psycho-biological perspective. In this context the exerciser's needs must be considered in the formula. What is the optimal exercise mode, intensity, frequency and duration, for example, and how can the exercise prescription be personalized within the restrictions of most delivery systems?

References

Bahrke, M.S. and Morgan, W.P. (1978). Anxiety reduction following exercise and meditation. *Cogn. Ther. Res.*, **2**, 323–334.

Bouchard, C. (1988). Gene–environment interactions in human adaptability. In *Physical Activity in Early and Modern Populations* (R.M. Malina and H.M. Eckert, eds), pp.56–66. Human Kinetics.

Bouchard, C., Shephard, R.J. and Stephens, T. (eds) (1994). *Physical Activity, Fitness, and Health*. Human Kinetics.

Brown, D. R., Morgan, W.P. and Raglin, J.S. (1993). Effects of exercise and rest on state anxiety and blood pressure of physically challenged college students. *J. Sports Med. Phys. Fitness*, **33**, 300–305.

Chaouloff, F. (1997). The serotonin hypothesis. In *Physical Activity and Mental Health* (W.P. Morgan, ed.), pp. 179–198. Taylor and Francis.

Cureton, T.K. (1963). Improvement of psychological states by means of exercise-fitness programs. *J. Assoc. Phys. Mental Rehab.*, **17**, 14–25.

Desharnais, R., Jobin, J., Coté, C., Lévesque, L. and Godin, G. (1993). Aerobic exercise and the placebo effect: A controlled study. *Psychosom. Med.*, **55**, 149–154.

DeCoverley Veale, D.M.W. (1987). Exercise dependence. *Br. J. Addiction*, **82**, 735–740.

Dishman, R.K. (1987). Exercise adherence and habitual physical activity. In *Exercise and Mental Health* (W.P. Morgan and S.E. Goldston, eds), pp. 57–82. Hemisphere Publishing.

Dishman, R.K. (ed.) (1988). *Exercise Adherence: Its Impact on Public Health*. Human Kinetics.

Dishman, R.K. (1994). Biological psychology, exercise, and stress. *Quest*, **46**, 28–59.

Dishman, R.K. and Buckworth, J. (1997). Adherence to physical activity. In *Physical Activity and Mental Health* (W.P. Morgan, ed.), pp. 63–80. Taylor and Francis.

Dishman, R.K. and Sallis, J.F. (1994). Determinants and interventions for physical activity and exercise. In *Physical Activity, Fitness and Health* (C. Bouchard, R.J. Shephard and T. Stephens, eds), pp. 214–238. Human Kinetics.

Grosz, H.J. and Farmer, B.B. (1969). Blood lactate in the development of anxiety symptoms. *Arch. Gen. Psychiatry*, **21**, 611–619.

Greist, J.H., Klein, M.H., Eischens, R.R., Faris, J., Gurman, A.S. and Morgan, W.P. (1979). Running as treatment for depression. *Compr. Psychiatry*, **20**, 41–54.

Haskell, W.L. (1987). Developing an activity plan for improving health. In *Exercise and Mental Health* (W.P. Morgan and S.E. Goldston, eds), pp. 37–55. Hemisphere Publishing.

Haskell, W.L. (1994). Dose–response issues from a biological perspective. In *Physical Activity, Fitness, and Health* (C. Bouchard, R.J. Shephard and T. Stephens, eds), pp. 868–882. Human Kinetics.

Hodgdon, R.E. and Riemer, D. (1960). Some muscular strength and endurance scores of psychiatric patients. *J. Assoc. Phys. Mental Rehab.*, 14, 38–44.

Hoffmann, P. (1997). The endorphin hypothesis. In *Physical Activity and Mental Health* (W.P. Morgan, ed.), pp. 163–177. Taylor and Francis.

Holden, C. (1984). The genetics of personality. *Science*, **237**, 598–601.

Hughes, J.R. (1984). Psychological effects of habitual aerobic exercise: A critical review. *Prev. Med.*, **13**, 66–78.

Ikai, M. and Steinhaus, A.H. (1961). Some factors modifying the expression of human strength. *J. Appl. Physiol.*, **16**, 157–163.

Jankowski, K., Andrejewska, E., Endicott, J. *et al.* (1976). Effect of psychotherapy, pharmacotherapy and sport therapy on emotionally disturbed adolescents. *J. Clin. Psychother.*, **24**, 251–255.

Johnson, W.R. (ed.)(1960). *Science and Medicine of Exercise and Sports*. Harper and Brothers.

Lader, M. (1985). Benzodiazepines, anxiety and catecholamines: A commentary. In *Anxiety and the Anxiety Disorders* (A.H. Tuma and J. Maser, eds), pp. 77–83. Erlbaum, Lawrence and Associates.

Landers, D.M. and Petruzello, S.J. (1994). Physical activity, fitness, and anxiety. In *Physical Activity, Fitness, and Health* (C. Bouchard, R.J. Shephard and T. Stephens, eds), pp. 868–882. Human Kinetics.

Layman, E. (1960). Physical activity as a psychiatric adjunct. In *Science and Medicine of Exercise and Sports* (W.R. Johnson, ed.), pp. 703–725. Harper and Brothers.

Martinsen, E.W. (1987a). The role of aerobic exercise in the treatment of depression. *Stress Med.*, **3**, 93–100.

Martinsen, E.W. (1987b). Exercise and medication in the psychiatric patient. In *Exercise and Mental Health* (W.P. Morgan and S.E. Goldston, eds), pp. 85–95. Hemisphere Publishing.

Martinsen, E.W. (1990). Benefits of exercise for the treatment of depression. *Sports Med.*, **9**, 380–389.

Martinsen, E.W., Medhus, A. and Sandvik, L. (1985). Effects of aerobic exercise on depression: A controlled study. *BMJ*, **291**, 109.

Martinsen, E.W. and Morgan, W.P. (1997). Antidepressant effects of physical activity. In *Physical Activity and Mental Health* (W.P. Morgan, ed.), pp. 93–106. Taylor and Francis.

Martinsen, E.W., Raglin, J.S., Hoffart, A. and Friis, S. (1998). Tolerance to intensive exercise and high levels of lactate in panic disorder. *J. Anxiety Disorders*, **12**, 333–342.

Martinsen, E.W. and Stanghelle, J.K. (1997). Drug therapy and physical activity. In *Physical Activity and Mental Health* (W.P. Morgan, ed.), pp. 81–90. Taylor and Francis.

McDonald, D.G. and Hodgdon, J.A. (1991). *The Psychological Effects of Aerobic Fitness Training: Research and Theory*. Springer-Verlag.

Meeusen, R. and DeMeirleir, K. (1995). Exercise and brain neurotransmission. *Sports Med.*, **20**, 160–188.

Mondin, G.W., Morgan, W.P., Piering, P.N., Stegner, A.J., Stotesbery, C.L., Trine, M.R. and Wu, M.-Y. (1996). Psychological consequences of exercise deprivation in habitual exercisers. *Med. Sci. Sports Exerc.*, **28**,1199–1203.

Morgan, W.P. (1968). Selected physiological and psychomotor correlates of depression in psychiatric patients, *Res. Quart. Exerc. Sport*, **39**, 1037–1043.

Morgan, W.P. (1969a). Physical fitness and emotional health: A review. *Am. Corrective Ther. J.*, **23**, 124–127.

Morgan, W.P. (1969b). A pilot investigation of physical working capacity in depressed and non-depressed psychiatric males. *Res. Quarterly*, **40**, 859–861.

Morgan, W.P. (1970a). Physical working capacity in depressed and non-depressed psychiatric females: A preliminary study. *Am. Corrective Ther. J.*, **24**, 14–16.

Morgan, W.P. (1970b). Physical fitness correlates of psychiatric hospitalization. In *Contemporary Psychology of Sport* (G.S. Kenyon, ed.), pp. 297–304. Athletic Institute.

Morgan, W.P. (1973). Efficacy of psychobiologic inquiry in the exercise and sport sciences. *Quest*, **20**, 39–47.

Morgan, W.P. (1974). Exercise and mental disorders. In *Sports Medicine* (A.J. Ryan and F.L. Allman, Jr, eds), pp. 671–679. Academic Press.

Morgan, W.P. (1977). Involvement in vigorous physical activity with special reference to adherence. In *Proceedings, National College Physical Education Association* (L.I. Gedvilas and M.E. Kneer, eds), pp. 235–246. Publications Office, University of Illinois - Chicago.

Morgan, W.P. (1979a). Anxiety reduction following acute physical activity. *Psychiatr. Ann.*, **9**, 36–45.

Morgan, W.P. (1979b). Negative addiction in runners. *Physician Sportsmed.*, **7**, 57–70.

Morgan, W.P. (1981). Psychological benefits of physical activity. In *Exercise, Health and Disease* (F.J. Nagle and H.J. Montoye, eds), pp. 299–314. Charles C. Thomas.

Morgan, W.P. (1982). Psychological effects of exercise. *Behav. Med.*, **4**, 25–30.

Morgan, W.P. (1984). Physical activity and mental health. In *The Academy Papers* (H. Eckert and H.J. Montoye, eds), pp. 132–145. Human Kinetics.

Morgan, W.P. (1985). Affective beneficence of vigorous physical activity. *Med. Sci. Sports Exerc.*, **17**, 94–100.

Morgan, W.P. (1993). Hypnosis and sport psychology. In *Handbook of Clinical Hypnosis* (J. Rhue, S.J. Lynn and I. Kirsch, eds), pp. 649–670. American Psychological Association.

Morgan, W.P. (1994a). Psychological components of effort sense. *Med. Sci. Sports Exerc.*, **26**, 1071–1077.

Morgan, W.P. (1994b). Physical activity, fitness and depression. In *Physical Activity, Fitness and Health* (C. Bouchard, R. J. Shephard and T. Stephens, eds), pp. 851– 867. Human Kinetics.

Morgan, W.P. (ed.) (1997a). *Physical Activity and Mental Health*. Taylor and Francis.

Morgan, W.P. (1997b). Methodological considerations. In *Physical Activity and Mental Health* (W.P. Morgan, ed.), pp. 145–160. Taylor and Francis.

Morgan, W.P., Brown, D.R., Raglin, J.S., O'Connor, P.J. and Ellickson, K.A. (1987). Psychological monitoring of overtraining and staleness. *Br. J. Sports Med.*, **21**, 107–114.

Morgan, W.P., Costill, D.L., Flynn, M.D., Raglin, J.S. and O'Connor, P.J. (1988). Mood disturbance following increased training in swimmers. *Med. Sci. Sports Exerc.*, **20**, 408–414.

Morgan, W.P. and Goldston, S.E. (eds)(1987). *Exercise and Mental Health*. Hemisphere Publishing.

Morgan, W.P. and O'Connor, P.J. (1987). Exercise and mental health. In *Exercise Adherence and Public Health* (R.K. Dishman, ed.), pp. 91–121. Human Kinetics.

Morgan, W.P. and O'Connor, P.J. (1989). Psychological effects of exercise and sports. In *Sports Medicine*, 2nd Edn (A.J. Ryan and F. Allman, eds), pp. 671–689. Academic Press.

Morgan, W.P., O'Connor, P.J. and Koltyn, K.F. (1990). Psychological benefits of physical activity through the life span: Methodological issues. In *Physical Education and Life-Long Physical Activity*. Reports of Physical Culture and Health, No. 73 (R. Telama, ed.), pp. 65–72. Jyvaskyla.

Morgan, W.P., Roberts, J.A., Brand, F.R. and Feinerman, A.D. (1970). Psychological effect of chronic physical activity. *Med. Sci. Sports Exerc.*, **2**, 213–217.

Morgan, W.P., Roberts, J.A. and Feinerman, A.D. (1971). Psychologic effect of acute physical activity. *Arch. Phys. Med. Rehab.*, **52**, 422–425.

Munõz, R.F., Holon, S.D., McGrath, E., Rehm, L.P. and VandenBos, G.R. (1994). On the AHCPR Depression in Primary Care Guidelines: Further considerations for practitioners. *Am. Psychol.*, **49**, 42–61.

Nelson, T. and Morgan, W.P. (1994). Acute effects of exercise on mood in depressed female students. *Med. Sci. Sports Exerc.*, **26**, S156.

North, T.C., McCullagh, P. and Tran, Z.V. (1990). Effects of exercise on depression. In *Exercise and Sport Sciences Reviews* (K.B. Pandolf, ed.), pp. 379–415. Williams and Wilkins.

O'Connor, P.J. (1997). Overtraining and staleness. In *Physical Activity and Mental Health* (W.P. Morgan, ed.), pp. 145–160. Taylor and Francis.

O'Connor, P.J., Aenchbacher, L.E. and Dishman, R.K. (1993). Physical activity and depression in the elderly. *J. Aging Phys. Activity*, **1**, 34–58.

O'Connor, P.J., Morgan, W.P. and Raglin, J.S. (1991). Psychobiologic effects of three days of increased training in female and male swimmers. *Med. Sci. Sports Exerc.*, **23**, 1055–1061

Pitts, F.N., Jr and McClure, J.N. (1967). Lactate metabolism in anxiety neurosis. *New Engl. J. Med.*, **227**, 1329–1336.

Polivy, J. (1994). Physical activity, fitness, and compulsive behaviors. In *Physical Activity, Fitness, and Health* (C. Bouchard, R.J. Shephard and T. Stephens, eds), pp. 868–882. Human Kinetics.

Raglin, J.S. (1990). Exercise and mental health: Beneficial and detrimental effects. *Sports Med.*, **6**, 323–329.

Raglin, J.S. (1997). Anxiolytic effects of physical activity. In *Physical Activity and Mental Health* (W.P. Morgan, ed.), pp. 107–126. Taylor and Francis.

Raglin, J.S. and Morgan, W.P. (1987). Influence of exercise and quiet rest on state anxiety and blood pressure. *Med. Sci. Sports Exerc.*, **19**, 456–463.

Rejeski, W.J. (1994). Dose–response issues from a psychosocial perspective. In *Physical Activity, Fitness, and Health* (C. Bouchard, R.J. Shephard and T. Stephens, eds), pp. 868–882. Human Kinetics.

Rice, D.C., Rosenberg, D. and Radzyminski, S.F. (1961). Physical fitness of the mentally ill: The effect of hospitalization. *J. Assoc. Phys. Mental Rehab.*, **15**, 143–144.

Roberts, J.A. and Morgan, W.P. (1971). Effect of type and frequency of participation in physical activity upon physical working capacity. *Am. Corrective Ther. J.*, **25**, 99–104.

Ross, C.E., and Hayes, D. (1988). Exercise and psychologic well-being in the community. *Am. J. Epidemiol.*, **127**, 762–771.

Simons, A.D., McGowan, C.R., Epstein, L.H., Kupfer, D.J. and Robertson, R.J. (1985). Exercise as a treatment for depression: An update. *Clin. Psychol. Rev.*, **5**, 553–568.

Sonstroem, R.J. (1984). Exercise and self-esteem. In *Exercise and Sport Sciences Reviews*, Vol. 12 (R.L. Terjung, ed.), pp. 123–155. Collamore.

Sonstroem, R.J. (1997). The effect of exercise on self-esteem: Recent models and measures. In *Physical Activity and Mental Health* (W.P. Morgan, ed.), pp. 127– 143. Taylor and Francis.

Sonstroem, R.J., and Morgan, W.P. (1989). Exercise and self-esteem: Rationale and model. *Med. Sci. Sports Exerc.*, **21**, 329–337.

Spielberger, C.D., Gorsuch, R.L. and Lushene, R.E. (1983). *Manual For the State–Trait Anxiety Inventory*. Consulting Psychologists Press, Inc.

Stephens, T. (1988). Physical activity and mental health in the United States and Canada: Evidence from four population surveys. *Prev. Med.*, **17**, 35–47.

Stern, M.J. and Cleary, P. (1981). Psychosocial changes observed during a low-level exercise program. *Arch. Int. Med.*, **141**, 1463–1467.

Stern, M.J. and Cleary, P. (1982). The national exercise and heart disease project: Long-term psychosocial outcome. *Arch. Int. Med.*, **142**, 1093–1097.

Taylor, C.B., Sallis, J.F. and Needle, R. (1985). The relation of physical activity and exercise to mental health. *Public Health Rep.*, **100**, 195–202.

Weinstein, W.S. and Meyers, A.W. (1983). Running as treatment for depression: Is it worth it? *J. Sport Psychol.*, **5**, 288–301.

Zung, W.W.K. (1965). Self-rating depression scale. *Arch. Gen. Psychiat.*, **12**, 63–70.

10

Psychological factors in sport performance

John S. Raglin

Sport scientists have long been interested in identifying the major determinants of sport performance (Bannister, 1956; Costill, 1994; Lincoln, 1997). While psychological factors have been acknowledged to contribute to success in sport, research has largely been focused on the influence of biological variables such as somatotype, maximum oxygen consumption or muscle fibre type. However, some sport psychologists contend that psychological factors are of primary importance, and claims such as: '60–90 per cent of success in sports is due to mental factors and psychological mastery' (p. 1, Garfield and Bennett, 1989) are not unheard of. Assumptions such as this have helped spur the development and implementation of a wide variety of intervention techniques including mental imagery, goal setting, relaxation, confidence enhancement and negative thought stopping (Martens *et al.*, 1990). Although such methods have gained a considerable degree of acceptance by applied sport psychologists, as well as by many athletes and coaches, it has been noted that supportive research is often lacking or seriously flawed (Dishman, 1989; 1991; Morgan, 1997; Meyers *et al.*, 1996).

The case of mental imagery, the most widely used sport psychology technique for performance enhancement (Vealey and Greenleaf, 1997), is useful to consider. Mental imagery, also referred to as mental practice or visualization, has been the subject of many investigations and has been employed in a variety of ways including confidence enhancement, injury rehabilitation and technique analysis. In reviews of the literature, effect sizes for the influence of mental imagery on motor skill tasks have been fairly consistent, ranging from .43 (Druckman and Swets, 1988) to .57 (Meyers *et al.*, 1996). While the magnitude of these effect sizes may initially seem impressive, it was noted by Feltz and Landers (1983) that the benefit of imagery on motor skill is only 'somewhat better than no practice at all' (p. 25). Moreover, mental imagery studies have rarely included appropriate experimental controls in order to determine the extent to which improvements can be attributed to confounding factors such as the Hawthorne effect or the tendency to improve performance as a result of the special attention inherent in participation in the experiment

(Dishman, 1991; Morgan, 1997). The inclusion of placebo conditions in tests of putative ergogenic aids is crucial because research has shown that performance measures such as maximum voluntary force of muscle contraction often fall short of the true physiological maximum (Enoka, 1997). A related concern is the Rosenthal effect, whereby subjects alter their behaviour in accordance with their expectations of the experimental result. Hence, in some cases apparent improvements in skill acquisition or performance may be the consequence of nothing more than the special attention or obvious demands of the experimental protocol (i.e. the Hawthorne or Rosenthal effects).

There are also concerns regarding the means by which imagery is assumed to operate. A variety of theoretical explanations have been forwarded, and those that involve neuromuscular responses to imagery are among the most widely accepted. Dishman (1991), however, has noted that because imagery techniques lack kinesthetic feedback and knowledge of results, there is 'no plausible explanation' (p. 45) for how neuromuscular changes could improve motor control in many if not all sport tasks.

Applied sport psychologists uniformly agree that, to be effective, mental images of sport tasks must be highly vivid and accurate (Suinn, 1993), yet no published evidence exists to indicate that athletes possess above-average ability in imagery. Moreover, sex differences favouring males have consistently been found in the mental rotation tasks commonly used to test imagery skill (Voyer *et al.*, 1995). This implies that imagery should be less effective for female athletes. In the case of accuracy, systematic errors in both speed and object deflection (e.g. angle of a bouncing ball) have been found to consistently occur with mental imagery (Malmstrom *et al.*, 1992; Malmstrom and Perez, 1992). Negative phrasing of imagery has not always been found to degrade a perceptual motor task, as should occur if accuracy is indeed crucial for imagery to benefit performance (Lippman, 1991).

Finally, the bulk of research has been limited to tests of imagery on skill acquisition in non-athletes or novices. Literature reviews have identified no more than four published studies examining the effects of imagery with elite athletes (Druckman and Bjork, 1991; Feltz and Landers, 1983). Aside from the obvious concern over the lack of external validity, it is possible that the content of mental imagery differs dramatically between unskilled and highly skilled athletes. For example, Mark Spitz, winner of 11 Olympic medals in swimming, was once asked by his coach, Doc Counsilman, to demonstrate on land the arm movements of his freestyle stroke as he imagined making the stroke in the water. Spitz made a straight arm pull, typical of what was illustrated in swimming manuals at the time. However, when films of Spitz's stroke were examined, he was found to make a far more complex sculling motion, which Counsilman later determined to work through the Bernoulli principle (Counsilman, 1971). Counsilman concluded that Spitz had no insight into the actual mechanics of his stroke or the reasons why it was so efficient. This may well be an example of implicit memory which occurs when tasks are so well-learned that they become essentially automatic and not subject to conscious recall. A similar phenomenon, referred to as automatic skill response, was described decades ago by the pioneering American sport psychologist, Coleman Griffith (Kroll and Lewis, 1970). In contrast, explicit memory occurs at the learning stage where the skill is governed by higher level control and is under conscious awareness. This finding would suggest that teaching skilled athletes methods of making literal images of well-learned motor skills could be counterproductive and actually interfere with efficient performance.

In the absence of empirical evidence it is sometimes argued that the acceptance of psychological techniques by coaches and athletes is itself sufficient to justify their use. However, social validity, as this phenomenon is referred to, is intended for comparing the relative degree of acceptance of interventions that have already been validated (Geller, 1991). Its use in sport is constrained in large part by the widespread use of unsubstantiated ergogenic aids, a recent case being the use of biomagnetic therapy to treat sport injuries (Downer, 1997).

Because of the failure of research to clearly support many popular sport psychology interventions, it has been argued by the sport psychologist Ranier Martens (1987) that applied sport psychologists should instead rely upon personal intuition. As Martens (1987) stated: '...practising sport psychologists who use tacit knowledge derived from experience have a stronger knowledge base than academic psychologists who rely exclusively on orthodox science' (p. 45). Unfortunately, the efficacy of such intuitive approaches has proven dubious. In a study by Mahoney et al. (1987), 16 sport psychologists of international reputation were asked to examine a questionnaire on sport issues completed by elite and non-elite athletes. The sport psychologists then completed the questionnaire according to how they thought the ideal athlete would answer. Substantial differences were found between the predictions of the sport psychologists and the elite athletes surveyed ($n = 126$). For example, 30 per cent of elite athletes responded 'true' to an item asking if they worried considerably about choking during an important competition, whereas the sport psychologists unanimously indicated that choking would not be a problem for elite athletes. Major discrepancies between the predictions of the sport psychologists and the responses of the elite athletes occurred with several other questionnaire items.

In summary, the empirical support for widely used sport psychology techniques is often seriously flawed or, in some cases, altogether absent. In a meta-analysis of sport psychology research on the performance effects of cognitive behavioural techniques, Meyers et al. (1996) found no studies of elite athletes, whereas 64 per cent (37/58) involved 'participants with little or no proficiency with the sport task' (p. 157). Given such limitations, it has been proposed that the acceptance of sport psychology techniques by athletes and coaches (i.e. social validity) or the personal expertise of applied sport psychologists can obviate the need for empirical evidence. However, social validity and intuitive approaches are often misleading and the need for well-conducted, controlled experimental studies remains.

The purpose of this chapter is to provide an overview of research on the relationship between selected psychological factors and sport performance. The organization of topics will progress from the discussion of constitutional variables such as personality to transient psychological variables experienced immediately prior to or during sport. Special attention will be given to methodological issues and research concerns such as external validity. Readers interested in reviews on other applied sport psychology topics may wish to consult other recent reviews (Dishman, 1991; Meyers *et al.*, 1996; Morgan, 1997).

Psychological traits and athleticism

Coaches and physical educators have long spoken about the importance of the character of the athlete in success on the playing field. In 1888, Dudley indicated that success in equally matched athletes is generally mediated by psychological factors: '...one man has the peculiar constitution of mind and nerves to make him successful which is lacking in the other' (p. 43). More recently a similar perspective was voiced by Roger Bannister (1956), who stated: '...psychological and other factors beyond the ken of physiology set the razor's edge of defeat or victory...' (p. 225). Following the development of validated psychological measures, research was soon initiated to test these suppositions and determine if associations exist between psychological factors and sport performance. Much of the initial work focused on personality measures. Personality traits are regarded as dispositions toward behaviour that are stable across time and context. The number of core personality factors has long been debated, but most measures include dimensions related to emotionality and social adaptability (Digman, 1990).

Initial reviews of the sport literature appeared in the 1960s and they consistently reported that the personality structure of athletes differed from the general population, with athletes scoring higher in the traits of extroversion and emotional stability (Cooper, 1969; Wartburton and Kane, 1966). However, several reviews published during the following decade failed to replicate earlier findings, concluding instead that personality was not associated with either sport participation or athletic success (Kroll, 1976; Martens, 1975; Singer *et al.*, 1975). Two general explanations were offered, one being that psychological traits did not contribute to sport behaviour. Researchers were instead encouraged to focus their efforts on the examination of other factors, particularly the influence of the social environment. The other conclusion was more circumspect and proposed that, in order to adequately examine the relationship between personality and athletic performance, it would be necessary to develop psychological measures specific to the sport context. General measures of personality developed with non-athletes in mind were regarded as too broad and non-specific to be useful in sport research.

The position that personality was regarded to have essentially no role in sport performance has since been described as the 'skeptical perspective' (Morgan, 1978), whereas the other extreme, the 'credulous perspective', indicated that personality factors were highly important to athletic success (Olgivie and Tutko, 1966). These antithetical perspectives were addressed in reviews by Morgan (1978, 1980), who found that much of the sceptical literature was marred by a variety of flaws which falsely led to negative results. One widespread problem was that much of the sport and personality research lacked adequate consideration of personality theory to guide it. In an example cited by Morgan, Rushall (1970) found no differences between successful and unsuccessful US swimmers or American football players with four of the personality factors assessed by the 16-Personality Factors (16-PF) (Catell, 1972), a widely used and validated instrument. This led him to conclude that 'personality is not a significant factor in sport performance' (p.164). A related study was conducted by the English psychologist, Kane (1970), who used the 16-PF to compare personality traits between university students majoring in physical education and general studies majors. Again, no differences were observed between groups for any of the 16 first-order factors. However, Kane then re-examined the results after combining the 16 factors to form more general higher-order personality factors according to the theory underlying the 16-PF. This analysis yielded significant relationships. Consistent with previous studies, it was found that extroversion and emotional stability were each positively related to sport participation. These results highlight the necessity of using established psychological theory to guide research efforts in personality research.

Another major factor identified by Morgan (1978, 1980) as being responsible for negative results was the rarely considered potential of response distortion. Response distortion refers to the tendency for some individuals to falsify their responses in psychological questionnaires, typically in a desirable manner. Special items or 'lie scales' included in many psychological measures can be used to detect the occurrence of such faking. Unfortunately, they have been infrequently employed in sport psychology research, often because it has been assumed that athletes seldom if ever respond falsely to psychological questionnaires. There is evidence, however, to the contrary. In a study that examined the association between personality and other psychological factors in success among candidates for the US Olympic freestyle wrestling team, Nagle *et al.* (1976) found the lie score alone accounted for 34 per cent of the variance associated with success, the highest level for any psychological variable examined. Specifically, wrestlers who did not make the Olympic team were found to be more apt to 'fake good'. Other studies have also found similar tendencies for less successful athletes to distort their psychological profiles in a positive manner (Morgan and Johnson, 1978; Newcombe and Bolye, 1995). Hence, in some cases null findings may result from less successful athletes falsifying their psychological responses to resemble emotionally healthy profiles common to successful athletes. Unfortunately, Morgan's (1978, 1980) early attention to this problem has been largely ignored in subsequent sport psychology research. A recent literature review of studies of mood state in athletes revealed that only about 10 per cent employed some means to control for response distortion (Rowley *et al.*, 1994).

In summary, there is evidence that the personality structure of athletes is unique. Athletes have been found to exhibit greater emotional stability and often score higher in extroversion compared with published norms for non-athletes. While sport-specific personality profiles have not consistently been noted, successful athletes have been found to possess relatively better mental health than their less successful counterparts. The magnitude of differences between successful and unsuccessful athletes has consistently been found to be modest, with the variance of performance accounted for by psychological measures falling within a narrow range from 45 per cent (Morgan *et al.*, 1987) to 53 per cent (Nagel *et al.*, 1976). These findings contrast with both the credulous and sceptical perspectives in support of a more moderate stance between these two extremes. Longitudinal research is limited (Morgan, 1978, 1980) but indicates that the personality structure found in athletes is present before participation in organized sport and is unaffected by subsequent participation. Several advantageous characteristics have been associated with personality traits found in athletes. For example, extroverts have greater pain tolerance and also give lower ratings of perceived exertion on standardized exercise tasks than introverts (Morgan, 1981). These findings have led Morgan (1985) to propose that the absence of introversion may be more crucial to successful performance than the presence of high levels of extroversion. Hence, a successful athlete could have a profile in which the extroversion score ranges anywhere from the population norm (i.e. ambivert) to very high.

The mental health model of sports performance

A significant contribution to our understanding of psychological factors in sport performance comes from the mental health model of sports performance developed by Morgan (1978, 1980, 1985). This model, simply stated, posits that psychopathology is inversely related to sport performance. In other words, the athlete who is depressed, anxious, neurotic or psychotic will tend to perform worse than the mentally healthy athlete. Successful athletes who develop mental health problems would also be predicted to exhibit a decline in sport performance. The model stems from the results of studies conducted by Morgan and colleagues (1985), who examined the efficacy of psychological profiles in distinguishing successful and unsuccessful athletes. Athletes in various sports were studied and several investigations involved samples of elite athletes who were attempting to qualify for positions on Olympic or international teams. The results of these studies provided support for the model. Successful athletes were generally found to score lower on standardized measures of anxiety, introversion, depression and neuroticism compared with unsuccessful athletes. The mood state profile of successful athletes was also revealed to be comparatively better, particularly at times when the athletes were training intensively. Specifically, successful athletes scored lower on measures of tension, depression, anger, fatigue and confusion and higher in psychic vigour compared with published norms for the Profile of Mood States (POMS) (McNair *et al.*, 1992). This combination of low scores on undesirable mood factors and high scores for the desirable factor of vigour, has been referred to as the 'iceberg profile' (Morgan, 1978, 1980). Figure 10.1 shows mood state profiles in successful and unsuccessful candidates for the 1972 United States Olympic freestyle wrestling team. The profile of the successful wrestlers is typical of an iceberg profile.

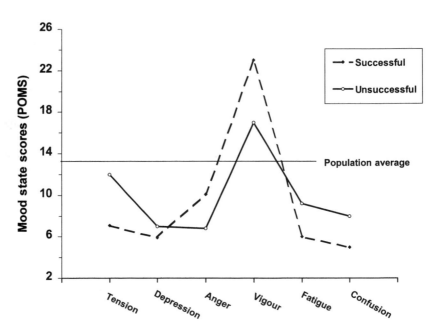

Figure 10.1. Mood state profiles in successful and unsuccessful candidates for the 1972 US Olympic freestyle wrestling team. (Adapted from Nagle *et al.*, 1975)

Although the absolute differences in psychological factors were often found to be quite small, on the basis of statistical methods such as discriminant function analysis or through clinical evaluations of the data, 70–85 per cent of successful and unsuccessful athletes could be correctly classified on average. This level of prediction was consistently better than chance but was judged insufficient to be used as a selection tool. In addition, virtually every study of the mental health model resulted in errant predictions, whereby some athletes with positive psychological profiles failed (i.e. false positives) and individuals with poor profiles were successful (i.e. false negatives). Even if the accuracy of the model was measurably improved, ethical concerns should preclude its use in selecting athletes for competition. The selection process would require the provision of psychological data on individual athletes to the coaching staff, and disclosure of confidential information is barred by professional psychological organizations such as the American Psychological Association. The pressure on athletes to participate in psychological evaluation against their will may remain present even when compliance is voluntary and disclosure provided only following written consent. For example, it has been speculated that Charlie Ward, American football player and winner of the Heisman trophy for the top college player, was not drafted to play professionally because he refused to participate in psychological evaluations used in selecting team members (Smith, 1997).

Dynamic psychological factors in the mental health model: mood state and sport training

Morgan (1985) noted that, although there was empirical support for the mental health model, its efficacy would probably be improved by incorporating dynamic assessments of psychological factors repeatedly over time. As he stated: 'There is evidence that an athlete's response to training, not his or her baseline characteristics, represents the most important issue' (p. 79). Subsequent research has provided strong support for the efficacy of serial assessments of mental health in athletes. In a summary of research conducted over a 10-year period in college swimmers and athletes in other sports, Morgan and associates (1987) found that mood state, as measured with the Profile of Mood States, or POMS, was consistently associated with the current level of training athletes were undergoing. The POMS is a 65-item questionnaire that measures the stable mood states of tension, depression, anger, vigour, fatigue and confusion. In sport research these factors are often combined to form a higher-order measure of global mood disturbance.

Studies of athletes in endurance sports such as swimming have shown that elevations in training load are associated with corresponding elevations in mood disturbance (Morgan *et al.*, 1987; Raglin *et al.*, 1992). Mood disturbances were generally alleviated following reduced training (i.e. tapers), and the profiles of athletes were found not to differ from baseline measures obtained at the beginning of the training season. This dose–response relationship between training load and mood state has since been replicated in studies of over a thousand athletes in endurance sports such as swimming and distance running (O'Connor, 1997). Research has also shown that athletes training for non-endurance sports respond similarly, provided that the training stimulus is sufficient (Raglin et al., 1995).

Rapid changes in training load can also result in significant shifts in mood state. O'Connor et al. (1991) assessed acute mood state responses in collegiate men and women swimmers who underwent an abrupt elevation in training volume from an average of 6800 to 12 075 m of daily training. Acute mood responses were determined by having the swimmers complete the POMS on the basis of how they felt 'right now'. Significant ($P < 0.05$) elevations in mood disturbance were observed within 2 days following increased training, and the magnitude of mood change did not differ between the men and women swimmers. Morgan et al. (1988) examined the efficacy of mood state in evaluating the ability of 12 male college swimmers to complete a 10-day period of intensified training. Each swimmer was to complete an average of 8900 m a day of swim training at a pace equal to 94 per cent of VO_{2max}, but three were unable to complete this regimen and their daily training loads were reduced. The POMS was completed on a daily basis and the swimmers were also evaluated physiologically. Total mood state for the entire sample increased linearly during the initial 5 days of training and then reached an asymptote. Inspection of the individual data revealed that four swimmers exhibited pronounced elevations in their total mood scores, and this subgroup included the three individuals unable to complete the training. These psychological responses corresponded closely with the physiological results (Costill et al., 1988). The three swimmers who could not complete the training had significantly lower muscle glycogen levels, and the overall agreement between psychological and physiological evaluations was 89 per cent.

The observation that mood state changes are consistently related to training load has potential practical implications concerning the staleness syndrome, a problem that affects approximately 10 per cent of endurance athletes who undergo intensive physical training (Morgan et al., 1987). Also known as the overtraining syndrome, staleness is a condition linked to chronically worsened athletic performance, medical problems such as infectious disorders and clinical depression (Fry et al., 1991; Kuipers and Keizer, 1988; O'Connor, 1997; Morgan et al., 1987). Staleness is regarded as a consequence of the failure to adapt to the rigorous training that many athletes must undergo in order to achieve their athletic potential. It is possible to avoid staleness by reducing the training load of athletes, but this is rarely a feasible option. As a consequence, efforts have been made to identify markers that can be reliably used to detect staleness in its early stages. Most research has focused on physiological variables (Fry *et al.*, 1991), and several potentially useful measures have been identified including testosterone and cortisol (Urhausen *et al.*, 1995). Unfortunately, physiological measures such as these are expensive and time-consuming to obtain, and require technical resources beyond those available to most athletes and coaches.

Because of these limitations it has been proposed that psychological assessments may serve as an alternative means of monitoring athletes who overtrain. Verde *et al.* (1992) found that, compared with putative physiological measures of overtraining, mood state assessment as measured by the POMS was more sensitive in identifying athletes at potential risk. Mood state has also been found to correlate with biological factors linked with training state (Morgan *et al.*, 1988; O'Connor *et al.*, 1989; Raglin *et al.*, 1996). With some exceptions (Hooper *et al.*, 1997) mood disturbances have consistently been found to be higher in athletes showing signs of staleness. There is also evidence that the patterning of mood disturbance differs between stale athletes and those who are able to tolerate heavy training. Research with college swimmers has revealed that POMS vigour and fatigue factor scores exhibit the largest shift for most athletes, whereas depression is relatively unaffected (Raglin *et al.*, 1991). In contrast, depression increases the most of all POMS factors in athletes who develop staleness.

Intervention studies

Some research has been conducted in an effort to determine the utility of mood state monitoring in preventing the development of staleness. Morgan *et al.* (reported in Raglin, 1993) assessed mood state on a daily basis in 40 collegiate female and male swimmers during the most intense training cycle. Training load was titrated based on deviations in mood from the team average. Individual swimmers with excessive mood disturbance had their training load reduced until their mood scores did not differ appreciably from the other athletes. The intervention operated in both directions, and training was increased in swimmers who exhibited mood state scores lower than their team mates. Raising the training load in understressed athletes is consistent with the mental health model, as athletes possessing good mental health should be capable of tolerating and benefiting from greater overload. The results indicated that none of the swimmers developed staleness, whereas in the previous 10 seasons there were no instances in which the entire team was free of staleness.

Berglund and Säfström (1994) used a similar intervention in race canoeists who were training for Olympic competition. Mood state (POMS) was assessed weekly during the training season and training load was adjusted on the basis of mood state scores. In cases in which an individual athlete's POMS total mood disturbance scores exceeded her or his own baseline value by 50 per cent or more, training was reduced until the mood score responded favourably. Training was increased when mood was within 10 per cent of the baseline value. None of the athletes developed staleness, leading the authors to conclude that altering training on the basis of mood state was useful in minimizing the risks associated with overtraining.

Unfortunately, appropriate control conditions were absent in each of the previous examples, so there remains a need to test this approach utilizing greater experimental rigour and larger samples. If these results can be replicated and generalized to other sports, then mood state monitoring, combined with selected physiological assessments, could provide an effective means of preventing the occurrence of staleness in athletes who must overtrain. Theoretically this same approach may also assist in optimizing the adaptive consequences of intensive training on sport performance.

Treatment of the staleness syndrome

As noted earlier, staleness is commonly associated with a host of symptoms, some quite serious. Along with sufficient rest from training, it is important for affected individuals to undergo medical evaluation. Appropriate attention to potential psychological problems is also warranted. Morgan *et al.* (1987) have noted that approximately 90 per cent of stale athletes are clinically depressed. These athletes typically require counselling or psychotherapy, sometimes in conjunction with antidepressant medication. There is evidence that the depression seen in stale athletes may have a biological basis. O'Connor *et al.* (1989) found elevations in mood disturbance and salivary cortisol levels during overtraining in female collegiate swimmers. Cortisol and POMS depression scores were even higher ($P < 0.05$) during overtraining in swimmers identified by the coach as stale. This finding is notable, as hypercortisolism has been used as a marker of clinical depression associated with dysregulation of the hypothalamic-pituitary-adrenal axis. Some sport psychologists have proposed that techniques such as mental imagery or relaxation can be effective in treating staleness (Henschen, 1997). However, research has not been conducted to examine the efficacy of these or other sport psychology interventions in the case of staleness. Given this lack of evidence, it is recommended that stale athletes receive conventional medical and psychological treatment until there is compelling evidence to indicate otherwise.

In summary, empirical support exists for the mental health model. The accuracy of predictions based on static aspects of the model for either athletic success or failure range from 70 to 85 per cent. While this degree of accuracy is better than chance, it is not sufficient for the purpose of selection of athletes. These findings do, however, reinforce the importance for the well-being of athletes of attending to both physical and mental health. Research has also provided support for the dynamic aspect of the mental health model. Mood state has been found to be closely associated with training load in a linear, dose–response fashion. These findings have led to proposals that mood state assessment may provide a means of reducing the risks of overtraining (i.e. the staleness syndrome). There is preliminary evidence (see, for example, Berglund and Säfström, 1994) in support of this approach, but further research is needed. The selective use of both psychological and physiological measures may ultimately provide the most efficacious approach to preventing staleness.

The mental health model is not without its critics and several recent reviews have reached unfavourable conclusions about its efficacy (Renger, 1993; Rowley *et al.*, 1994; Terry, 1993). Unfortunately, these reviews did not include mental health model research that employed a variety of psychological measures. Instead, they were limited strictly to POMS research and the mental health model was defined solely on the basis of the iceberg profile. It has been noted that these reviews included studies which did not consider the dynamic aspects of the mental health model (Raglin, in press). The results of monitoring studies consistently indicate that the stress of intense physical training results in mood disturbances in athletes, including those of elite calibre, and the failure of some research-ers to incorporate this finding has apparently led to false conclusions regarding the efficacy of the model. In contrast, results consistent with the mental health model have been reached in studies (Mahoney, 1989; Newcombe and Boyle, 1995) and reviews (Vander Auweele *et al.*, 1992) that properly distinguished its static and dynamic features.

Acute psychological factors prior to sport performance: anxiety

Research has found that acute psychological states resulting from the stress of impending competition can also have a significant impact on athletic success. State anxiety responses experienced immediately before and during competition have been considered among the most important psychological factors in athletic performance. State anxiety is defined as the level of anxiety an individual is experiencing at a given moment (Spielberger *et al.*, 1983). Psychological states are transitory and can change dramatically in intensity from one moment to the next. In contrast, trait anxiety is a more stable factor that assesses the general tendency for an individual to experience elevations in state anxiety when exposed to stressors such as sport competition.

Sport psychologists generally believe that high levels of anxiety are harmful to performance (LeUnes and Nation, 1996; Martens *et al.* 1990; Taylor, 1996). As a consequence, performance enhancement interventions have focused almost exclusively on means to reduce rather than raise anxiety (Taylor, 1996). Techniques commonly used to alleviate anxiety include hypnosis, progressive relaxation, visualization, biofeedback, autogenic training, meditation, negative thought stopping and confidence enhancement (Martens *et al.*, 1990).

The perspective that anxiety interferes with sport performance was originally developed in the field of general psychology. Among the concepts introduced, the inverted-U hypothesis, otherwise known as the Yerkes–Dodson law, has become perhaps the most widely accepted hypothesis in all of sport psychology. Yet, despite the pervasiveness of the inverted-U hypothesis, its origins lie far from sport. Yerkes and Dodson (1908) examined the effect of stimulus intensity on the speed of habit formation in mice during maze running. Electrical shocks of different strength were used and the illumination of the maze was varied to alter the difficulty of the task. It was found that higher intensity shocks exerted a detrimental effect in the most difficult maze conditions, whereas less intense stimulation aided learning. In other words, in most cases moderate intensity shocks generally resulted in the quickest learning.

Although the findings of Yerkes and Dodson concern the effects of stimulus intensity, they have since become more closely linked with arousal and anxiety (Teigen, 1994). Arousal has been defined as a generalized state of physiological activation that may range from very low (i.e. sleep) to extremely high. The physiological responses to arousal are assumed to closely co-vary and be closely tied to dysphoric emotional states, particularly anxiety (Duffy, 1957). Accordingly, the hypothesis is often interpreted in the context of anxiety: optimal performance should occur when anxiety is moderate, whereas deviations above or below this range should result in progressively worsening performance. Hence, anxiety and performance should also exhibit a relationship describing an inverted-U.

The inverted-U hypothesis has been modified for athletes to account for the task demands of different sporting events and skill levels. According to Oxendine (1970), sports that require a high degree of motor precision and minimal physical effort should be performed at a relatively lower level of anxiety or physiological arousal. Conversely, activities that require greater physical effort but less motor skill should benefit from a relatively higher anxiety. In every case the inverted-U function is maintained. It also has been hypothesized that as one's skill and experience in a sporting activity increase, so does the optimum anxiety range (LeUnes and Nation, 1996). For any given sporting event, the more skilled athletes should benefit from a relatively higher level of anxiety than less skilled individuals. With these modifications it should then be possible to establish an inverted-U for any individual, given information about the athlete's sport and skill level (Landers and Boutcher, 1997).

Anxiety has been hypothesized to reduce performance by taking up crucial cognitive (Humphreys and Revelle, 1984) and attentional resources (Easterbrook, 1959). It has been proposed that increasing anxiety or arousal will result in a concomitant reduction in the span of attentional aware-ness. As anxiety grows, cues relevant to successful performance even-tually become neglected, leading to a degradation in performance (Easterbrook, 1959). Related explanations indicate that high levels of arou-sal or anxiety interfere with cognitive memory retrieval (Eysenck and Calvo, 1989; Humphreys and Revelle, 1984). Purely physiological expla-nations have been proposed, the most common being that high anxiety leads to elevated muscle tension which in turn interferes with perfor-mance. Although elevated muscle tension is one of the most consistent physiological symptoms of chronic anxiety disorders (Hoen-Saric *et al.*, 1989), it is far less common in non-pathological conditions or in acute anxiety responses of 'normals'. Moreover, as noted by Eysenck and Calvo (1992), 'arousal, as it is assessed by physiological measures of acti-vation, seems to make no more than a minor contribution to the anxiety–performance relationship' (p. 413).

Problems with the inverted-U hypothesis

Despite the long popularity of the inverted-U hypothesis in sport psychol-ogy, and the number of interventions based on its tenets, the hypothesis has received considerable criticism. It has been noted that physiological measures (e.g. heart rate) commonly associated with arousal were not assessed in the original work of Yerkes and Dodson (1908) nor in much of the follow-up research (Teigen, 1994). Morever, the concept of global arousal has been found to be flawed. Research indicates that physiological activation is complex and not a broad and undifferentiated response (Lacey, 1971). Considerable variability also exists in central nervous sys-tem responses. Neurotransmitter systems associated with activation (e.g. dopamine, noradrenaline) have been found to exhibit 'rather different, sometimes context-dependent, functions in arousal-like processes' (p. 67, Robbins, 1997). Variables long-associated with arousal (e.g. heart rate, respiration, muscle tension) are often unchanged even during the intense anxiety experienced during panic attacks (Aronson *et al.*, 1989). More importantly, reviews of the literature have consistently found a lack of empirical support for the inverted-U hypothesis (Näätänen, 1973; Neiss, 1988). Reviews of sport research have reached similar conclusions about its validity (Fazey and Hardy, 1988; Morgan and Ellickson, 1989; Raglin, 1992). These reviews also indicated that the inverted-U hypothesis fails to account for potential individual differences in the effects of anxiety on sport performance.

Sport-based theories of anxiety and performance

As a result of the failure of the inverted-U hypothesis to adequately explain the association between anxiety and sport performance, some researchers have developed theoretical perspectives specific to athletic performance. One of the most promising comes from the work of the Russian psychologist, Yuri Hanin. The model stems from research in which Hanin assessed anxiety prior to competition in several thousand Russian athletes across a wide range of sports and settings. The Russian language version of the State–Trait Anxiety Inventory (STAI), a measure of general anxiety, was used in this work. Hanin's findings led to the development of his 'zone of optimal functioning' theory, now referred to as the individual zones of optimal functioning (IZOF) model (Hanin, 1978, 1986, 1997). The IZOF model posits that anxiety is associated with sport performance, with each athlete possessing an optimal zone or range of anxiety that is most beneficial for performance. Perhaps the most important distinguishing feature of the IZOF model is that it indicates that the optimum range of anxiety is individualized and may be low, moderate or high depending upon the athlete. Another important distinction to the model is that neither the type of sporting event nor an athlete's skill level systematically alters the optimum level of anxiety. This contrasts with the inverted-U hypothesis whereby optimum performance anxiety is dependent both on the task demands inherent in the sport and on the skill level of the individual.

The IZOF model provides two means to establish the optimal anxiety range of an athlete. In the direct method, pre-competition anxiety is assessed until an athlete has a personal best performance. Four anxiety units (approximately one-half standard deviation) are added and subtracted from this value to establish the limits of the optimal anxiety zone. Because many assessments of anxiety, sometimes over a period of years, may be required before an athlete has a best performance, Hanin developed an alternative retrospective method. In this case, athletes complete the STAI on the basis of how they recall feeling prior to their own best past performances. As with the direct method, the optimal anxiety range is established by adding and subtracting one-half standard deviation from the recalled best value. Hanin has examined the accuracy of this method and reported correlations between actual and recalled anxiety values ranging from .60 to .80. These findings have been replicated by other researchers who have found coefficients of similar magnitude ($r =$ .70 to .86) in recalls of past pre-competition anxiety after intervals of 3–4 months (Imlay *et al.*, 1995; Raglin and Morris, 1994; Raglin and Turner, 1993) to up to 22 months (Turner and Raglin, 1996). Hence, there is evidence that the recall method for establishing optimal pre-competition anxiety is sufficiently accurate for the majority of athletes, although cases of inaccurate recall have been reported (Imlay *et al.*, 1995; Raglin and Morris, 1994).

IZOF research with US athletes also supports Hanin's supposition that optimal athletic performance can occur with high anxiety for many athletes. In studies of Olympic calibre distance runners, Morgan and colleagues (1987, 1988) found that 30 per cent of women reported performing best at high levels of anxiety (i.e. one standard deviation above the mean).

Other research has found that similar percentages (30–51 per cent) of young and adult athletes in track and field events (Raglin and Turner, 1993; Wilson, and Raglin, 1997) as well as other sports (Raglin and Morris, 1994) report performing best with high anxiety levels.

Some research has been conducted to determine the impact of pre-competition anxiety on sport performance based on the IZOF model. In a study of adolescent female swimmers, Raglin et al. (1991) examined the influence of anxiety on performance. Pre-competition anxiety was assessed 1 h prior to easy and difficult competitions, and these values were contrasted with recalled-best anxiety scores. Using performance ratings made by the head coach, the swimmers were categorized as either successful or unsuccessful. In the case of the difficult meet, it was found that the successful swimmers possessed pre-competition anxiety levels closer to the optimum as established by recall than did the athletes judged to have performed poorly. Similar group differences did not occur in the easy competition, leading the authors to propose that possessing optimal anxiety may not be as crucial to performance when less is at stake. This was later confirmed by Salminen et al. (1995), who also found that optimum pre-competition anxiety had a significant impact on performance only in the case of difficult competitions.

Imlay et al. (1995) conducted a study with 16 collegiate track and field athletes in an attempt to determine if above-average performances were related to optimal anxiety zones established via the direct method. Pre-competition anxiety was assessed prior to seven competitions and performances for each meet were categorized using national collegiate standards for different events. A trend supporting the IZOF model was found. Sixty-one per cent of the athletes had their best performance when pre-competition anxiety was within the optimum zone, whereas only 31 per cent were within this zone when a poor performance was produced.

Raglin and Turner (1993) attempted to determine the net impact of anxiety on the performances of collegiate track and field athletes by comparing the IZOF model to the inverted-U hypothesis. Optimal anxiety was assessed using the STAI with the recall method and actual pre-competition anxiety was assessed prior to three indoor meets. Individual performances were recorded for each meet and were transformed using four methods: (1) International Amateur Athletic Federation (IAAF) points; (2) a percentage based on qualifying standards for national competition for the same event; (3) a percentage based on the personal-best performance of each athlete; and (4) a percentage based on the recent average performance of each athlete. These transformations allowed performance to be analysed without regard to the event or sex of the athletes. Mean performance was contrasted between cases in which pre-competition anxiety was within or outside the optimal zone established via recall. Comparisons between groups that possessed either optimal or non-optimal anxiety based on the inverted-U hypothesis were also conducted.

Performance was revealed to be better ($P < 0.05$) for cases possessing anxiety within the IZOF for contrasts based on national qualifying standards. This trend approached significance ($P = 0.06$) for contrasts based on IAAF standards. None of the tests of the inverted-U variants yielded significant differences.

In a follow-up study Turner and Raglin (1996) again examined the influence of anxiety on sport performance on the basis of the IZOF and inverted-U models in track and field athletes. Performances in three outdoor meets were transformed using three of the four methods previously described. Differences ($P < 0.05$) were found that conformed to the IZOF model for each of the three standards, and performance averaged approximately 2.0 per cent higher in cases in which pre-competition anxiety was inside the optimal range for the IZOF. Tests of the inverted-U hypothesis were conducted, but the findings were either not significant or were contrary to expectations. Contrasts were also made for cases in which anxiety levels fell below or exceeded IZOF by varying degrees, and it was revealed that performance decrements were greatest when anxiety was either just above or below the optimal zone (Figure 10.2). Larger deviations from optimal anxiety (i.e. > 1 SD) were associated with smaller decrements in performance.

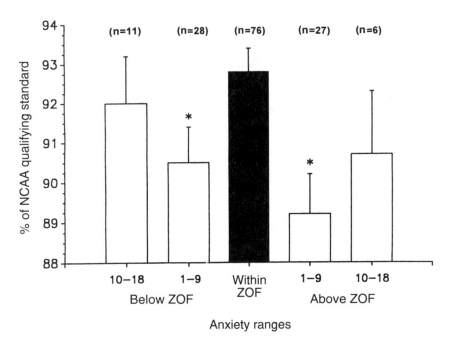

Figure 10.2. Mean performance (SE) of subjects with anxiety levels either within the optimal zone or at selected ranges above or below optimal (*$P < 0.05$). (From Turner and Raglin, 1996, Variability in precompetition anxiety and performance in collegiate track and field athletes. *Medicine and Science in Sports and Exercise*, **28**, 378–385, with permission)

Salminen *et al.* (1995) examined the efficacy of the IZOF model in Finnish track athletes, rhythmic gymnasts and ice skaters. All athletes completed retrospective recalls of best performance and assessments of anxiety within 2 h of several competitions via the Finnish language version of the STAI. Relative performance success was determined after each competition using a 10-point scale. Significantly ($P < 0.05$) better performances were found in athletes whose pre-competition anxiety fell within their own IZOF for difficult competitions. A similar trend in performance was noted for easier competitions but the difference did not reach significance.

Despite empirical support for various aspects of the IZOF model, it has been criticized for not explicitly providing theoretical explanations for why anxiety harms performance for some individuals yet improves it for others (Gould and Tuffey, 1996; Jones, 1995). While it is true that IZOF research published to date has largely focused on testing major tenets of the model rather than seeking explanations for interindividual variability in optimal anxiety, theoretical speculation may be premature given the status of the IZOF as a model. Moreover, it has been argued that the field of sport psychology has been hampered by the application of theory in the absence of an adequate data base (Kane, 1970; Morgan, 1980). As stated by Kane (1978), this may result in 'the facile shifting of theoretical perspectives to accommodate all the contemporary moods and "mini-theories" in psychology' (p. 236). Recent examples of this trend are evident. For example, the multidimensional anxiety theory of sport performance has undergone considerable changes since its inception by Martens *et al.* (1990), having recently been reconceptualized within the framework of the IZOF model (Krane, 1993) and catastrophe theory (Krane *et al.*, 1994). The substantial empirical support for the IZOF model represents an exception to this trend and this 'bottom-up' approach may avoid difficulties that can arise from premature theorizing.

In more recent work, Hanin (1997) has extended the IZOF model to incorporate the influence of both negative and positive affect on performance. Instead of using an existing measure of affect, Hanin has turned to the use of ideographic methods in which each athlete selects items from an array that he/she determines are personally relevant. This approach diverges from the trend in sport psychology to develop sport-specific psychology scales for use by all athletes. Preliminary findings from several studies indicate there is considerable variability in the profiles of positive and negative affect experienced by athletes prior to optimal performance (Hanin, 1997). Hanin has also extended the IZOF model to include emotions occurring during performance in an effort to determine if emotional states experienced during long sporting events interact with performance.

Other more individualized anxiety and performance theories for sport contexts have been recently developed. Primary among these are reversal theory and catastrophe theory. Consistent with the IZOF model, these theories each indicate that anxiety can either facilitate or harm sport performance. However, both reversal and catastrophe theory incorporate specific anxiety or self-reported arousal scales rather than the more general measures used in most IZOF research. Reversal theory (Kerr, 1989) contends that self-reported arousal is important to performance, in spite of problems noted in the literature. Arousal is interpreted on the basis of the individual's current hedonic or emotional state, which in turn is governed by the interaction of 'meta-motivational states' that exist in opposition. These meta-motivational paratelic (high arousal preferring) and telic (low arousal preferring) states can be measured through self-report questionnaires. In summarizing studies that have tested reversal theory in several sports, Kerr and Cox (1991) conclude that more successful athletes report higher levels of arousal than less successful athletes but experience these as less stressful.

Catastrophe theory involves measures of self-confidence and cognitive and somatic anxiety (Fazey and Hardy, 1988). Assessments of these factors are made using a version of the Cognitive–Somatic Anxiety Inventory (CSAI-2) (Martens *et al.*, 1990), a sport anxiety questionnaire that has been modified to assess facilitative and debilitative aspects of anxiety (Jones, 1995). Somatic anxiety and performance are assumed to form an inverted-U shaped function. In contrast, cognitive anxiety is posited to be negatively related to performance, whereas self-confidence exhibits a positive relationship. These dimensions are considered conjointly, and together combine in a complex three-dimensional form referred to as a butterfly or catastrophe cusp. Perhaps the most important prediction based on this function is that once anxiety exceeds a specific point, the decrement in performance should be immediate and severe. Also, recovery of performance requires an anxiety reduction below the level where the drop-off initially occurred. Research involving various aspects of catastrophe theory has been conducted (Jones, 1995) but, in a review of this work, Landers and Boutcher (1997) conclude that the results 'have not provided very consistent support for the catastrophe cusp model' (p. 211). The lack of evidence for catastrophe theory may be due in part to its inherent complexity which has been likened to 'a nightmare' by Gill (1994). Landers and Boutcher (1997) also contend that the theory is unnecessarily complex.

In summary, it has become recognized that traditional theories of anxiety and sport performance theories have suffered from a lack of empirical support. Moreover, the external validity of theories based on non-athlete samples has been questioned. As a consequence, researchers have recently developed models and theories of anxiety that are specific to athletes. These approaches differ and further research is needed before a decision can be made about their relative efficacy, but they each recognize the precedence of individual differences in explaining the relationship between anxiety and performance. Most important, each of these theories and models indicates that high levels of anxiety can be beneficial for performance in many athletes. Moreover, they each have progressed from assessing the single emotional state of anxiety performance to examining the influence of multiple emotional states.

Acute psychological factors prior to sport performance: cognitive strategies

A related issue concerns the influence of cognitive states experienced immediately prior to performance. Cognitive strategies such as 'psyching-up' have long been regarded as a crucial element for optimum performance. One of the earliest and most influential studies on this topic was conducted by Shelton and Mahoney (1978). These investigators had contestants at a weight lifting meet complete maximum efforts at handgrip ergometry under the condition where subjects utilized their own usual method for mentally preparing for a maximum muscular effort. Subjects were randomly assigned to either a control or experimental condition. All subjects completed a baseline trial followed by one in which they were instructed to count backwards in fours before making another maximum effort. This was done in an effort to distract subjects from employing any cognitive strategies. In the final trial the subjects in the experimental group were asked to 'psych themselves up' using their own preferred method, whereas the control subjects were instructed to count backwards in sixes. Upon completion of the study the subjects were each asked to describe the method they used to psych themselves up. The analysis revealed a significant ($P < 0.05$) difference in the ergometer value from trial two to three, with the experimental group exhibiting a 6.3 per cent improvement. In contrast, the performance of the control group decreased by 2.9 per cent. On the basis of these results the authors concluded that the psyching-up instructions favourably influenced performance. Unfortunately, a placebo group was not employed in this study, and the possibility exists that some or all of the improvement noted was a consequence of the Hawthorne effect (i.e. any treatment is better than no treatment). Post-test interviews indicated that the subjects used a variety of psyching-up methods and over half (54 per cent) used more than one strategy. Because of this it was not possible to determine if the various psyching-up methods had an equal effect on grip strength. Despite these concerns, the findings of this study have been uncritically accepted, so far as being referred to as the 'seminal paper on psyching-up' (p. 100, LeUnes and Nation, 1996). Subsequent research has provided mixed support for the efficacy of psyching-up strategies. In a review of this literature, Meyers *et al.* (1996) found that psyching strategies were superior to distraction in increasing strength, but not beneficial for tasks involving speed or balance. They also indicated that no evidence existed that such strategies resulted in elevations in measures of physiological activation, as has been hypothesized.

A recent training study paints an even more complex picture of the influence of psyching-up strategies on sport performance. Tenenbaum and colleagues (1995) examined the influence of the most commonly used cognitive strategies on strength performance. Following 3 weeks of resistance training, 45 male physical education students were randomly assigned to either a non-treatment control or one of two interventions. Subjects in the cognitive condition received training in the use of positive self-statements. The somatic condition involved practice in relaxation with visualization of best performance along with autogenic training. Subjects in the experimental groups met with instructors for 30-min training sessions held once a week for 4 weeks. Sessions were taped for home practice and subjects were also given additional assignments to complete on their own. These assignments were also used as a manipulation check to ensure

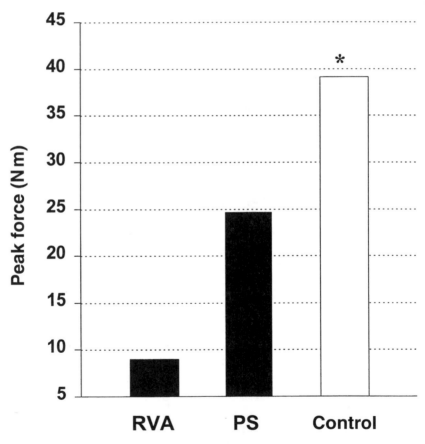

Figure 10.3. Increases in isokinetic strength following psychological intervention. RVA = relaxation/visualization and autogenic training; PS = positive; * = significantly ($P < 0.05$) different from the experimental conditions. (Adapted from Tenenbaum *et al.*, 1995)

that the subjects were practising outside of the training sessions. Knee extension strength was assessed prior to and following the 4-week intervention by means of an isokinetic dynamometer. Significant ($P < 0.05$) improvements in peak power were observed for each condition (control: 39.1 per cent; positive statement: 24.6 per cent; relaxation–visualization: 9.0 per cent) (see Figure 10.3). *Post hoc* analysis indicated that the improvement was significantly ($P < 0.05$) greater for the control group than for the performance enhancement conditions. This occurred despite the fact that baseline peak force was highest ($P < 0.05$) in the control group. This unexpected finding led the authors to hypothesize that the novelty of the isokinetic testing device required a considerable degree of concentration and may also have elicited anxiety in the subjects. However, anxiety was not assessed and, based on this hypothesis, it should follow that the relaxation condition would be more effective than the other conditions. A more tenable explanation offered was that the mental effort required by the cognitive techniques acted to divert needed attentional resources away from the task. The authors concluded by stating: 'For inexperienced weight trainers, mental preparation techniques may hinder strength improvement after relatively short periods of practice' (p. 6).

The results of this training study indicate that cognitive strategies such as imagery and positive self-statements can actually inhibit performance improvements in recreational athletes. While it was implied that more skilled athletes may yet benefit from such procedures, replication with appropriate samples is necessary. Given that the motor skills of elite athletes are highly learned and likely to involve implicit rather than explicit memory, the use of highly involved cognitive techniques may also prove counterproductive. Moreover, the generalizability of single techniques such as 'arousal enhancement' is limited because it has been found that athletes employ a wide variety of divergent cognitive techniques (e.g. relaxation or arousal). The reasons for this interindividual variability have yet to be been determined but a tenable explanation comes from the IZOF model. Athletes may employ cognitive techniques that help them to recreate the emotional state they experience prior to outstanding performances. Hence, individual differences in optimal anxiety may contribute to the considerable variation found in the types of so-called psyching techniques observed in athletes competing in the same sport. This hypothesis should be examined in future research.

Cognitive strategies during performance: association–dissociation

Athletes have been found not only to employ cognitive techniques prior to competition but also during performance. One of the most important examples of this comes from research by Morgan and Pollock (1977). Interviews with 20 participants in the Boston marathon revealed that the runners consistently employed cognitive strategies during the race, particularly during difficult or painful stages of the race such as 'the wall'. The content of the cognitive strategies used differed across athletes, but each was used to distract or divert their attention from the sensations of exertion associated with the running. Examples of methods used included imagining writing letters to friends and acquaintances, designing and constructing a house, making complex mathematical calculations, and reliving past experiences. Morgan used the term dissociation to describe these strategies and defined it as a cognitive technique intended to distract athletes from the physical discomfort, pain and exertion of intense physical work.

Support for the ergogenic effect of dissociation was found in a controlled laboratory experiment by Morgan and colleagues (1983). Maximum oxygen consumption was determined in 27 adult male non-athletes and this was later followed by a treadmill run to volitional exhaustion at 80 per cent VO_{2max}. Prior to a second run to exhaustion at this intensity the subjects were randomly assigned to either a non-treatment control or dissociation condition. Subjects in the dissociation group were instructed to silently repeat the word 'down' with each step and to synchronize their foot pace and respiration, modelling a dissociative technique used by Tibetan monks. Endurance time did not differ across trials in the control group, but the dissociation condition resulted in an 28 per cent increase ($P < 0.05$) in endurance time. The physiological responses during exercise did not differ between the control and dissociation groups, indicating that the increase in endurance time in the experimental group was directly related to the diversionary aspects of dissociation.

While recreational runners report dissociating to distract them from the dysphoric sensations associated with marathons, and non-athletes can significantly increase running time to exhaustion by dissociating, elite runners have been found to use a different cognitive strategy. In a study of 19 international calibre runners and eight non-elite runners, Morgan and Pollack (1977) found the elite runners did not dissociate during competitions. Instead they indicated paying close attention to bodily sensations such as muscle tension, fatigue and respiration. They reported using this information to gauge their pace, and they made alterations based on bodily feedback toward the goal of optimizing running economy. This cognitive strategy, defined as association, represents the conscious effort to monitor all the signs of physical exertion and moderate pace on the basis of this information. Unfortunately, the concept of association has since been grossly oversimplified in the literature. Heil (1993), for example, has referred to it as 'a widely held fallacious assumption regarding the relationship between performance and pain' (p. 167). The elite runners in the study possessed significantly higher VO_{2max} values than the non-elite athletes, and exhibited lower values on physiological factors such as heart rate and ventilation during treadmill runs at 10 and 12 miles per hour (16 and 19 km h^{-1}). But perceived exertion ratings did not differ between the elite and non-elite groups during the 10 mile an hour pace, despite the fact that indicators of physiological strain were higher in the non-elite runners.

A similar trend for some athletes to underrate physical effort has been found by Nagle *et al.* (1975). Wrestlers who were unsuccessful in making the US freestyle team had higher exercise heart rates during leg ergometry exercise at a standardized workload compared with athletes who made the team, suggesting there were fitness differences in favour of the successful wrestlers. However, perceived exertion ratings did not differ between groups. Morgan (1997) has hypothesized that these might indicate that elite athletes are more likely to use association on a routine basis. It is also possible that some athletes consistently underrate perception of effort, similar to the tendency for unsuccessful athletes to be more apt to 'fake good' on standardized psychological measures compared with elite athletes. Research will be needed to determine the reasons for these differences and to see if they generalize to other athlete groups.

Research indicates that the use of association by elite athletes during competition does not generalize to practice. Elite runners consistently indicate that they use dissociation to a far higher degree during training runs than during competition (Morgan *et al.*, 1987, 1988). Anecdotal reports of elite athletes in other sports support the previous findings regarding the use of cognitive strategies in competition and training. O'Connor (1992) reported the case of Greg LeMond, who won the Tour de France in 1989 by making up a 50 sec deficit on the final day of the race. LeMond indicated to his support crew that he did not want them to provide split times or any information on his relative position because it 'would only detract from his concentration' (p. 139). A similar sentiment was offered by the five-times Tour de France winner, Miguel Indurain, who reported not using heart rate monitors during races because 'his body acts as its own monitor' (p. 118, Elder, 1992). The example of heart rate monitors is significant. These devices are employed in the effort to optimize training and performance by assisting athletes in accurately gauging their physiological responses to physical work. Yet some professional cyclists have indicated heart rate monitors to be of little use in road races and report using them in a manner suggestive of dissociation. For example, the professional rider Neil Stevens indicated wearing a heart rate monitor not to maximize performance but to 'keep control of himself' in race stages in which his task was to maintain position rather than attempt to win. Stevens went on to state: 'If you happen to be feeling good, then the next thing you know, you're flying' (p. 118, Elder, 1992).

Empirical and anecdotal findings indicate that the cognitive strategies of association and dissociation are commonly used by athletes in endurance sports. Recreational runners have been found to dissociate in order to distract themselves from the unpleasant sensations of hard physical effort. There is also evidence that the use of a dissociative strategy can increase treadmill running endurance time in non-athletes. While these findings suggest that dissociation can aid performance, the exclusive use of this strategy may be counterproductive and increase the risk of injury because serious warning signs and symptoms are ignored. In contrast, elite athletes report relying on association during competition in an effort to gauge their pace, whereas they report using dissociation more frequently in training. Morgan (1997) has provided anecdotal accounts of athletes judiciously using both strategies in the effort to maximize performance. However, controlled research will be needed to quantify the potential benefit of this approach.

General summary

Research has confirmed the long-held view that psychological factors play a role in sport performance. Personality studies indicate that athletes are more extroverted and emotionally stable in comparison with population norms. Successful athletes possess healthier emotional profiles than less successful competitors, and are better able to adapt to the psycho-biological stress of intense training. While there are a number of reasons why psychological assessments should not be used in selecting athletes for positions on teams, these findings do underscore the importance of maintaining the psychological health of athletes.

The psychological responses to stressors associated with sport competition and training have also been found to affect performance, but in a more individualized fashion. For example, while sport psychology interventions generally involve alleviating anxiety to combat the stress of sport competition, studies indicate that between 30 and 45 per cent of athletes in many sports report performing best when anxiety is high. Physiological stressors associated with intensive physical effort result in a variety of unpleasant sensations, and recreational runners have been found to use various dissociative techniques to alleviate this discomfort. In contrast, elite runners generally pay close attention to these sensations during competition, and report using this information to optimize their pace. The stress of intensive training also has psychological consequences. Research indicates that training load and mood disturbance exhibit a dose–response relationship, but individual differences have been observed. Approximately 10 per cent of athletes who train intensively develop the staleness syndrome, whereas some individuals appear to benefit from having even greater training loads imposed upon them.

These findings have implications for many psychological techniques commonly used in attempts to enhance sport performance. In the field of applied sport psychology it is generally assumed that stress and its emotional consequences are inherently harmful for athletic performance. As a consequence, many sport psychologists employ techniques such as relaxation or confidence enhancement to reduce stress-related emotions such as anxiety. These interventions are often presented to groups of athletes or all members of a team under the assumption that each individual will benefit equally. While this perspective is intuitively attractive and likely to appeal to many athletes, research indicates that the influence of stress on performance is far more complex. Both the nature of the stressor and the athlete's responses to it must be considered, and in many cases reducing stress can be counterproductive. Moreover, the counterintuitive nature of these findings raises serious concerns regarding sport psychology practices based on personal expertise or group acceptance (i.e. social validity). The reasons why this substantial heterogeneity exists in athletes are not well understood and remain to be uncovered in future research.

References

Aronson, T.A., Carasiti, I., McBane, D. and Whitaker-Axmitia, P. (1989). Biological correlates of lactate sensitivity in panic disorder. *Biol. Psychiat.*, **26**, 463–477.

Bannister, R.C. (1956). Muscular effort. *Br. Med. Bull.* **12**, 222–225.

Berglund, B. and Säfström, H. (1994). Psychological monitoring and modulation of training load of world-class canoeists. *Med. Sci. Sports Exerc.*, **26**, 1036–1040.

Costill, D.L. (1994). Applied exercise physiology. In *American College of Sports Medicine: 40th Anniversary Lectures*, pp. 69–79. American College of Sports Medicine.

Costill, D.L, Flynn, M.G., Kirwan, J.P., Houmard, J.A., Mitchell, J.B., Thomas, R. and Park, S.H. (1988). Effects of intensified training on muscle glycogen and swimming performance. *Med. Sci. Sports Exerc.*, **20**, 249–254.

Counsilman, J.E. (1971). Application of Bernoulli's principle to human propulsion in water. In *Biomechanics in Swimming, Water Polo, and Diving* (L. Lewillie and J. Clarys, eds), pp. 59–71. Universite Libre de Bruxelles.

Digman, J.M. (1990). Personality structure: emergence of the five-factor model. *Ann. Rev. Psychol.*, **41**, 417–440.

Dishman, R.K. (1989). Psychology of sports competition. In *Sports Medicine* (A.F. Ryan and F. Allman, eds), pp.129–164. Academic Press.

Dishman, R.K. (1991). *The failure of sport psychology in the exercise and sport sciences*. American Academy of Physical Education Paper No.24, pp. 40–47. Human Kinetics.

Downer, J. (1997). What's the attraction? *Time Magazine*, 11 August, p. 81.

Duffy, E. (1957). The psychological significance of the concept of 'arousal' or 'activation'. *Psychol. Rev.*, **64**, 265–275.

Easterbrook, J.A. (1959). The effect of emotion on cue utilization and the organization of behavior. *Psychol. Rev.*, **66**, 183–201.

Elder, D. (1992) Racing with a heart-rate monitor. *Velo News*, **2**, 10 August, p. 118.

Enoka, R.M. (1997). Neural adaptations with chronic physical activity. *J. Biomech.*, **30**, 447–455.

Eysenck, H.J., Nias, K.B.D. and Cox, D.N. (1982). Personality and sport. *Adv. Behav. Res. Ther.*, **1**, 1–56.

Eysenck, M.W. and Calvo, M.G. (1992). Anxiety and performance: the processing efficiency theory. *Cognit. Emot.*, **6**, 409–434.

Fazey, J. and Hardy, L. (1988). *The Inverted-U Hypothesis: A Catastrophe for Sport Psychology?* White Line Press.

Fry, R.W., Morton, A.R. and Keast, D. (1991). Overtraining in athletes: an update. *Sports Med.*, **12**, 32–65

Garfield, C. and Bennett, H.Z. (1989). *Peak Performance Training*. Jeremy P. Tarcher.

Geller, E.S. (1991). Where's the validity in social validity? *J. Appl. Behav. Anal.*, **24**, 179–184.

Gill, D.L. (1994). A sport and exercise psychology perspective on stress. *Quest,* **44**, 20–27.

Gould, D. and Tuffey, S. (1996). Zones of optimal functioning research: a review and critique. *Anxiety Stress Coping,* **9**, 53–68.

Hanin, Y.L. (1978). A study of anxiety in sports. In *Sport Psychology: An Analysis of Athletic Behavior* (W.F. Straub, ed.), pp. 236–249. Mouvement Publications.

Hanin, Y.L. (1986). State–trait research on sports in the USSR. In *Cross-Cultural Anxiety,* Vol. 3 (C.D. Spielberger and R. Diaz-Guerrero, eds), pp.45–64. Hemisphere Publishing.

Hanin, Y.L. (1997). Emotions and athletic performance. Individual Zones of Optimal Functioning Model. In *European Yearbook on Sport Psychology,* Vol.1 (R. Seiler, ed.), pp. 30–70. FEBSAC.

Heil, J. (1993). Mental training in injury management. In *Psychology of Sport Injury,* pp.151–174. Human Kinetics.

Henschen, K.P. (1997). Athletic staleness and burnout: diagnosis, prevention and treatment. In *Applied Sport Psychology: Personal Growth to Peak Performance,* 3rd Edn (J.M. Williams, ed.), pp. 398–408. Mayfield.

Hoehn-Saric, R., McLeod, D.R. and Zimmerli, W.D. (1989). Psychophysiological response patterns in panic disorder. *Acta Psych. Scand.,* **83**, 4–11.

Hooper, S.L., Traeger-MacKinnon, L. and Hanrahan, S. (1997). Mood states as an indication of staleness and recovery. *Int. J. Sport Psychol.,* **28**, 1–12.

Imlay, G.J., Carda, M.E., Stanbrough, M.E., Dreiling, A.M. and O'Connor, P.J. (1995). Anxiety and athletic performance: a test of zone of optimal functioning theory. *Int. J. Sport Psychol.,* **26**, 295–306.

Jones, G. (1995). More than just a game: research developments and issues in competitive anxiety in sport. *Brit. J. Psychol.,* **86**, 449–478.

Kane, J.E. (1970). Personality and physical abilities. In *Contemporary Psychology of Sport* (G.S. Kenyon, ed.), pp. 131–141. Athletic Institute, Chicago.

Kane, J.E. (1978) Personality research: the current controversy and implications for sports studies. In *Sport Psychology: An Analysis of Athlete Behaviour* (W.F. Straub, ed.), pp. 228–240. Mouvement Publications.

Kerr, J.H. (1989). Anxiety, arousal, and sport performance. In *Anxiety in Sports: An International Perspective* (D. Hackfort and C.D. Spielberger, eds), pp. 137–151. Hemisphere.

Kerr, J.H. and Cox, T. (1991). Arousal and individual differences. *Person. Indiv. Diff.,* **12**, 1075–1085.

Krane, V. (1992). Conceptual and methodological considerations in sport anxiety research: from the inverted-U to catastrophe theory. *Quest,* **44**, 72–87.

Krane, V., Joyce, D. and Rayfield, J. (1994). Competitive anxiety, situational criticality, and softball performance. *Sport Psychol.,* **8**, 58–72.

Kroll, W. (1976). Current strategies and problems in personality assessment of athletes. In *Psychology of Sport: Issues and Insights* (A.C. Fisher, ed.), pp. 371– 389. Mayfield.

Kroll, W. and Lewis, G. (1970). America's first sport psychologist. *Quest,* **13**, 1–4.

Kuipers, H. and Keizer, H.A. (1988). Overtraining in athletes: review and directions for the future. *Sports Med.,* **6**, 79–92.

Lacey, J.I. (1967). Somatic patterning and stress: Some revisions of the activation theory. In *Psychological Stress* (M.H. Appley and R. Trumbell, eds), pp. 14–37. Appleton-Century-Crofts.

Landers, D.M. and Boutcher, S.H. (1997). Arousal–performance relationship. In *Applied Sport Psychology: Personal Growth to Peak Performance,* 3rd Edn (J.M. Williams, ed.), pp. 197–218. Mayfield.

LeUnes, A.D. and Nation, J.R. (1996). *Sport Psychology: An Introduction.* Nelson-Hall.

Lincoln, T. (1997). Mostly in the mind. *Nature,* **389**, 911–912.

Lippman, L.G. (1991). Positive versus negative phrasing in mental practice. *J. Gen. Psychol.,* **117**, 255–265.

Mahoney, M.J. (1989). Psychological predictors of elite and non-elite performance in olympic weight lifting. *Int. J. Sport Psychol.,* **20**, 1–12.

Mahoney, M.J., Gabriel, T.J. and Perkins, T.S. (1987). Psychological skills and exceptional athletic performance. *Sport Psychol.*, **1**, 181–199.

Malmstrom, F.V.and Perez, W.A. (1992). Imagining a bouncing ball. *Bull. Psychonomic Soc.*, **30**, 417–420.

Malmstrom, F.V., Perez, W.A., Fulero, S.M. and Weber, R.J. (1992). Measuring the speed of mental images. *Bull. Psychonomic Soc.*, **30**, 229–232.

Martens, R. (1975). The paradigmatic crisis in American sport psychology. *Sportwissenschaft*, **5**, 9–24.

Martens, R. (1987). Science, knowledge, and sport psychology. *Sport Psychol.*, **1**, 29–55.

Martens, R., Vealey, R.S. and Burton, D. (1990). Anxiety in sport. In *Competitive Anxiety in Sport*, pp. 3–10. Human Kinetics.

McNair, D.M., Lorr, M. and Dropplemann, L.F. (1992). *Profile of Mood States Manual.* Educational and Testing Service.

Meyers, A.M., Whelan, J.P. and Murphy, S.M. (1996). Cognitive behavioral strategies in athletic performance enhancement. In *Progress in Behavioral Modification*, Vol 30 (M. Hersen, R.M. Eisler and P.M. Miller, eds), pp. 137–164. Brooks/Cole Company.

Morgan, W.P. (1978). The credulous–skeptical argument in perspective. In *An Analysis of Athlete Behavior* (W.F. Straub, ed.), pp. 218–227. Mouvement Publications.

Morgan, W.P. (1980). The trait psychology controversy. *Res. Quart. Exerc. Sport*, **50**, 50–76.

Morgan, W.P. (1981). Psychophysiology of self-awareness during vigorous physical activity. *Res. Quart. Exerc. Sport*, **52**, 385–427.

Morgan, W.P. (1985). Selected psychological factors limiting performance: a mental health model. In *Limits of Human Performance* (D.H. Clarke and H.M. Eckert, eds), pp. 70–80. Human Kinetics.

Morgan, W.P. (1997). Mind games: the psychology of sport. In *Perspectives in Exercise Science and Sport Medicine: Optimizing Sport Performance*, Vol. 10 (D.R. Lamb and R. Murray, eds), pp. 1–62. Cooper Publishing.

Morgan, W.P. and Ellickson, K.A.(1989). Health, anxiety, and physical exercise. In *Anxiety in Sports: An International Perspective* (D. Hackfort and C.D. Spielberger, eds), pp. 165–182. Hemisphere Publishing.

Morgan, W.P. and Johnson, R.W. (1978). Personality characteristics of successful and unsuccessful oarsmen. *Int. J. Sport Psychol.*, **9**, 119–133.

Morgan, W.P. and Pollock, M.L. (1977). Psychological characterization of the elite distance runner. *Ann. N.Y. Acad. Sci.*, **302**, 382–403.

Morgan, W.P., Brown, D.L., Raglin, J.S. O'Connor, P.J. and Ellickson, K.A. (1987). Psychological monitoring of overtraining and staleness. *Brit. J. Sports Med.*, **21**, 107–114.

Morgan, W.P., Costill, D.L., Flynn, M.G., Raglin, J.S. and O'Connor, P.J. (1988). Mood disturbance following increased training in swimmers. *Med. Sci. Sports Exerc.*, **20**, 408–414.

Morgan, W.P., Horstman, D.H., Cymerman, A. and Stokes, J. (1983). Facilitation of physical performance by means of a cognitive strategy. *Cogn. Ther. Res.*, **7**, 251–264.

Morgan, W.P., O'Connor, P.J., Ellickson, K.A. and Bradley, P.W. (1988). Personality structure, mood states, and performance in elite male distance runners. *Int. J. Sport Psychol.*, **19**, 247–263.

Morgan, W.P., O'Connor, P.J., Sparling, P.B. and Pate, R.R. (1987). Psychological characterization of the elite female distance runner. *Int. J. Sports Med.*, **8** (Suppl.), 124–131.

Näätänen, R. (1973). The inverted-U relationship between activation and performance: a critical review. In *Attention and Performance IV* (S. Kornblum, ed.). Academic Press.

Nagle, F.J., Morgan, W.P., Hellickson, R.O., Serfas, R.C. and Alexander, J.F. (1975). Spotting success traits in Olympic contenders. *Physic. Sports Med.*, **3**, 31–34.

Neiss, R. (1988). Reconceptualizing arousal: psychobiological states in motor performance. *Psychol. Bull.*, **103**, 345–366.

Newcombe, P.A. and Boyle, G.L. (1995). High school students' sports personalities: variations across participation level, gender, type of sport, and success. *Int. J. Sport Psychol.*, **26**, 277–294.

O'Connor, P.J. (1997). Overtraining and staleness. In *Physical Activity and Mental Health* (W.P. Morgan, ed.), pp. 145–160. Hemisphere Publishing.

O'Connor, P.J., Morgan, W.P. and Raglin, J.S. (1991). Psychobiologic effects of three days of increased training in female and male swimmers. *Med. Sci. Sports Exerc.*, **23**, 1055–1061.

O'Connor, P.J., Morgan, W.P., Raglin, J.S., Barksdale, C.M. and Kalin, N.H. (1989). Mood state and salivary cortisol changes following overtraining in female swimmers. *Psychoneuroendocrinology*, **14**, 303–310.

Ogilvie, B.C. and Tutko, T.A. (1966). *Problem Athletes and How to Handle Them.* Pelham.

Oxendine, J.B. (1970). Emotional arousal and motor performance. *Quest*, **13**, 23–32.

Raglin, J.S. (in review). Personality and sport performance: the mental health model revisited.

Raglin, J.S. (1992). Anxiety and sport performance. In *Exercise and Sport Sciences Reviews*, Vol. 20 (J.O. Holloszy, ed.), pp. 243–274. Williams and Wilkins.

Raglin, J.S. (1993). Overtraining and staleness: Psychometric monitoring of endurance athletes. In *Handbook of Research in Sport Psychology* (R.N. Singer, M. Murphey and L.K. Tennet, eds), pp. 840–850. Macmillan.

Raglin, J.S. and Turner, P.E. (1993). Anxiety and performance in track and field athletes: a comparison of the inverted-U hypothesis with ZOF theory. *Pers. Indiv. Diff.*, **14**, 163–172.

Raglin, J.S., Eksten, F. and Garl, T. (1995). Mood state responses to a pre-season conditioning program in male collegiate basketball players. *Int. J. Sport Psychol.*, **26**, 214–225.

Raglin, J.S., Morgan, W.P. and O'Connor, P.J. (1991). Changes in mood states during training in female and male college swimmers. *Int. J. Sports Med.* **12**, 585–589.

Raglin, J.S., Morgan, W.P. and Wise, K.J. (1990). Pre-competition anxiety and performance in female high school girl swimmers: a test of optimal function theory. *Int. J. Sports. Med.*, **11**, 171–175.

Renger, R. (1993). A review of the Profile of Mood States (POMS) in the prediction of athletic success. *J. Appl. Sport Psychol.*, **5**, 78–84.

Robbins, T.W. (1997). Arousal systems and attentional processes. *Biol. Psychol.*, **45**, 57–71.

Rowley, A.J., Landers, D.M., Kyllo, L.B. and Etneir, J.L. (1994). *J. Sport Exerc. Psychol.*, **17**, 185–199.

Rushall, B.S. (1970). An evaluation of the relationship between personality and physical performance categories. In *Contemporary Psychology of Sport* (G.S. Kenyon, ed.), pp. 157–165. Athletic Institute.

Shelton, T.O. and Mahoney, M.J. (1978). The content and effect of 'psyching-up' strategies in weightlifters. *Cogn. Ther. Res.*, **38**, 263–273.

Singer, R.N., Harris, D., Kroll, W., Martens, R. and Sechrest, L. (1977). Psychological testing of athletes. *J. Physical Ed. Rec.*, **48**, 30–32.

Smith, T.W. (1997). Punt, pass and ponder the questions. *The New York Times*, 20 April, p. F-11.

Spielberger, C.D., Gorsuch, R.L., Lushene, P.E., Vagg, P.R. and Jacobs, G.A. (1983). *Manual for the State–Trait Anxiety Inventory* (Form Y). Consulting Psychologist Press.

Suinn, R. (1993). Imagery. In *Handbook of Research on Sport Psychology* (R.N. Singer, M. Murphey and L.K. Tennent, eds), pp. 492–510. Macmillan.

Taylor, J. (1996). Intensity regulation and athletic performance. In *Exploring Sport and Exercise Psychology*, pp. 75–106. American Psychological Association.

Tenenbaum, G., Bar-Eli, M., Hoffman, J.R., Jablonovski, R., Sade S. and Shitrit, D. (1995). The effect of cognitive and somatic psyching-up techniques on isokinetic leg strength performance. *J. Strength Conditioning Assoc.*, **9**, 3–7.

Terry, P. (1993). The efficacy of mood state profiling with elite performers: a review and synthesis. *Sport Psychol.*, **9**, 309–324.

Turner, P.E. and Raglin, J.S. (1996). Variability in precompetition anxiety and performance in collegiate track and field athletes. *Med. Sci. Sports Exerc.*, **28**, 378–385.

Urhausen, A., Gabriel, H. and Kindermann, W. (1995). Blood hormones as markers of training stress and overtraining. *Sports Med.*, **20**, 251–276.

Vanden Auweele, Y., De Cuyper, B., Van Mele, V. and Rzenicki, R. (1993). Elite performance and personality: from description and prediction to diagnosis and intervention. In

Handbook of Research on Sport Psychology (R.N. Singer, M. Murphey and L.K. Tennent, eds), pp.257–289. Macmillan.

Vealey, R.S. and Greenleaf, C.A. (1997). Seeing is believing: understanding and using imagery in sport. In *Applied Sport Psychology: Personal Growth to Peak Performance,* 3rd Edn (J.M. Williams, ed.), pp. 237–260. Mayfield.

Verde, T., Thomas, S and Shepard, R.J. (1994). Potential markers of heavy training in highly trained distance runners. *Brit. J. Sports Med.*, **26**, 167–175.

Voyer, D., Voyer, S. and Bryden, M.P. (1995). Magnitude of sex differences in spatial abilities: a meta-analysis and consideration of critical variables. *Psychol. Bull.*, **117,** 250–270.

Winton, W.M. (1987). Do introductory textbooks present the Yerkes–Dodson law correctly? *Am. Psychol.* **42**, 202–203.

Yerkes, R.M. and Dodson, J.D. (1908). The relation of strength of stimulus to rapidity of habit-formation. *J. Compar. Neuro. Psychol.*, **18**, 459–482.

11

Training for endurance and for strength and speed (power)

N.C. Craig Sharp and Yiannis Koutedakis

Aspects of training including its terminology are considered in this chapter, as is the periodization of the training year and its formatting into training units, microcycles, mesocycles and macrocycles. Training for endurance involves two quite different aspects of endurance, based on the two main metabolic pathways which meet the energy demands of muscular work: the aerobic pathway of Krebs and the anerobic pathway of glycolysis. Aerobic endurance training involves sustained work at OBLA (onset of blood lactate accumulation), while anaerobic endurance training involves interval methods of work and rest at maximal levels of effort, or resistance training with relatively low loads and high numbers of repetitions.

Training for strength involves high loading with consequently low numbers of repetitions (reps) in a training set. Training for speed involves intermediate loading, with higher rep numbers, performed fast. The product of muscle strength and speed, or of force and velocity, is power, a collective attribute which is sought by many athletes working hard in the weights room. Plyometrics may be considered as a form of power training, but as it involves high eccentric loading, which is a potent stimulus for delayed-onset muscle soreness, it has to be entered into with cautious progression. In all training schedules, the importance of adequate and appropriate rests at all stages cannot be over-emphasized.

Training for endurance

Introduction to training

Training in general for sport involves a broad spectrum of factors, involving the coaching of techniques, motor skills and tactics, backed up by psychology, biochemistry, nutrition, physiology and biomechanics, supported by medicine, surgery, physiotherapy, podiatry and osteopathy, with appropriate team selection, management and financial back-up – and in all of this physical fitness is a central component. Physical fitness for sport may be defined as the adaptation of the relevant body systems to the anticipated demands of the sport. Such fitness may be said to encompass six areas: cardiorespiratory or aerobic fitness, local muscle endurance or anaerobic fitness, muscle strength, muscle speed (the product of the latter two being muscle power), flexibility and appropriate body composition. This chapter will briefly look at aspects of endurance, aerobic and anaerobic, and of muscle power, in terms of strength and speed.

For training purposes, the sporting year may be divided into several periods, each of which contains greater or smaller subdivisons, the macro-, meso- and microcycles, the last consisting of 'training units'. Such 'periodization' has long since been formalized (e.g. Matveyev, 1966), but over the past half-century some form of scheduling has increasingly been part of serious training, especially for more complex events such as rowing, canoeing, gymnastics and racket sports. Periodization sets out the format and the time-scale of the complete training and competition plan.

Martin and Coe (1997) identify four primary aspects of the entire adaptation to training:

- An initial tissue fatigue (and even tissue breakdown) as a response to the training load (weights, anaerobic shuttles etc.). This may cause an initial reduction in performance.
- Adaptation to the training stress as a result of tissue recovery. This often results in an improved mental outlook.
- Retention and improvement of performance following a tapering of the training.
- Reduction in performance if training is decreased for too long (i.e. detraining).

Thus Martin and Coe see the training life of an athlete as a 'constant cycle of hard work (with fatigue), recovery (with regeneration), improvement in performance (for a brief period) and brief lay-off (for mental and physical rest) to permit another cycle to repeat'.

The modern competitor will often consider 1 year as a 'period', within which are contained the major championships and relevant training, although many competitors utilize 'double periodization', whereby the year is divided effectively into two competition seasons. A few outstanding competitors (and those who eschew commercialism) may operate on a quadriennial periodization, i.e. working in Olympiad blocks of 4 years, superb examples of which are quadruple Olympic champions Lasse Viren and Steve Redgrave.

The object of organizing the training year is both to optimize training improvement and to target the major and secondary competitions, in terms of tapering the training and peaking for performance. This embraces three periods (Dick, 1997): preparation, competition and transition. In phase one of the preparation period, the competitor is 'training to train', and this may last for 4 months, during which the quantity of general mixed training is progressively increased in order to be able to cope with the higher quality and intensity of work in phase two. The object of this second preparation phase is to 'train to compete', and it runs into the competiton period. Thus it aims to focus on more specific training components, matched with increasing attention to the techniques of the sport.

The competition period has three phases. Dick (1997) notes that in the first of these the competitor is 'competing to learn', and is developing and stabilizing competition performance. In the second phase, the competitor is 'training to win', and in the final phase the object is to 'compete to win'.

The third period is one of transition, in which the object is to recharge, physically and mentally, in order to go into a higher plateau preparation phase for the next half-year or year.

All training schedules are organized around the **training unit** which is a training assignment aimed at a specific aspect, such as upper body strength or leg speed. Two to several such units may be dovetailed into a training **session**, and a number of sessions form a microcyle which usually for convenience lasts 1 week (or possibly 2 weeks). A leading gymnast, for example, may incorporate 35 units into a 12-session microcycle, in a 35-h training week. The microcycle is planned so that the optimum effect is gained from each unit; for example attention is paid to alternating muscle groups, or balancing skill work with flexibility training etc. The appropriate choice of rest times, and even rest days, is just as important as training, and the art of the coach (as opposed to the technical science) is to mix and match the elements in the microcycle (and then to phase the microcycles into the longer mesocycles and then move on to the macrocycles and into the phases and ultimately the periods themselves – and beyond!).

The original concept of the macrocycle was that it was not usually shorter than 4 weeks nor much longer than 6 weeks (although some coaches think in terms of up to a 1-year macrocycle). Their end is often characterized by a need to move to a different form of training – possibly a reduction in volume and increase in intensity. The mesocycle is an intermediate period with a specific overall goal. For example, a squash second-phase preparation period may cover a 12-week macrocycle, with three 4-week mesocycles, aiming respectively at aerobic endurance, anaerobic endurance and court speed, each divided into four single-week microcycles. The training would be progressive, with the training volume or loading being increased through a microcycle and then the intensity being increased, then the volume again, in a rhythmic see-saw pattern. Each mesocycle would include training units which dovetail back to the previous mesocycle – and dovetail forward to the next mesocycle.

Training principles

All programmes must be flexible enough to cope with illness, injury, emergency, weather, work, change of location and individual lifestyles.

It is important to note some general principles which apply to all training regimens:

- **Specificity.** The effect of training is reasonably specific to its type, which means that it should be geared to the relevant energy systems and to relevant muscle groups, with their appropriate forces, speeds, fatigue patterns and ranges of movement.
- **Reversibility.** Training effects are reversible, due to either injury or illness and bedrest, or too infrequent or insufficiently intensive training, as may occur during the competiton season through lack of maintenance training (Koutedakis *et al.*, 1992). Competition edge lost by a week's injury or a few days of bed-rest should be restored in 2–3 training weeks.
- **Overload.** Adaptation to training is dependent on overload, and thus training volume and load progressively increase as indicated above. As fitness with respect to a particular component increases, a higher quality of exercise stress is needed to create 'overload'.
- **Monitoring.** This is part of progression; the programme should be sampled quantitatively, possibly by appropriate simple fitness tests or time trials, to assess progress and reset training goals and intensity.

A training programme will comprise a number of elements such as:

- **Reps** (repetitions) – specific exercises repeated a fixed number of times.
- **Sets** – a number of reps, e.g. 'three sets of 10 reps'.
- **Duration** – the length of time of the set, including any rest intervals.
- **Rests** – the time between reps and sets. Often to aid recovery such rests are 'active', i.e.the exercise is continued, but at 50 per cent of the training effort.
- **Training type** – continuous and interval are the main types, each containing a wide variety of training modes, from long, steady runs to plyometrics, or from bench presses to squash court speed 'ghosting'.

Endurance: aerobic

This depends on: (1) central delivery of oxygen, involving the lungs, blood, heart and circulation; and (2) uptake of oxygen by muscle. Let us turn first to point (1).

Following long periods of intensive aerobic training, little change is noted in lung parameters. The haemoglobin may fall to the low end of the normal range (the so-called 'sports anaemia') due to a relative plasma expansion of up to 25–30 per cent (just as occurs in pregnancy). The maximum cardiac output may increase by some 25–30 per cent, mainly through an increase in maximum stroke volume. The vascular shunt of blood from abdominal and pelvic viscera may occur quicker at the beginning of exercise (and be far less associated with the hepatic form of 'stitch', i.e. referred pain at the right shoulder), and there may be a more rapid increase in the muscle microcirculation.

If we now consider point (2), the uptake of oxygen by muscle, this involves the muscle capillary bed, myoglobin and mitochondria.

Following such training as described above, the capillary density may increase by some 50 per cent or more, as may the mitochondria, which multiply in number and increase their enzyme acitivity. Myoglobin may also increase (Reynafarje, 1962). The importance of these aerobic changes in muscle may be seen by the effects of a month of one-legged cycle ergometer training, followed by a $\dot{V}O_{2max}$ test with the trained and untrained legs respectively (Saltin, 1985). The maximum oxygen uptake when using the trained leg may be 10 per cent or more higher, with very little change in the untrained leg.

Overall, these central and peripheral muscle factors combine to determine the maximum oxygen uptake ($\dot{V}O_{2max}$), which rigorous training may increase by up to ~ 25 per cent. They also determine the proportion of the $\dot{V}O_{2max}$ which may be utilized continuously throughout the duration of the sport, from the few minutes of the middle-distance runner, canoeist or rower, to the extended periods required for team games and by the squash or badminton player or the long-distance walker, swimmer and runner or triathlete.

In general, $\dot{V}O_{2max}$ is an indication of potential aerobic endurance, but the OBLA point (the onset of blood lactate accumulation, otherwise known as the lactate threshold or anaerobic threshold) is a better guide to the current aerobic endurance status of the competitor. OBLA may occur at a 30 per cent or higher rate of oxygen intake following extensive training. After 2 weeks of bed-rest, it is not uncommon for the $\dot{V}O_{2max}$ to decline by some 20 per cent, with a corresponding drop in the OBLA point, which may take 4 or 5 weeks of training to restore. During bed-rest or lay-off there is usually a loss of lean body mass and often an increase in body fat, although body weight may not change.

The most appropriate intensity of aerobic training for sport varies according to the initial fitness level. Many modern competitors use various forms of exercise pulse-meters and, very roughly, the training-zone heart rate should just exceed the sum of the resting heart rate and 60 per cent of the difference between resting and maximal heart rates, with age-related maxima being roughly estimated as 220 less the age in years.

For general aerobic sports fitness, the duration at this intensity should not normally be below 15 or much above 40 min of continuous effort. It may be better to do interval aerobic training, for example by running a training unit consisting of a set of three repetition miles, each in, say, 6 min with a 5-min rest between each. During the rest the heart rate should fall to around 100–120 beats per minute (bpm). If it does not, then the rest intervals should probably be increased. Such aerobic intervals should be run at a constant pace, i.e. without a finishing sprint, with from three to five such training units per weekly microcycle.

Examples (for a team game or racket sport) of aerobic endurance training by running are:

Distance	Reps	Sets	Intensity	Rest interval or warm-down
600 m	8	1	2 min	2 min jog
800 m	6	1	3 min	3 min jog
1 mile	3	1	6 min	5 min jog
3 miles	1	1	20 min	6 min jog or walk
5 miles	1	1	38 min	6 min jog or walk

For health-related fitness of the general population, some of the above could be adapted to give a unit of approximately 20 min of exercise at an intensity that just makes normal talking difficult, performed three times per week. It is worth noting that the energy cost of brisk walking may well be greater than that of slow jogging, so one could be substituted for the other. Also, it is probable that two 10-min training units in a day are as effective as one 20-min unit. For women around the menopause who are keen on aerobic fitness, it should be noted, additionally, that running, walking, aerobics, dance and racket sports are better for *bone* health, in terms of postponing osteoporosis, than are non-weight-bearing aerobic activities such as swimming and cycling. Also, for the upper body skeleton, ergometer rowing, canoeing, weights or the multigym or other fixed-resistance apparatus should be employed.

Endurance: anaerobic

This usually refers to local muscle endurance which, apart from very short-lasting (up to 4 or 5 s) bursts of maximum phosphagen (creatine phosphate) effort, is a mix of both aerobic and anaerobic endurance. Anaerobic energy may be derived from creatine phosphate or from glycolysis. Training of the former is usually part of speed or power training, as creatine phosphate is the major energy source for the impulse sports and actions. Comparatively, in approximate terms, if one unit of power is the maximum aerobic contribution, then three to four units would be released from glycolysis, and up to nine units from the creatine phosphate source. Aerobic sources are often noted as being 'highly efficient' in terms of extracting energy from glycogen, and at an aerobic 37 moles of ATP per mole of glycogen-derived glucose, compared to only 3 anaerobic moles of ATP, this would appear to be true. However, muscle can derive energy at a much higher rate by metabolizing glucose anaerobically, so that it can generate three to four times as much power anaerobically, for some 20–30 s. This can be seen on a cycle ergometer, where an average young male PE student might be able to work at 250 watts aerobically, but can average 750 watts or more for 30 s mainly on glycolysis – and perhaps peak at 1400–1500 watts in the first 2 or 3 s of an all-out effort.

Because anaerobic work, energized by glycolysis, uses only glucose and extracts only about 8 per cent of the energy from the glucose molecule, glycolysis metabolizes glucose some 1200 per cent faster than if it is used aerobically. Thus, if there is of the order of 2 h of (aerobically metabolized) glycogen stored in muscle, then that same store could be depleted by some 10 min of anaerobic work. This has nutritional implications that need to be borne in mind by those engaging in micro- or meso-cycles of heavy anaerobic training.

Given that muscle relies principally on anaerobic sources of ATP when the power output puts an energy demand on the muscle greater than its more limited aerobic capacity can handle, the intensity of work for anaerobic training must be high, of the order of 80–95 per cent of maximum, in each rep. At the lower end of these figures will be competitors who may have higher levels of fast, type II fibres (especially the more glycolytic type IIb fibres); at the upper end would be those richer in type I fibres (or the more aerobic type IIa fibres). The length of the reps should be about 20–45 s to engage glycolysis maximally. Reps which are short rely too much on creatine phosphate, and those which are too long (say over 60 s) rely principally on the aerobic energy supply.

Anaerobic training is almost invariably done in an interval mode, with appropriate *active* rest periods, which may occur in a time ratio of some 1:3 work/rest at the beginning of an anaerobic mesocycle, progressively changing to 1:1 two or three microcycles later, and possibly finishing on 2:1 work/rest. The training mode usually takes the form of shuttle runs on court, pitch, gym or track; or it may involve skipping or even step-ups – or appropriate reps of swimming, cycling, rowing or canoeing. Specialized sports such as dinghy sailing or skiing or equine flat-racing have their own dry-land hiking benches, ski-agitators or mechanical horses respectively, and wrestlers work with weighted leather mannikins. On all of these, interval work is done based on similar principles of work and active rest. It is very important that the quality (intensity) of the work is not allowed to diminish through attempts to attain an over-optimistic target number. Especially in the later stages of the mesocycle, it is usually better to perform less work of higher quality.

Examples of anerobic interval training in various modes are:

Training mode	Reps	Sets	Intensity	Rests
200 m runs	6	2	30–35 s	2 min jog between reps 10 min jog/walk between sets
Skipping	10 × 3 s1		180 skips min^{-1}	2 min jog between reps
Step-ups	5 × 1 min 1		50–60 steps min^{-1}	2 min jog between reps
'Ghosting' (squash)	10–20 × 30 s	1–2	90% effort	30 s jog 5 min jog between reps
Weights	60–70	1–3	40–60% 1-RM	Perform to a rhythm, one lift every 2 ss

Anaerobic endurance may be improved by at least 20–50 per cent, depending on initial fitness levels and on the severity of the training regimen. It should be noted that most 'anaerobic' training regimens also improve aerobic fitness. For example, a training programme consisting of six reps of ergometer cycling for 20 s at an intensity equivalent to 170 per cent of $\dot{V}O_{2max}$ with 10 s rest, resulted in an improvement (over 6 weeks of four units per week) in $\dot{V}O_{2max}$ of 13 per cent, although this would be regarded very much as high-intensity anaerobic work (Tabata *et al.*, 1997). Comparing the anaerobic demands (in terms of accumulated oxygen deficit) of six reps of 20 s work at 170 per cent $\dot{V}O_{2max}$ intensity and 10 s rests, as above, with a second regimen of four reps of 30 s work at 200 per cent $\dot{V}O_{2max}$ and 120 s rests, Tabata *et al.* noted that the oxygen deficit was 69 ml O_2 kg^{-1} after the first regimen and only 46 ml after the second. The first regimen's deficit, at 69 ml O_2 kg^{-1}, was at the limit of the subject's previously measured anaerobic capacity (of 69 ml O_2 kg^{-1}), while the second regimen, at 46 ml, was well below that capacity. Interestingly, the oxygen uptake in the first regimen amounted to 55 ml.kg^{-1}, and 47ml kg^{-1} in the second. So the first regimen was the better, both for glycolysis and, as a secondary effect, for aerobic training. Nevertheless, the second regimen allowed more of the higher intensity work in total and allowed greater time for creatine phosphate recovery, and so may have been a better speed session, for which one is looking at supramaximal intensity effort for very short time periods, say 5–10 s (see 'Speed' below). This experiment is included to illustrate the potential usefulness of laboratory testing in trying to set the absolute and relative intervals for anaerobic training. As found in working very closely with squash squads (and less closely with team games), a given regimen may provoke completely different effects in sports such as squash, where the squads do not consist of the same type of relative metabolic 'clones' as, say, a rowing eight or a kayak four or a track relay squad. Following the *same* intervals of work/rest in elite squash players of similar standard, working at similar subjective intensities, near 10-fold variations in blood lactate were found between different players (Sharp, 1997), presumably reflecting very different muscle fibre profiles. Obviously, the resulting training stimuli were very different, although the schedule, on paper, was the same for all. One should beware of common training schedules for squads of individuals.

Training for strength

Strength training has been part of athletes' preparation for at least 2500 years. Archaeological reports have confirmed that the carved stones of varying sizes found in the ancient stadium of Olympia were used by Greek athletes for their strength training. During the last 60 years, strength training has been widely reintroduced, as scientific information on the development of effective programmes has become available.

Strength is generally understood to be the ability of an athlete to overcome external resistance, or to counter external forces, by using muscle. Therefore, muscle strength can be simply defined as the maximum force that can be exerted in a single voluntary contraction. However, since many of the individual movements in sport last for up to a few seconds, the entire force–time continuum, and not just the force at an instant of time, is the information required by competitors and coaches.

Strength-training principles

Strength training entails exposing muscle to exercise stimuli of sufficient intensity and duration to produce a desirable and lasting training effect. In the case of sport competitors, these stimuli should also derive from exercises that are mechanically as similar as reasonably possible to the sport in question. As for endurance training above, the main strength-training principles are overload, specificity and reversibility.

Overload

Milo of Croton was the first known athlete who, perhaps unwittingly, implemented the principle of progressive muscle overloading as early as the late sixth century BC. He carried a bull calf on his back each day until the animal reached maturity. This practice was resurrected by DeLorme and Watkins (1948) who suggested that, in order to improve strength, exercise resistance (or load) must be periodically increased. By ensuring that the magnitude of the training load is above the habitual level, the overload principle is also applicable to untrained individuals and novice athletes. Pregnancy may be regarded as a form of progressive resistance training, for both leg strength and aerobic endurance.

Specificity

The specific pattern of neuromuscular activation required to perform a resistance exercise (Häkkinen, 1989) includes aspects such as the particular muscles mobilized, types of muscle action, training loads and training velocities. In turn, this activation stimulates other systems (e.g. hormonal) which modulate the biological changes (Kraemer, 1992). In line with this concept of specificity, Komi and Häkkinen (1988) proposed a training model according to which training loads are relatively low, but the velocity of the muscle actions is high (Figure 11.1).

In general, strong similarities should exist between the training conditions and those required in the field during competition (Ackland and Bloomfield, 1995). Low-intensity strength training, for example, does not prepare the muscle for situations in which high muscle force is required. This conforms to current training strategies employed by world-class shot-putters and javelin throwers, both of whom aim to

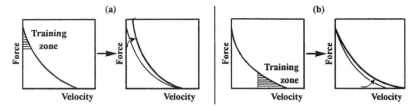

Figure 11.1. The force–velocity relationship (redrawn from Komi and Häkkinen, 1988). If the aim is to increase force levels, exercises should be characterized by high loads and low velocities (a). Alternatively, if speed of movement is the intended adaptation, then low exercise loads should be coupled with high velocity muscular actions (b).

impart maximum velocity to their implements. Nevertheless, they utilize different exercise velocities in the weight-training room (Zatsiorsky, 1995), partly because the javelin is usually released at much higher velocities (~ 30 m s^{-1}) than the shot (~ 14 m s^{-1}). It has also been found that training at low or intermediate isokinetic velocities results in peak-power improvements at low, intermediate and to some extent high test velocities, but training at relatively high velocities may demonstrate improvements only at high test velocities (Kanehisa and Miyashta, 1983). Nevertheless, it should be noted that Bell *et al.* (1989) found little advantage in adopting a velocity-specific pattern of resistance training.

Reversibility

One of the basic tenets of strength training is that of reversibility or detraining, which is a deconditioning process caused by the reduction or cessation of optimal strength-training stimuli. However, strength gains decline more slowly than the rates at which they increased (Fleck, 1994; Zatsiorsky, 1995) and several factors may affect the rate of reversibility.

The first such factor is the duration of the strength training prior to its reduction. As a general rule, the longer the training period, the slower the detraining (Moritani and deVries, 1979). A second factor is the type of muscle action. A combination of concentric and eccentric strength training, for example, will result in a slower reduction of the mean fibre area during detraining than will concentric-only exercises (Dudley *et al.*, 1991). Third is muscle fibre type. A period of 3 months without training resulted in a 12 per cent decrease in type II muscle fibre area compared to the peak training value, but no size changes were found in type I fibres (Häkkinen *et al.*, 1985). The final item is the duration of the detraining period, where it has been found that 4 weeks of reduced training or inactivity resulted in very minor reductions in muscular strength (i.e. force production) but in a dramatic decline in the ability to generate power (velocity and force combined) (Neufer *et al.*, 1987). However, a 12-week period of detraining resulted in a mean strength reduction of 18 per cent (Houston *et al.*, 1983).

Strength-training components

A single formula for strength training to satisfy the needs of all individuals of varying age, gender and fitness levels may not exist (DiNubile, 1991; Kraemer *et al.*, 1996). However, scientists and coaches agree that a well-conceived training programme should incorporate at least four distinct components: (1) optimum exercise intensity, i.e. load; (2) appropriate volume; (3) specific rest periods between sets; and (4) adequate recovery time from training (Fitts and Widrick, 1996; Powers and Howley, 1994).

Exercise intensity (or exercise load)

Table 11.1 illustrates various training intensities and their most common training effects. When an adult muscle is forced to contract at intensities which exceed 60 per cent of its maximal force-generating capacity, adaptations occur which result in increases in strength and cross-sectional area (MacDougal, 1992). Such strength-training loads may also increase fast muscle contraction patterns, possibly due to more rapid recruitment of motor units (Schmidtbleicher, 1992) and possibly better synchronization of motor unit activation.

A universal method for assessing the strength of a muscle or muscle group is by noting the maximum weight which can be lifted successfully in a single effort. This, the single-repetition-maximum (1-RM), can subsequently be used in a training prescription. For children and untrained

Table 11.1.   Strength-training intensities and training effects

Intensity (% 1-RM)	Training effect
81–100	1. Strength 2. Hypertrophy
61–80	1. Hypertrophy 2. Strength 3. Explosive strength (power)
41–60	1. Strength endurance 2. Explosive strength (power)
21–40	1. Strength endurance 2. General conditioning
1–20	No strength training effects

individuals, the 1-RM may also be estimated from the maximum weight which can be lifted 10 times (10-RM) (American Academy of Pediatrics, 1983). A table is then consulted from which their 1-RM is read off. More recently, the use of a higher number of repetitions (10–20) has been successfully used to predict the 1-RM (Mayhew *et al.*, 1992).

Volume

The **volume of training** for a given exercise may be defined as the product of the number of sets, the number of repetitions and the load (sets × reps × load). In elite athletes the relative magnitudes of these three individual load–volume components are critical. While weight lifters and body builders both attain very high training volumes, the former meet their training demands by performing many sets of low repetitions, but with near maximal load (Garhammer and Takano, 1992). In contrast, body builders usually exercise in fewer sets of many repetitions with lower loads (Tesch, 1992b), such that their most common training method consists of three to five sets (per muscle group) of eight to ten repetitions in each set at 80 per cent 1-RM. However, whether such training *is* the most effective strategy for building muscle mass is not clear from the studies to date.

Rest periods between exercises

Since the ability to generate high dynamic tensile forces in muscle appears to be the primary stimulus for strength gains, the optimization of rest periods in order to enhance the effect of subsequent bouts of muscular work is important (Baker *et al.*, 1993; Edman and Lou, 1992). Both experimental (Bilcheck *et al.*, 1993; Robinson *et al.*, 1995) and anecdotal evidence support the use of longer (~ 3 min) rather than shorter (< 1 min) rest intervals between strength-training exercises, although it has also been argued that the development of fatigue, through the reduction or elimination of rest intervals, may enhance strength development (Rooney *et al.*, 1994; Schott *et al.*, 1995). More research is needed in this area.

Recovery from exercise

Tesch (1992b) has proposed that two work-outs per week per muscle group is sufficient to induce an optimum adaptive response and that more frequent sessions may 'overtrain' muscle. This is supported by Ackland and Bloomfield (1995) who proposed a recovery period of 48–72 h between intensive resistance-training sessions.

Such positions may stem from the fact that most of the physiological adaptations to strength training are time- and energy-dependent and, in order to meet these requirements, recovery is essential.

Adaptations to strength training

Muscular

Strength gains are related to muscle hypertrophy following intensive strength training, undertaken for at least 2–3 months and accompanied by an adequate protein diet. Hypertrophy mainly occurs as a result of an increase in fibre size, but may also be due to an increase in interstitial connective tissue and in the capillary vascular bed, and arguably to a small increase in fibre number.

Force development at subcellular levels reaches a peak when there is optimum overlap and cross-bridge activation between myosin and actin; hence, the more of these contractile proteins, the greater the force development. Indeed, synthesis of actin, myosin and other proteins is a response to resistance training (MacDougal, 1992; Goldspink, 1992), particularly in type II fibres (Häkkinen *et al.*, 1985), although type I fibres do have the capability to hypertrophy following such training (MacDougal *et al.*, 1984).

Maximal eccentric actions produce greater hypertrophy than exercise consisting mainly of concentric contractions (Komi and Buskirk, 1972). It is thought that the higher forces experienced during eccentric exercises (Westing *et al.*, 1988) may provide greater physiological training stimuli, possibly by fracturing sarcomere Z lines. It should also be noted that muscle hypertrophy may not always be equally distributed throughout the whole muscle following strength training (Narici *et al.*, 1989). Finally, as with endurance training, dynamic strength-training programmes may also lead to increased type IIa and decreased type IIb size and numbers in both men and women (Andersen and Henriksson, 1977; Kraemer *et al.*, 1995). However, while transformation within the type II muscle fibre subtypes may occur with training, no transformations between type I and type II fibres have yet been reported as a consequence of exercise.

Neural

In some cases, the magnitude of strength increases following appropriate high-intensity training regimens is up to 50 per cent greater than would seem to be explained by fibre hypertrophy alone (Narici *et al.*, 1989). Many researchers have concluded that an elevated neural involvement may account for some of the exercise-induced changes in muscular strength (Häkkinen *et al.*, 1985; Ploutz *et al.*, 1994), suggesting that, at least in the early stages (2–8 weeks) of training, hypertrophy is not a prerequisite for strength gains. However, in part this may be because the combination of high intensities (> 80 % 1-RM) and low volumes of work often used in the early stages of strength-training programmes, may not provide optimal stimuli for muscle growth (Sale, 1992). As training proceeds and work volumes increase and/or change, hypertrophy may then become more dominant. Neural component change has also been invoked to explain increases in strength and power in Olympic weight lifters associated with little or no change in their muscle fibre size (Häkkinen and Pakarinen, 1993). However, it seems that strength and power increases are bounded by a genetic upper limit of neuromuscular adaptations (Häkkinen, 1994).

Metabolic (oxidative)

Apart from the expected anaerobic changes (Kraemer *et al.*, 1996), strength training may also promote adaptations related to aerobic function at fibre level. Favourable changes may include: increased capillary density (Frontera *et al.*, 1990; Tesch *et al.*, 1990), raised percentage of the more oxidative type IIa fibres (Staron *et al.*, 1991), increased levels of oxidative enzymes (Ploutz *et al.*, 1994) and elevated muscle glycogen stores (Tesch *et al.*, 1990). Protocols of moderate intensity (e.g. 8–12-RM), high volumes (i.e. many sets) and short rests (i.e. > 1 min between exercises) normally result in high lactate concentrations (Kraemer *et al.*, 1987), and an increased capillary density facilitates perfusion and lactate removal. In general, high-repetition, lower-load weight training protocols are thought to be more appropriate for such changes (Kraemer *et al.*, 1996; Tesch, 1992a).

Muscle performance: peak force and power output

The performance of some athletes (e.g. in judo, wrestling and rugby forwards in the scrum) is based on the ability to demonstrate high levels of static (i.e. isometric) force; that of others (throws, jumps and weight lifting) on dynamic (explosive or impulse) forces; and still others (running) on dynamic isotonic forces. The peak force and power output of a muscle depend on a clutch of central (neural), peripheral (muscular), mechanical and other factors (Table 11.2). Alterations in any of these factors may affect the levels of force and power output. For instance, according to the size principle, at low force motor units with a low threshold (and low fibre:neurone ratios) are recruited (Henneman *et al.*, 1965). As more force is required, motor units with higher thresholds (and higher fibre:-neurone ratios) are mobilized.

When peak force is expressed in Nm cm^{-2}, little or no difference has been observed between different muscle fibre types at zero or very low velocity (Fitts *et al.*, 1982). Training studies have shown that isometric or low velocity–high torque training results in greater improvements in peak force than high velocity–low torque muscular work (Fitts and Widrick, 1996). Low velocity–high torque resistance training also improves peak power output by promoting both intramuscular (i.e. the relationship between excitatory and inhibitory mechanisms within a muscle) and inter-muscular co-ordination (Schmidtbleicher, 1992).

Table 11.2. Selected factors that affect human muscle performance

Neural	Excitation of the motor pool	Co-ordination	Recruitment	Synchronization frequency
Muscular	Cross-sectional area	Fibre-type ratio	Architecture and shortening velocity	Type of contraction and pre-stretched state
Mechanical	Lever arm	External torque	Inertia	Momentum
Miscellane-ous	Age, gender	Temperature	Fatigue	Motivation and drugs

Practical considerations

Strength

The most popular form of resistance training is probably weight lifting. Exercises are designed to strengthen specific muscles by causing them to overcome a fixed resistance, usually barbells, dumb-bells or weight plates. Weight lifting is usually conducted according to the 'split' system, whereby a single work-out focuses on two or three major muscle groups. With this system, athletes may include all muscle groups within a 3- or 4-day interval.

It has been noted above that, in order to demonstrate muscular strength and size gains, the training load must be progressively increased (DeLorme and Watkins, 1948; Häkkinen, 1994), in at least three evenly spread training sessions per week. However, satisfactory gains of strength can be *maintained* by as little as one session of resistance training per week (Bell *et al.*, 1993), allowing the main focus of training to be shifted to the development of other performance-related parameters, such as endurance, flexibility and/or technique and competition tactics. However, it should be emphasized that strength training should not be ignored during the competition cycle.

The importance of periodization for strength training increases with the level of training (Häkkinen, 1989; Häkkinen and Pakarinen, 1993). It has been suggested that periodized training provides differential recovery for muscle fibres – according to whether light, moderate or heavy resistance is used – and may therefore provide a better stimulus for strength improvements (Ploutz *et al.*, 1994). Furthermore, by altering the intensity and volume of exercise over time, the deleterious effects of overtraining may be avoided (Fry *et al.*, 1994; Koutedakis *et al.*, 1990).

Apart from the concept of periodization, seasonal variations of strength have also been observed (Koutedakis *et al.*, 1992). It is not clear whether these variations are the direct result of specific training programmes or due to uncontrolled biological developments (Koutedakis, 1995). However, maintaining optimum muscle strength levels and agonist:antagonist ratios is generally recognized as a major component in injury prevention and in successful sports performance. For example, in moderate-velocity isokinetic knee flexion and extension (hamstring: quads), peak muscle force ratios of less than 50 per cent have been associated with low-back pain and/or injury in athletes (Knapik *et al.* 1991; Koutedakis *et al.* 1997). Hazeldine (1992) provides a good practical introduction to strength-training regimens.

Speed

In weight training for speed, loading of the order of 70 per cent of the 1-RM is heavy enough to recruit even recalcitrant type IIb fibres, but light enough to be moved fast. The number of lifts would be up to 20, done as fast as possible, rhythmically, every 5 s.

For running speed, apart from leg work in the weights room, there are various forms of interval sprint training, best done on a running track or firm, smooth grass. Some such training may be done 'overspeed', i.e. down a slight incline or even appropriately towed by a bungee behind a vehicle. Alternatively, the mode may involve sports hall shuttle-runs, or on-court ghosting for squash or badminton, with equivalents in canoeing and rowing. The work periods should last for a minimum of 5 s, but not more than 10 s. Adequate rest is extremely important, as such speed training demands the highest muscle power output, mainly based on creatine phosphate and, to a lesser extent, glycolytic energy. Hence a work/rest ratio of about 1:5 is advised, in sets of up to 10, with some 5–10 min of moderately active rest between sets.

An example of a running or squash 'ghosting' speed schedule is:

Exercise mode	Reps	Sets	Intensity	Rest
50 m sprint	5	3	Maximum	45 s walk between reps 5 min jog between sets
Court ghosting	10 × 10 s	3	Maximum	50 s jog between reps 5 min jog between sets

Other speed-training methods involve speed drills, such as running on the spot with high knee lift and exaggerated arm movements, say 20 s of 50 per cent effort with 1 min active recovery, then at 75 per cent effort with the same recovery, and finally at maximal effort with 90 s recovery. This would form one set, which may be repeated two to five times, depending on the fatigue status. *Speed work should always be done when the athlete is fresh* and thoroughly warmed up. This is the reason for the proportionately long rest periods, and also why, in mixed training sessions, the speed work should always be done first. It is also the reason why speed sessions should be halted as soon as the quality begins to fall. Improvements in speed are not dramatic, ranging from 10–20 per cent, but this can lead to an important increase in muscle power, in which speed of course is an important component. Although speed is one of the qualities that deteriorates first following lay-off, it can also be regained comparatively quickly, within weeks. Most authorities agree that a mesocycle of strength training should precede a mesocycle of speed training, and especially before plyometrics is introduced. As described below, plyometrics is an especially forceful training mode, and hence it is important that muscle and the junctions of tendon with both muscle and bone have been rendered capable of withstanding the high forces generated.

Power – plyometrics

This is a muscle conditioning system geared specifically to power. It involves stretching the muscle groups immediately prior to contraction, as occurs naturally when the volleyball spiker dips before leaping high. This prestretch induces a myotactic or stretch reflex which phases in to the contraction. The high-velocity high-loading is thought to maximize the stimuli both biochemically in terms of protein synthesis (and possibly metabolically) and physiologically in terms of possibly synchronizing motor unit activation within progressively smaller windows of time, together with a faster muscle spindle response (Sale, 1992). Plyometrics may also favourably alter the energy-storage properties of collagen, and hence of tendon, ligament and fascia (Zernicke and Loitz, 1992).

The classic plyometric exercise is the depth-jump. For example, three boxes of appropriate height (from 30 to 60+ cm) are placed 1 m apart on a sprung surface. The subject should stand on the first with knees slightly flexed and arms down, then jump down and immediately up onto the next box with a strong arm swing, and so on for up to 10 reps in a set. Up to five sets may be done in a training unit, with perhaps two units per week. However, to avoid injury it is absolutely vital to progress into plyometrics very gradually over several weeks, as the high eccentric work on landing induces unusual amounts of delayed-onset muscle soreness. Plyometric training further includes bounding and one- or two-legged hopping and fast catching and trunk twisting exercises, often with various weights of medicine ball. The important factors are maximum speed and effort, i.e. maximum intensity. Details of plyometric exercises for all muscle groups are to be found in appropriate texts (e.g. Radcliffe and Farandos, 1985).

Conclusions

The vital aspect of all training regimens is that they should be well planned, as in the case of periodized schedules, that they should contain adequate provision for rest and that they should be monitored for correct progression. Training keynotes are overload, specificity and reversibility. Aerobic training involves optimizing pulmonary, cardiac, haematological and vascular elements to optimize delivery of blood to muscle. It also involves muscle capillarization, myoglobin and mitochondria so that maximum sustained oxygen extraction is achieved, together with removal of both metabolites and heat. Anaerobic training involves optimizing both the glycolytic provision of energy and the dispersal, whether by buffer systems or removal, of the resultant lactic acid.

Strength and speed combine to give power. Strength training has been part of the athlete's preparation regimen for the last 60 years. Optimal intensity (load) of exercise, appropriate volumes, specific rest periods between sets and recovery from training constitute the main components of such training. Well-conceived strength-, speed- and power-training programmes may result in positive muscular, neural and metabolic adaptations which can be maintained for as long as there is a steady flow of stimuli. However, an all-embracing formula for strength and power training which satisfies the needs of all individuals according to their age, gender and fitness levels has yet to be found.

Two excellent practical texts relating to training are those by Dick (1997) and Martin and Coe (1997).

Acknowledgement

NCCS would like to express great gratitude to his early coaches George Munro, Bill Armour and Andy Forbes of Victoria Park AAC Glasgow, and Haydn Davies of the Edinburgh Sports Club. He would also like to express his admiration and gratitude to five modern coaching greats, John Atkinson, John Anderson, Harry Wilson, Frank Dick and the late Ron Emes. So good are they, that with them he has always felt more than a nagging doubt that 'the sports physiologist rides in the dung cart of progress, telling the world the way it has gone' (to paraphrase Humphrey Lyttelton). At the least, he hopes that a little of their remarkable collective wisdom is reflected above.

References

Ackland, T.R. and Bloomfield, J. (1995). Applied anatomy. In *Science and Medicine in Sport* (J. Bloomfield, P.A. Fricker and K.D. Fitch, eds), pp. 2–31. Blackwell.

American Academy of Pediatrics (1983). Weight training and weight lifting: information for the pediatrician. *Phys. Sportsmed.*, **11**, 157–161.

Andersen, P. and Henriksson, J. (1977). Training induced changes in the subgroups of human type II skeletal muscle fibres. *Acta Physiol. Scand.*, **99**, 123–125.

Baker, A.J., Kustov, K.G., Miller, R.G. and Weiner, M.W. (1993). Slow force recovery after long duration exercise: Metabolism and activation factors in muscle fatigue. *J. Appl. Physiol.*, **74**, 2294–2300.

Bell, G.J., Syrotiuk, D.G., Attwood, K. and Quinney, H.A. (1993). Maintenance of strength gains while performing endurance training in oarswomen. *Can. J. Appl. Physiol.*, **18**, 104–115.

Bell, G.J., Patersen, S.R., Quinney, H.A. and Wenger, H.A. (1989). The effect of velocity specific strength training on peak torque and anaerobic rowing power. *J. Sports Sci.*, **7**, 205–214.

Bilcheck, H.M., Kraemer, W.J., Maresh, C.M. and Zito, M.A. (1993). The effects of isokinetic fatigue on recovery of maximal isokinetic concentric and eccentric strength in women . *J. Str. Cond. Res.*, **7**, 43–50.

Davies, C.T.M. (1985). Strength and mechanical properties of muscle in children and young adults. *Scand. J. Sports Sci.*, **7**, 11–15.

DeLorme, T. and Watkins, A. (1948). Techniques of progressive resistance exercise. *Arch. Phys. Rehab. Med.*, **29**, 263–266.

DiNubile, N. (1991). Strength training. *Clin. Sports Med.*, **10**, 33–63.

Dudley, G.A., Tesch, P.A., Miller, B.J. and Buchannan, P. (1991). Importance of eccentric actions in performance adaptations to resistance training. *Aviat. Space Environ. Med.*, **62**, 543–550.

Edman, K.A.P. and Lou, F. (1992). Myofibrillar fatigue versus failure of activation during repetitive stimulation of frog muscle fibres. *J. Physiol.*, **457**, 655–673.

Fitts, R.H. and Widrick, J.J. (1996). Muscle mechanisms: adaptations with exercise training. *Exerc. Sport Sci. Rev.*, **24**, 427–473.

Fitts, R.H., Courtright, J.B., Kim, D.H. and Witzmann, F.A. (1982). Muscle fatigue with prolonged exercise: contractile and biochemical alterations. *Am. J. Physiol.*, **242**, C65–C73.

Fleck, S.J. (1994). Detraining: Its effects on endurance and strength. *J. Str. Cond. Res*, **16**, 22–28.

Frontera, W.R., Meredith, C.N., O' Reilly, K.P. and Evans, W.J. (1990). Strength training and determinants of $\dot{V}O_2$ max in older men. *J. Appl. Physiol.*, **68**, 329–333.

Fry, A.C., Kraemer, W.J., van Borselen, F. *et al.* (1994). Catecholamine responses to short-term, high intensity resistance exercise overtraining. *J. Appl. Physiol.,* **77,** 941–946.

Garhammer, J. and Takano, B. (1992). Training for weightlifting. In *The Encyclopaedia of Sports Medicine: Strength and Power* (P. Komi, ed.), pp. 357–369. Blackwell.

Goldspink, G. (1992). Cellular and molecular aspects of adaptation in skeletal muscle. In *The Encyclopaedia of Sports Medicine: Strength and Power* (P. Komi, ed.), pp. 211–229. Blackwell.

Häkkinen, K. (1994). Neuromuscular adaptation during strength training, detraining and immobilisation. *Crit. Rev. Phys. Rehabil. Med.,* **6,** 161–198.

Häkkinen, K. (1989). Neuromuscular and hormonal adaptations during strength and power training. A review. *J. Sports Med.,* **29,** 9–26.

·Häkkinen, K. and Pakarinen, A. (1993). Muscle strength and serum testosterone, cortisol and SHBG concentrations in middle-aged and elderly men and women. *Acta Physiol. Scand.,* **148,** 199–207.

Häkkinen, K., Alen, M. and Komi, P.V. (1985). Changes in isometric force- and relaxation-time, electromyographic and muscle fibre characteristics of human skeletal muscle during strength training and detraining. *Acta Physiol. Scand.,* **125,** 573–585.

Henneman, E., Somjen, G. and Carpenter, D.O. (1965). Functional significance of cell size in spinal motoneurons. *J. Neurophysiol.,* **28,** 560–580.

Houston, M.E., Froese, E.A., Valeriote, P. *et al.* (1983). Muscle performance, morphology and metabolic capacity during strength training and detraining: a one leg model. *Eur. J. Appl. Physiol.,* **51,** 25–35.

Kanehisa, H. and Miyashita, M. (1983). Specificity of velocity in strength training. *Eur. J. Appl. Physiol.,* **52,** 104–106.

Knapik, J.J., Bauman, C.L., Jones, B.H. *et al.* (1991). Preseason strength and flexibility imbalances associated with athletic injuries in female collegiate athletes. *Am. J. Sports Med.,* **19,** 76–81.

Komi, P.V. and Häkkinen, K. (1988). Strength and power. In *The Encyclopaedia of Sports Medicine: The Olympic Book of Sports Medicine, Volume 1* (A. Dirix., H.G. Knuttgen and K. Tittel, eds), pp. 181–193. Blackwell.

Komi, P.V. and Buskirk, E.R. (1972). Effect of eccentric and concentric muscle conditioning on tension and electrical activity of human muscle. *Ergonomics,* **15,** 417–434.

Koutedakis, Y. (1995). Seasonal variations in fitness parameters in competitive athletes. *Sports Med.,* **19,** 373–392.

Koutedakis, Y., Frischknecht, R. and Murphy, M. (1997). Knee flexion to extension peak torque ratios and low-back injuries in highly active individuals. *Int. J. Sports Med.,* **18,** 290–295.

Koutedakis, Y., Budget, R. and Faulmann, L. (1990). Rest and under-performing elite competitors. *Br. J. Sports Med.,* **24,** 248–252.

Koutedakis, Y., Boreham, C., Kabitsis, C. and Sharp, N.C.C. (1992). Seasonal deterioration of selected physiological variables in elite male skiers. *Int. J. Sports Med.,* **13,** 548–551.

Kraemer, W.J. (1992). Endocrine responses and adaptations to strength training. In *The Encyclopaedia of Sports Medicine: Strength and Power in Sport* (P. Komi, ed.), pp. 291–304. Blackwell.

Kraemer, W.J., Fleck, S.J. and Evens, W.J. (1996). Strength and power training: Physiological mechanisms of adaptation. *Exerc. Sport Sci. Rev.,* **24,** 363–397.

Kraemer, W.J., Patton, J., Gordon, S.E. *et al.* (1995). Compatibility of high intensity strength and endurance training on hormonal and skeletal muscle adaptations. *J. Appl. Physiol.,* **78,** 976–989.

Kraemer, W.J., Noble, B.J., Clark, M.J. and Culver, B.W. (1987). Physiologic responses to heavy-resistance exercise with very short rest periods. *Int. J. Sports Med.,* **8,** 247–252.

MacDougal, J.D. (1992). Hypertrophy or hyperplasia. In *The Encyclopaedia of Sports Medicine: Strength and Power* (P. Komi, ed.), pp. 230–238. Blackwell.

MacDougall, J.D., Sale, D.G., Alway, S.E. and Sutton, J.R. (1984). Muscle fiber number in biceps brachii in bodybuilders and control subjects. *J. Appl. Physiol.,* **57,** 1399–1403.

Matveyev, L.P. (1966): quoted in Dick, F. (1997). *Sports Training and Coaching*, p. 255. A. and C. Black.

Mayhew, J.L., Ball, T.E., Arnold, M.D. and Bowen, J.C. (1992). Relative muscular endurance performance as a predictor of bench press strength in college men and women. *J. Appl. Sports Sci. Res.*, **6**, 200–206.

Moritani, T. and deVries, H. (1979). Neural factors versus hypertrophy in the time course of muscle strength gain. *Am. J. Phys. Med.*, **158**, 115–130.

Narici, M.V., Roi, G.S., Landoni, L. *et al.* (1989). Changes in force cross-sectional area and neural activation during strength training and detraining of the human quadriceps. *Eur. J. Appl. Physiol.*, **59**, 310–319.

Neufer, P.D., Costill, D.L., Fielding, R.A., Flynn, M.G. and Kirwan, J.P. (1987). Effect of reduced training on muscular strength and endurance in competitive swimmers. *Med. Sci. Sports Exerc.*, **19**, 486–490.

Ploutz, L.L, Tesch, P.A., Biro, R.L.and Dudley, G.A. (1994). Effect of resistance training on muscle use during exercise. *J. Appl. Physiol.*, 76, 1675–1681.

Powers, S.K. and Howley, E.T. (1994). *Exercise Physiology: Theory and Application to Fitness and Performance*, 2nd Edn. Wm. C. Brown Communications, Inc.

Reynafarje, B. (1962). Myoglobin content and enzymatic activity of muscle and altitude adaptation. *J. Appl. Physiol.*, **9**, 301–305.

Robinson, J.M., Stone, M.H., Johnson, R.L. *et al.* (1995). Effects of different weight training exercise/rest intervals on strength , power and high intensity exercise endurance. *J. Str. Cond. Res.*, b, 216–221.

Rooney, K.J., Herbert, R.D.and Balnave, R.J. (1994). Fatigue contributes to the strength training stimulus. *Med. Sci. Sport Exerc.*, **26**, 1160–1164.

Sale, D.G. (1992). Neural adaptations to strength training. In *The Encyclopaedia of Sports Medicine: Strength and Power* (P. Komi, ed.), pp. 249–265. Blackwell.

Saltin, B. (1985). The physiological and chemical basis of aerobic and anaerobic capacities in man: effect of training and range of adaptation. *Proc.5th Biennial Conference on Exercise, Nutrition and Performance* (P. Russo and G. Gass, eds), pp. 41–78. Cumberland College of Health Sciences.

Schmidtbleicher, D. (1992). Training for power events. In *The Encyclopaedia of Sports Medicine: Strength and Power* (P. Komi, ed.), pp. 381–395. Blackwell.

Schott, J., McCully, K. and Rutherford, O.M. (1995). The role of metabolites in strength training: Short versus long isometric contractions. *Eur. J. Appl. Physiol.*, **71**, 337–341.

Sharp, N.C.C. (1997). Physiological aspects of squash. In *Science and Racket Sports* (T. Reilly and R.E. Eston, eds). F.N. Spon.

Staron, R.S., Leonardi, M.J., Karapondo, D.L., Malicky, E.S., Falkel, J.E., Hagerman, F.C. and Hikida, R.S. (1991). Strength and skeletal muscle adaptations in heavy-resistance trained women after detraining and retraining. *J. Appl. Physiol.*, **70**, 631–640.

Tabata, I., Irishawa, K., Kuzaki, M., Nishimura, K., Ogita, F. and Miyachi, M. (1997). Metabolic profile of high intensity exercises. *Med. Sci. Sports Exerc.*, **29**(3), 390–395.

Tesch, P.A. (1992a). Short- and long-term histochemical and biochemical adaptations in muscle. In *The Encyclopaedia of Sports Medicine: Strength and Power* (P. Komi, ed.), pp. 239–248. Blackwell.

Tesch, P.A. (1992b). Training for body building. In *The Encyclopaedia of Sports Medicine: Strength and Power* (P. Komi, ed.), pp. 370–380. Blackwell.

Tesch, P.A., Thorsson, A., and Colliander, E.B. (1990). Effects of eccentric and concentric resistance training on skeletal muscle substrates, enzyme activities and capillary supply. *Acta Physiol. Scand.*, 140, 575–580.

Westing, S.H., Seger, J.Y., Karlson, E. and Ekblom, B. (1988). Eccentric and concentric torque–velocity characteristics of the quadriceps femoris in man. *Eur. J. Appl. Physiol.*, **58,** 100–104.

Zatsiorsky, V.M. (1995). *Science and Practice of Strength Training*. Human Kinetics.

Zernicke, R.F. and Loitz, B.J. (1992). Exercise-related adaptations in connective tissue. In *Strength and Power in Sport* (P.V. Komi, ed.), pp. 77–95. Blackwell.

Further reading

Dick, F. (1997). *Sports Training Principles*, 3rd Edn. A. and C. Black.

Hazeldine, R. (1990). *Strength Training for Sport*, 2nd Edn. The Crowood Press.

Komi, P.V. (ed.) (1992). Strength and Power in Sport. Blackwell.

Martin, D.E. and Coe, P. (1997). *Better Training for Distance Runners*. Human Kinetics.

Maughan, R., Gleeson, M. and Greenhaff, P.L. (1997). *Biochemistry of Exercise and Training*. Oxford University Press.

Radcliffe, J.C. and Farantinos, R.C. (1985). *Plyometrics: Explosive Power Training*. Human Kinetics.

Shephard, R.J. and Astrand, P.-O. (eds) (1992). *Endurance in Sport*. Blackwell.

12

Guidelines for laboratory and field testing of athletic potential and performance

John A. Hawley

The outstanding performances of the modern-day athlete are the product of the integration of many physiological, biomechanical, nutritional and psychological variables. While sport scientists acknowledge the major factor ultimately determining athletic potential is genetic endowment (Bouchard, 1986), there is no doubt that the majority of individuals have the capacity to improve their performances with appropriate physical training.

The attainment of sporting excellence requires careful systematic planning, the application of the most appropriate training and nutritional strategies, an injury-free build-up to a competitive peak, sound tactical acumen and, on the day of competition, optimum environmental conditions coupled with a fair degree of fortune (Hawley and Burke, 1998). The final outcome of any planned training programme is an athlete's or team's performance on a specified day in a given competitive situation. Thus, most sporting endeavours lend themselves to objective scientific analysis because measures of success, such as winning or losing, or improving a personal best performance time, are easily observed and can be accurately quantified. During training and competition, the athlete and coach should aim to identify the most important factor(s) which have an effect on performance and then, if practicable, systematically manipulate these variables in an attempt to improve subsequent performance. As such, it has become popular for many athletes to seek input from qualified sport scientists in an attempt to reach their full potential.

During the past 25 years the governments of several nations have committed considerable financial and human resources in an effort to identify and enhance sporting talent. A major feature of the sporting systems in many of these countries has been the establishment of national and regional Sports Institutes. At these venues athletes undergo sophisticated physiological and biomechanical testing and receive the latest nutritional and medical information, in an attempt to optimize training programmes and maximize subsequent performance. Although the pharmacological techniques used by many of the sport scientists on athletes from several Eastern bloc countries remain of doubtful ethical and scientific credibility, the establishment of centres of sporting excellence in other nations has been associated with improved athletic success. For example, since the establishment of the Australian Institute of Sport in Canberra in 1980, the performances of that nation's athletes have improved significantly. At the 1976 Montreal Olympic Games Australia won a total of five medals, but did not win a single Olympic title. At the 1992 Barcelona Olympics they won 27 medals, including seven golds. At the 1996 Atlanta games, Australia won a total of 41 medals, of which nine were gold.

It has been suggested that those nations which are not competitive in the sports sciences will ultimately become uncompetitive in those international sports identified for scientific study by other nations (Hawley and Burke, 1997). Future success in sport at the highest level is likely to be strongly influenced by the ability of sport scientists to identify individuals with special talents and to initiate the appropriate research programmes to foster the specific human factors that determine success in that sport. Accordingly, the purposes of this chapter are: (1) to give a synopsis of the aims and benefits of physiological testing of the athlete; (2) to provide guidelines for the construction of an effective athlete testing programme; and (3) to describe several standard laboratory and field tests for the identification of athletic potential and performance.

The aims and benefits of physiological testing programmes

Laboratory testing of athletes to identify athletic potential and predict sporting performance is not a modern phenomenon. Scientific interest into some of the physiological factors that determine athletic success dates back to the turn of the century when researchers from Scandinavia and Germany measured oxygen uptake ($\dot{V}O_2$) in runners and swimmers. These pioneering studies established that $\dot{V}O_2$ increased with the speed of running (Herbst, 1928) and swimming (Liljestrand and Stenstrom, 1920a; Liljestrand and Stenstrom, 1920b). They also showed that trained runners had the highest $\dot{V}O_2$ values when running, rather than swimming (Herbst 1928). These and subsequent investigations (Astrand, 1952; Robinson, 1937) were the first to identify the important role of maximum oxygen uptake ($\dot{V}O_{2max}$) for the successful performance of endurance events. They also highlighted the importance of testing athletes in their chosen sport for test results to be valid.

Since then many laboratory and field tests have been developed to evaluate the physiological status of athletes from a variety of sports (for reviews, see Maud and Foster, 1995; MacDougall et al., 1991). Regardless of an athlete's chosen event, the primary objectives of any physiological testing programme are to:

1. Aid in talent identification.
2. Determine the physiological and health status of an athlete.
3. Construct a sports-specific physiological profile of an individual athlete or team.
4. Provide baseline data for individual training programme prescription.
5. Indicate each athlete's or player's strengths and weaknesses relevant to their sport and/or position.
6. Monitor selected physiological and performance changes in an athlete.
7. Provide scientific feedback to coaches so that they can evaluate the efficacy of their training interventions.
8. Act as a motivational and educational process whereby the athlete and coach better understand the physiological components of their sport.

Any testing battery needs to be repeated at regular intervals, ideally before and after each different phase of the athlete's training. The results of these tests should be interpreted directly to the coach and athlete, and the sports scientist should then discuss with the coach the most suitable and practical methods of implementing specific training interventions. For any testing programme to be effective, a number of scientific criteria must be fulfilled.

Guidelines for the construction of an effective athlete testing programme

When a sport scientist constructs a battery of physiological tests for the assessment of an athlete's fitness, there are several methodological criteria that must be strictly adhered to. Ideally, all tests should have been previously reported in the sports science literature as reliable and valid, they should be sufficiently sensitive to detect small changes in the athlete's state of fitness, and be as sports-specific as practically possible.

Reliability of laboratory tests of exercise capacity

The reliability or reproducibility of a laboratory test when it is administered to the same athlete on more than one occasion is a crucial issue in deciding on the utility of that test. Reproducibility determines the power of a test to detect changes in physiological status and/or performance. Yet, until recently, studies of the reliability of many commonly employed laboratory and field tests have been absent from the literature.

The variability of a test can arise from two main sources: technological variability and biological variability. Technological variability includes the variable errors of laboratory instruments, calibration errors, human errors in data recording, and uncontrolled environmental conditions. For

Table 12.1. The biological and technological variability of some frequently used laboratory tests

Test measure	Total variability (%)	Biological (%)	Technological (%)	Reference
Peak torque (30 sec)	6.7	76.1	23.9	Coggan and Costill, 1984
Peak torque (60 sec)	5.6	71.4	28.6	Coggan and Costill, 1984
Anaerobic power (30 sec)	5.4	68.5	31.5	Coggan and Costill, 1984
Anaerobic power (60 sec)	5.4	71.4	28.6	Coggan and Costill, 1984
Time to exhaustion (~ 100 sec)	5.3	90.0	10.0	Coggan and Costill, 1984
Time to exhaustion at 150% of PPO	1.7	–	–	Lindsay et al., 1996
VO_{2max} (l min^{-1})	7.9	–	–	Kuipers et al., 1985
Peak workload at VO_{2max}	5.0	–	–	Kuipers et al., 1985
VO_{2max} (l min^{-1})	5.6	92.7	7.3	Katch et al., 1982
VO_{2max} (ml kg^{-1} min^{-1})	5.6	92.6	7.4	Katch et al., 1982
VO_{2max} (l min^{-1})	9.0	–	–	Graham and Andrew, 1973
VO_{2max} (l min^{-1})	2.4	99.0	1.0	Taylor et al., 1944

PPO, peak sustained power output; VO_{2max}, maximal oxygen uptake.

example, current rapid response gas analysers have errors of only ±0.01 per cent of full scale when properly calibrated (Jones, 1988; McConnell, 1988), while calibration gas concentrations should be known to within ±0.03 per cent (Cotes and Woolmer, 1962; Weber and Janicki, 1986). With regard to automated metabolic testing units, the accuracy of measurement of ventilation is around ±4 per cent when volume is measured over time (McConnell, 1988) with a 2 per cent deviation from linearity when flow is integrated over time (Harrison *et al.*, 1980). However, for most laboratory tests, the technological error is relatively constant and does not increase or decrease in proportion to the magnitude of the test value (Henry, 1959). More to the point, the extent of variability due to technological error is small in comparison to the biological variability, and usually inconsequential (Table 12.1).

Biological variability refers to the day-to-day variation in energy metabolism which is usually ascribed to changes in gross mechanical efficiency (Kuipers *et al.*, 1985) or other biological fluctuations. Early data (Henry, 1959; Taylor, 1944) and more recent studies (Coggan and Costill, 1984; Katch *et al.*, 1982) indicate that, under carefully controlled laboratory conditions, biological variability accounts for as much as 90 per cent of the total variation in an individual's response to a maximum exercise test. The impact of this variability must be considered by the sport scientist when interpreting the results of laboratory tests to the coach and athlete. For example, the coefficient of variation (CV) for both well-trained and moderately trained individuals undertaking three or more tests for the determination of $\dot{V}O_{2max}$ has been reported to be between 2.5 and 9 per cent (Table 12.1). It is of interest that the variability found for either exhaustive or fixed-duration 'anaerobic' tests is similar to that reported for tests of $\dot{V}O_{2max}$.

Reliability of laboratory tests of performance

Until recently, the use of continuous, fixed-load, submaximal testing protocols has been the most common form of 'performance' test used in the laboratory. In such tests, athletes are requested to exercise until exhaustion, which has typically been defined as the inability to sustain a given power output or speed. The most remarkable attribute of these tests is that they have survived for so long in the scientific literature! Athletes are rarely, if ever, asked to exercise until volitional fatigue at some externally defined and arbitrary work-rate. On the contrary, the athlete who wins a race is the person who can cover a set distance as quickly as possible, or produce the most power in a given amount of time. During some sports, such as cycling, there are random and variable changes in exercise intensity as riders change pace, climb or descend hills, or draft behind another competitor's wheel. Under these conditions, where athletes are free to regulate their power output on a moment-by-moment basis, greater physiological responses may be achieved in the field than when the work pattern is determined by laboratory protocols (Foster *et al.*, 1993; Padilla *et al.*, 1996; Palmer *et al.*, 1994).

Even allowing for the fact that tests of 'time to exhaustion' have no ecological validity, the reproducibility of such measures is, at best, poor. The variability in tasks of running and cycling to exhaustion in both well-trained and untrained individuals has been reported to be as high as 25 per cent (Table 12.2). However, with sufficient familiarization to a task, this variability can be reduced substantially (Maughan *et al.*, 1989).

On the other hand, when athletes are required to perform a given amount of work, or cover a set distance as quickly as possible, the reliability of performance is quite low (Table 12.2). Jeukendrup *et al.* (1996) reported a CV of ~ 3.4 per cent for well-trained cyclists or triathletes performing either as much work as possible in a given time or a time-trial. Palmer *et al.* (1996) found even lower variability (~ 1 per cent) in timed rides over 20 and 40 km when subjects were able to ride their own bikes on an air-braked ergometer, while Hickey *et al.* (1992) reported similar day-to-day variation for the time taken for well-trained cyclists to complete ~ 1600 kJ of work. Schabort *et al.* (1997a) have recently reported a CV of only 0.7 per cent for trained rowers completing three 2000 m time-trials on a sports-specific ergometer. Taken collectively, these data suggest that trained athletes are able to optimize their pace and effort for simulated time-trials and reduce the variability of repeated performances to within ~ 1 per cent. Such low variability is essential if sport scientists are to avoid missing small but worthwhile effects of training on the performance of competitive athletes.

Today, laboratory measures of performance are being more frequently utilized by sport scientists as reliable, valid and practical methods of evaluating the effects of various nutritional and training interventions on the physiological responses of competitive athletes to the demands of their event (Juekendrup *et al.*, 1977; Hawley *et al.*, 1977b; Palmer *et al.*, 1997; Schabort *et al.*, 1997a). The use of simulated time-trial tasks are often preferable to laboratory measures of exercise capacity in that they allow the athlete to determine their own pace throughout an exercise bout and provide a true measure of performance (Schabort *et al.*, 1998a). In the final analysis, the results of laboratory performance tests should be complementary to the observations of the coach, and neither should ever be considered a replacement for the other.

Validity of laboratory tests of exercise capacity

Studies conducted over 75 years ago established that, when expressed relative to body weight, $\dot{V}O_{2max}$ was highest in the best endurance athletes (Herbst, 1928; Liljestrand and Strenstrom, 1920b), leading to a popular belief that $\dot{V}O_{2max}$ would be a good predictor of athletic potential in all endurance events (Costill, 1967; Foster, 1983). However, although $\dot{V}O_{2max}$ is a good predictor of endurance potential when a group of ath-

Table 12.2. The reproducibility of some laboratory tests of performance

Sport	n	Performance test	CV (%)	Reference
Cycling	8T	Time to complete 14 kJ (~ 60 sec)	2.43	Hickey et al., 1992
	8T	Time to complete 200 kJ (~ 12 min)	0.95	Hickey et al., 1992
	8T	Time to complete 1600 kJ (105 min)	1.0	Hickey et al., 1992
	10T	20 km time-trial	1.1	Palmer et al., 1996
	10T	40 km time-trial	1.0	Palmer et al., 1996
	8T	100 km time-trial	1.7	Schabort et al., 1998b
	30T	Time to exhaustion at 75% of maximal power	26.6	Jeukendrup et al., 1996
	30T	As much work as possible in 15 min	3.49	Jeukendrup et al., 1996
	30T	Time to complete a set amount of work (~ 1 hr)	3.35	Jeukendrup et al., 1996
Running	15UT	Time to exhaustion at 80% of VO_{2max}	17.3	McLellan et al., 1995
	8T	Distance covered in 60 min	2.7	Schabort et al., 1998a
	8T	Time to exhaustion at 'maximal aerobic speed'	26.5	Billat et al., 1994
Rowing	8T	2000 m time-trial	0.6	Schabort et al., 1999

CV, coefficient of variation; T, trained; UT, untrained; VO_{2max}, maximal oxygen uptake.[tfmr]

letes with vastly different performance capabilities are studied, it is a relatively poor predictor when athletes of similar ability are evaluated (Conley and Krahenbuhl, 1980; Costill and Winrow, 1970; Pollock, 1977). For example, correlations between $\dot{V}O_{2max}$ and race pace in marathon runners range from 0.63 to 0.91 (Sjodin and Svedenhag, 1985).

Part of the reason that the $\dot{V}O_{2max}$ of an athlete is not the single best predictor of athletic potential is because it is only one of many physiological variables positively related to successful endurance performance. In this regard, the maximum speed or power output an athlete can attain during a maximum test has also been shown to be an important predictor of athletic performance. For example, in runners, the peak treadmill speed attained during a progressive, maximum test has been shown to be as good a predictor of running performance over races at distances longer than 10 km as any physiological variable currently measured in the laboratory (Morgan et al., 1989; Noakes et al., 1990). For cyclists, the highest power output attained during an exhaustive test is a valid predictor of both 20 km (Hawley and Noakes, 1992) and 40 km time-trial performance (Hawley et al., 1997a; Lindsay et al., 1996). In swimming, measurements of maximum arm power have been used to predict sprint and middle-distance performance (Hawley and Williams, 1991; Hawley et al., 1992; Miyashita and Kanshisa, 1979; Sharp et al., 1992). Thus, although $\dot{V}O_{2max}$ still remains the test of choice for assessing the upper limit of aerobic exercise capacity, sport scientists should also determine the highest work-rate that the athlete reaches during such a test.

Validity of laboratory tests of performance

Several investigations have examined the validity of various laboratory tests of performance. For cycling, Coyle et al. (1991) reported that the average absolute work-rate (W) sustained during a 1 h laboratory performance test was highly correlated ($r = -0.88$) with 40 km time-trial performance in the field. Unfortunately, as no standard error of the estimate was provided by these authors, it is impossible to assess the magnitude of the predictive value of this zero-order correlation coefficient. Palmer et al. (1996) assessed the validity of the relationship between the average of three 40 km laboratory simulated time-trials with two road races. Regression analysis revealed a high correlation between laboratory and field times ($r = 0.98$). Of practical significance was that, in the absence of air resistance, the times recorded in the laboratory were, on average, 8 per cent faster than the road race performances.

In sports where the body mass of the athlete is supported in a seated position, the average $\dot{V}O_2$ sustained during simulated competitive efforts has been found to be a better predictor of performance than, for example, an athlete's $\dot{V}O_{2max}$. In rowing, correlations of > 0.95 have been reported between average $\dot{V}O_2$ during a 6 min all-out effort and on-water rowing performance, compared to correlations of less than 0.86 for $\dot{V}O_{2max}$ and performance (for review, see Hagerman, 1994).

The reason for such a good relationship between various laboratory tests and performance is because successful competitive efforts rely on an athlete being able to sustain a high power output for the duration of an exercise bout. Indeed, one of the most impressive attributes of outstanding rowers and cyclists is their ability to sustain an extremely high percentage of absolute $\dot{V}O_{2max}$ (Coyle et al., 1988; Hagerman et al., 1978; Mickelson and Hagerman, 1982). In rowing, one of the major criteria used to predict successful performance at the international level is the ability of a rower to sustain an average $\dot{V}O_2$ that is very close (98 per cent) to the peak $\dot{V}O_2$ measured during a simulated time-trial (Hagerman, 1994). Recent data gathered from an elite cyclist riding at world-record pace for 1 h (56.375 km h^{-1}) reveal that this subject sustained an average power output of 442 W or 6.4 W kg^{-1} for the duration (Hawley and Burke, 1997; Peter Keen, personal communication).

Standardized testing procedures

If the results of various physiological tests are to be comparable between different laboratories, then all testing should be conducted under standardized conditions. This applies to both the environment (laboratory equipment, ambient temperature etc.) and the athlete (similar pre-test dietary and training regimens). The following pre-test criteria have been suggested for sport scientists when undertaking laboratory and field testing (British Association of Sports Sciences, 1988; Hawley and Burke, 1997; Sports Science Institute of South Africa, 1995).

The laboratory environment and equipment:

1. Select a dedicated area which is free from other influences or disturbances.
2. Conduct tests in a well-ventilated area with the laboratory temperature between 20 and 22°C, and the relative humidity less than 60 per cent.
3. Conduct all tests without peripheral personnel who may influence the performance.
4. Ensure that the same practitioner is employed in subsequent testing.

The athlete:

1. Check the athlete is not suffering from any condition which may adversely affect performance, such as a cold or an injury.
2. Do not allow any athlete to perform any test with a viral infection, no matter how mild the condition may be considered.

3. Ensure that the athlete has not undertaken any intensive training or competition for 48 h prior to a test, nor performed a similar test within the previous 72 h.
4. Ensure that the athlete has not eaten for 2 h before a maximal test. Fluids such as carbohydrate–electrolyte solutions or water may be taken *ad libitum* in the hours before the test. However, some individuals are susceptible to reactive hypoglycaemia if they ingest beverages with a high sugar content in the 30–60 min before strenuous exercise. Thus, in these athletes, this practice should be avoided.
5. Prior to any test procedure, allow the athlete to perform their own warm-up routine, which must then be standardized for subsequent tests.
6. Ensure that the athlete uses the same equipment that they utilize during training and/or competition, such as racing shoes and clothing or other specialized gear.

Test procedures:

1. Ensure that the athlete is familiar with the all test equipment before starting any tests.
2. Explain, in detail, all test procedures to each athlete, particularly those tests with which the athlete is unfamiliar.
3. Allow the athlete to become habituated to all test procedures. This can take several performances of the criterion test before the results reflect true performance. However, in the case of some laboratory tests of performance, there appears to be little or no learning effect (Hickey *et al.*, 1982; Jeukendrup *et al.*, 1996; Palmer *et al.*, 1996).
4. For the most valid and reliable results, schedule physiological tests during the mid- to late afternoon or early evening period when strength and endurance are at their maximum.

Laboratory tests to measure athletic potential

Peak oxygen uptake and peak sustained power output or speed

Perhaps the single most commonly employed procedure in exercise physiology is the test for peak oxygen uptake, simply referred to as the athlete's $\dot{V}O_{2max}$. The determination of $\dot{V}O_{2max}$ determines an athlete's ability to take in, transport and utilize oxygen and is a measure of an athlete's maximum aerobic power production.

The laboratory protocols for assessing an athlete's $\dot{V}O_{2max}$ involve progressive, incremental exercise tests to exhaustion on either a cycle ergometer, a motor-driven treadmill or a rowing ergometer, or in a swimming pool or flume. Although testing protocols will vary between different laboratories, an athlete will usually be required to exercise for 10–15 min while the intensity (either the speed of movement or power output) is progressively increased until they become exhausted. The sport scientist has several objective and subjective criteria for determining whether or not the athlete has produced a true maximal effort (Hawley and Noakes, 1992; Shephard, 1984).

$\dot{V}O_{2max}$ values in endurance athletes from weight-bearing sports are usually well in excess of 75 ml kg^{-1} min^{-1} for males and > 70 ml kg^{-1} min^{-1} for females (Table 12.3; for reviews, see Maughan, 1994; Wells and Pate, 1988). In sports such as rowing and time-trial cycling the absolute $\dot{V}O_{2max}$ (l min^{-1}) of an athlete often provides a better indicator of athletic potential. Values of > 6.0 l min^{-1} for males and > 4.0 l min^{-1} for females would be expected for athletes from these sports (Hagerman, 1994; Inigo Mujika, personal communication).

In conjunction with the direct assessment of $\dot{V}O_{2max}$, a measurement of the athlete's peak power output (PPO) or peak speed should be determined. Obviously, the value for oxygen uptake measured at an athlete's peak work-rate will depend on their economy of motion (to be discussed subsequently). The fact remains that for some sports, the peak speed or power output that an athlete attains during a progressive, incremental maximal test lasting 10–20 min is just as good a predictor of athletic potential as any other physiological variable currently measured (Noakes, 1988). PPO values should be expressed relative to body mass to allow comparisons between athletes from the same sport. In cycling and rowing, power:weight ratios > 5.5 W kg^{-1} are considered the minimum values necessary for success at the elite level (Hagerman, 1994; Hawley and Noakes, 1992). For world class competitors, power:weight ratios > 6.5 W kg^{-1} are not uncommon (Peter Keen, personal communication; Inigo Mujika, personal communication).

Economy of motion

Economy of motion, or efficiency, is a major predictor of athletic performance in events lasting more than a few seconds (Conley and Krahenbuhl, 1980). The factors which determine an athlete's economy are not clear, but are probably related to a number of variables such as the number of years of training (Coyle et al., 1991), the volume of training (Pate et al., 1987; Scrimgeour et al., 1986) and the capillary density and oxidative enzyme activity of the active musculature (Coyle et al., 1991; Weston et al., 1997).

Even among elite competitors there may be large differences in the oxygen cost of motion. For example, Pollock et al. (1980) reported that the oxygen cost of running at 19 km h^{-1} ranged from 60.5 to 70.0 ml kg^{-1} min^{-1} in a group of world class runners. Coyle et al. (1991) have shown that the $\dot{V}O_2$ during submaximal cycling can vary by as much as 15 per cent in a group of well-trained competitive cyclists. For swimming, the single best predictor of performance is the stroke index, a surrogate measure of economy, defined as the distance covered

Table 12.3. Maximal oxygen uptake values of athletes from several endurance sports and of players from a variety of team sports (adapted from Hawley and Burke, 1997)

Sport	n	$\dot{V}O_{2max}$ $(ml\ kg^{-1}\ min^{-1})$
Cross-country skiing:		
Olympic/World Champions (males)	5	83.8
Cycling:		
Australian national team (male)	17	68.4
US national team (male)	23	74.0
Running:		
Elite female middle-distance (5000 m)	6	68.0
Elite female long-distance (10 000 m)	9	66.4
Elite male US middle-distance runners	11	78.8
Elite male US distance runners	20	76.9
Rowing:		
Australian 'highly ranked' (male)	8	63.5
Australian 'highly ranked' (female)	12	53.3
1992 US Olympic team (females)	25	58.6
1992 US Olympic team (males)	35	70.9
Swimming:		
US Collegiate (male)	12	56.2
Triathlon:		
Elite male	10	75.4
Elite female	10	65.6
Cricket:		
South African squad (pre-season)	17	60.5
English county batsmen	12	54.0
English county bowlers	13	51.7
Field hockey		
Australian state level (females)	6	50.1
Australian state level (males)	14	60.7
UK national team (males)	20	62.2
Soccer:		
Danish professionals	8	60.4
English First Division team (in season)	10	66.0
English First and Second Division (pre-season)	122	60.4

each stroke multiplied by the velocity of movement (Costill *et al.*, 1985; Hawley and Williams, 1991).

Whenever possible, longitudinal measures of an athlete's economy of motion should be determined. For good distance runners, $\dot{V}O_2$ at a submaximal steady-state pace of 16.0 km h^{-1} should be measured. Excellent economy would be indicated by a $\dot{V}O_2$ of < 50 ml kg^{-1} min^{-1}, while moderate economy would correspond to an oxygen cost of between 50 and 55 ml kg^{-1} min^{-1}. For elite distance runners, the submaximal $\dot{V}O_2$ at a speed of 19.0 km h^{-1} (or marathon- race pace) should be determined. For cyclists, $\dot{V}O_2$ corresponding to the highest average power output sustainable for 1 h provides a good measure of economy. Cycling economy can be determined by either the average work rate (W) divided by the average $\dot{V}O_2$ (l min^{-1}), or by conventional gross mechanical efficiency equations. For the former, an economy of > 75 W l^{-1} would be considered excellent (range 65–80 W l^{-1}), while for the latter, a mechanical efficiency of higher than 23 per cent is superior (range 18–25 per cent).

Anaerobic power

Because it is very difficult to sprint on a motorized treadmill at speeds faster than 25 km h^{-1}, the most widely used laboratory test to assess an athlete's anaerobic power is usually undertaken on a cycle ergometer. The Wingate anaerobic power test (WAT) was developed and validated in Israel at the Wingate Research Institute. The test–retest reliability of the WAT has ranged between 0.89 and 0.98, but is typically of the order of 0.94 (Bar-Or, 1987). With regard to the validity of the WAT, correlations between a variety of 'anaerobic' sporting tasks and an athlete's power output are usually > 0.80 (for review, see Bar-Or, 1987).

The WAT consists of 30 s of all-out cycling against a workload which is determined by the body mass and training status of the athlete. The workload is such that the athlete is completely fatigued at the end of the 30 s test. Most laboratories interface their cycle ergometer to a computer system which can sample the athlete's power output at regular time intervals, usually every 0.5 s. Three parameters can be determined from the WAT:

1. The athlete's peak power.
2. The athlete's mean power.
3. An index of the athlete's fatigue profile over the duration of the test.

The athlete's peak power is the highest power output they can sustain for any 5 s period of the test. The average power is the total work performed by the athlete divided by the time (30 s) of the test. A fatigue index measures the decay in power during the test (or simply the rate at which the athlete slows down). Most scientific studies tend to report only an individual's peak and mean power outputs from the WAT. Such values should always be expressed relative to an athlete's body mass to allow comparisons between individuals from different sports, and also

Table 12.4. Anaerobic indices of athletes from a variety of sports, as determined by the Wingate 'anaerobic' test (adapted from Hawley and Burke, 1997)

Sport	n	Peak power (W)	Peak power (W kg^{-1})	Mean power (W)	Mean power (W kg^{-1})
Cycling:					
US national road (male)	7	994	13.9	804	11.2
US national road (females)	6	784	12.2	615	9.6
Swimming:					
Age-group (males, upper body)	12	266	4.9	204	3.7
Age-group (females, upper body)	10	205	3.7	159	2.8
Age-group (males)	12	585	10.8	449	8.3
Age-group (females)	10	534	9.5	370	6.6
Soccer:					
English First and Second Division	122	1123	14.6	748	9.7
Rugby League:					
Forwards	13	1111	12.1		
Backs	12	1114	13.9		
Rugby Union:					
International (props)	5	1342	13.1	992	9.7
International (back row)	6	1388	13.8	1144	11.3
International (backs)	5	1336	15.7	1013	11.9

n refers to the number of athletes or players tested.

between individuals within the same sport or playing position. Table 12.4 shows the 'anaerobic' power of individuals from both endurance and team sports.

Field tests to measure athletic potential

Maximum endurance tests

Although the direct determination of an athlete's $\dot{V}O_{2max}$ in the laboratory provides the most accurate assessment of aerobic power, such a measurement requires expensive equipment and trained personnel. Consequently, sport scientists have developed several field tests which can provide an estimate of an athlete's $\dot{V}O_{2max}$. The best known of these is the 12 or 15 min run, as originally proposed by Balke (1954) and modified by Cooper (1968). In motivated individuals the correlation between running speed and $\dot{V}O_{2max}$ has been reported at 0.90 (Cooper, 1968), although correlations ranging from 0.04 to 0.89 have been noted (for review, see Shephard, 1982). The accuracy of maximum running tests is highly dependent on the willingness of athletes to perform an all-out effort, and also their ability to judge the optimum pace. While runners may be able to judge the most appropriate pace to produce the maximum running distance, inexperienced athletes will often start too fast and fatigue prematurely. Such a strategy may result in an underestimation of their true aerobic capacity.

Maximum swimming tests have also been proposed for the assessment of aerobic capacity (Cooper and Cooper, 1972). However, the validity of such an estimate is poor (Conley *et al.*, 1991). This is hardly surprising since the mechanical efficiency of swimming can be increased three- to four-fold by improvements in technique, rather than fitness. Indeed, the major determinant of success in middle-distance swimming is the distance covered with each stroke (Costill *et al.*, 1985; Craig *et al.*, 1985).

Multi-stage shuttle run

Tests requiring continuous, steady-state activity in which the body is translated horizontally in one plane are not representative of the physiological demands of team sports. In soccer, rugby (union and league), field hockey, lacrosse and basketball, players need a high level of aerobic fitness, but are also subject to frequent changes in both the pace and direction of running. In addition, players in team sports have to accelerate from a standing start many times during a match. For this reason, the multistage shuttle run test for aerobic fitness assessment was developed as a more valid test for players from a variety of team sports (Leger *et al.*, 1988; Ramsbottom *et al.*, 1988). The test–retest reliability of this protocol has been reported to be 0.95 (Leger *et al.*, 1988).

For the multi-stage shuttle run test, players are required to run back and forth for a distance of 20 m at a pace determined by the frequency of a sound signal. The running speed is increased by 0.5 km h^{-1} every 60 s. With a starting speed of 8.5 km h^{-1}, the first few minutes of the test act as a good warm-up for fit players, and allow them to get used to accelerating from a stationary position, decelerating, turning, and then accelerating once more. Each stage of the shuttle lasts exactly 60 s and, as the speed of each successive shuttle is increased, so is the number of runs (called levels) within that time. The test is terminated when the player is no longer able to reach a 20 m line at the prescribed time despite two verbal warnings. The last completed stage is defined as the maximum shuttle run speed. A player's $\dot{V}O_{2max}$ can then be predicted immediately upon termination of the test from validated tables (see Leger *et al.*, 1988). Table 12.5

displays the maximum shuttle run stage and level along with the predicted $\dot{V}O_{2max}$ values of players from a number of different team sports and playing positions. It is clear that the $\dot{V}O_{2max}$ varies between players from different sports and also between players from the same sport. The implication of this finding is that training programmes for team players must be individualized to the specific fitness requirements of each playing position (Hawley and Burke, 1997).

Although the WAT is the most commonly used laboratory procedure for estimating an athlete's 'anaerobic' power, many athletes will not have access to facilities to undertake such a test. In addition, a strong case could be made that a cycling test is not the most appropriate manner in which to

Table 12.5. Predicted values for maximal aerobic power from the multi-stage shuttle run (adapted from Hawley and Burke, 1997)

Sport	n	Maximal shuttle	$\dot{V}O_{2max}$ $(ml\ kg^{-1}\ min^{-1})$
Rugby Union:			
New Zealand 'A' (pre-season)			
Forwards	50	L 12–S 3	54.6
Backs	43	L 13–S 9	58.6
New Zealand 'B' (pre-season)			
Forwards	19	L 12–S 8	55.6
Backs	19	L 12–S 9	55.6
New Zealand under 19			
Forwards	29	L 11–S 6	52.6
Backs	24	L 11–S 11	54.6
South African squad (pre-season)			
Props and locks	6	L 11–S 2	51.1
Loose forwards	5	L 12–S 6	55.5
Fly-halves and centres	4	L 12–S 6	55.5
Full-backs and wings	4	L 12–S 8	56.0
English national squad (end of season)			
Forwards	3	L 12–S 10	58.0
Backs	9	L 13–S 13	59.6
South African under 19 (pre-season)			
Props and locks	10	L 11–S 9	53.3
Loose forwards	13	L 13–S 2	57.5
Fly-halves and centres	4	L 12–S 11	56.9
Full-backs and wings	6	L 12–S 8	56.1
Soccer:			
South African squad (early season)	13	L 13–S 4	58.0

n refers to the number of players tested.

evaluate the physiology of athletes from sports other than cycling. As a result, several field tests have been developed which allow the sport scientist to better assess the speed, agility and fatigue resistance of their players under more sports-specific conditions.

Maximum running speed and acceleration

A high maximum aerobic power is now a prerequisite for most players participating in team sports at a high level. Additionally, all outfield players are required to sprint at maximum speed and to accelerate from stationary positions throughout the duration of a game. Therefore, any test battery for evaluating the physiological status of players involved in team sports should include a measure of maximum sprint speed and acceleration.

For these tests, which can be conducted on a level field, or in a gymnasium, an electronic sprint timer with photo-electric sensors is set at chest height and placed at 10, 20, 30 and 40 m intervals from a start line. After a thorough warm-up and some acceleration runs of increasing speed, the player positions himself, in a standing start position, close to the start line without breaking the beam of the start sensor. Upon an auditory count-down signal, the player sprints maximally for 40 m, passing through the sensors. The player completes two flat-out runs separated by a 3–5 min recovery period. The elapsed time at 10, 20 and 40 m are recorded for each run and the fastest split and total time attained during either run recorded. Some coaches also like to determine the speed of their players over a short distance from a moving or rolling start. Such a test negates some of the disadvantage that the heavier players have when commencing the sprint run from a stationary position. Table 12.6 displays sprint times for players from a variety of team sports and playing positions.

Repeated shuttle run

The ability to attain a high maximum running speed over a short distance is obviously a necessary attribute in athletes participating in explosive running events, and in most playing positions in a variety of team sports. However, just as important for team sport players is the ability to perform repeated sprints over varying distances throughout the duration of a match. Thus, a measure of repeated sprint ability should always be included in a test battery for evaluating team sport players or indeed the participants in any event which requires the athlete to exercise at or near maximum speed for a short duration with incomplete recovery between work bouts. For this test, six cones are placed 5 m apart in a straight line on a level surface, as shown below:

Table 12.6. Sprint-run times from stationary starts for players from a variety of team sports (adapted from Hawley and Burke, 1997)

Sport	n	10 m (sec)	30 m (sec)	40 m (sec)
Soccer:				
German professionals	20	1.79	4.19	
German amateurs	19	1.88	4.33	
South African squad (early season)				
Defenders	2	1.77	4.13	5.30
Mid-field	5	1.79	4.16	5.34
Forwards	4	1.72	4.09	5.20
Rugby League:				
Elite British (end of season)				
Forwards	13			5.61
Backs	12			5.30
Rugby Union:				
English national squad (off-season)				
Forwards	9		4.4	
Backs	9		4.1	
English national squad (in-season)				
Forwards	9		4.3	
Backs	9		3.9	
New Zealand 'A' (pre-season)				
Forwards	45		4.5	
Backs	37		4.3	
New Zealand 'B' (pre-season)				
Forwards	12		4.8	
Backs	12		4.5	
New Zealand under 19 (pre-season)				
Forwards	29		4.6	
Backs	24		4.4	
South African squad (pre-season)				
Props and locks	6	1.83		5.52
Loose forwards and scrum-halves	5	1.86		5.53
Fly-halves and centres	4	1.80		5.21
Full-backs and wings	4	1.81		5.19

n refers to the number of athletes or players tested.

A ↔ B ↔ C ↔ D ↔ E ↔ F

← **5 m** →

Players begin the test at point A and, upon an auditory signal, sprint to cone B, touch the base of the cone, turn, return to point A, reach down to touch the base, and then sprint to point C. The player continues in this manner sprinting to the remaining cones (D, E and F), making sure to return to the start (A) between each outward shuttle. If a very fit player can run the entire shuttle (A to F and back) in under 30 s, then they begin the cycle again. An auditory signal after 30 s of the test indicates the end of that stage of the shuttle run. The number of stages is recorded while the player takes a 35 s rest, during which they make their way back to the start point (A). After 35 s they begin the run again. The test is repeated on six occasions and the distance covered during each run recorded. Two variables are determined from this test:

1. The total distance covered by a player during the six shuttle runs.
2. A fatigue index, determined as the difference between the maximum distance covered by the player during any single shuttle run minus the shortest distance covered during a run, usually the last shuttle.

As the total distance covered by a player during the entire test is a combined measure of their anaerobic and aerobic power systems, most laboratories tend only to report this value and disregard any measure of fatigue. To cover a total distance > 750 m requires excellent basic speed, the ability to turn at pace and accelerate, and an excellent aerobic system for a rapid recovery between the runs.

Physiological testing: how often and when?

One of the questions most frequently asked by athletes is how often they need to undergo physiological testing. The simple answer is 'as frequently as practically possible' bearing in mind the constraints of regular training and competition, and the financial implications of such testing. Since each athlete will differ in their responses to training it is important that their physiological status be regularly evaluated so that exercise prescription can be individually modified and optimized. With endurance-trained athletes, a full battery of physiological tests should be undertaken a *minimum* of twice a year. Ideally, the first testing session should take place at the end of the athlete's pre-season, with the subsequent evaluation taking place immediately prior to or during their competitive phase.

For players involved in team sports such as rugby, cricket or soccer, it is more difficult to prescribe the frequency at which physiological testing should be undertaken. Although players need to be assessed regularly, the competition schedule is often demanding, particularly in the modern era of professionalism. Today's international team players are expected to participate in a greater number of games with each passing season. This sometimes means that their off-season can be as short as 4–6 weeks. In such cases, it is recommended that physiological testing be incorporated into the early season fitness training of players. This approach to testing has the advantage of being time-effective for both players and coaching staff, as well as providing the coach with on-the-spot feedback as to the current fitness status of their squad.

Summary

Recently it has become popular for athletes to seek input from qualified sports scientists to assist them to reach their full athletic potential. This input should incorporate, but not be confined to, extensive physiological testing and monitoring of the athletes on a longitudinal basis. For the results of such tests to be meaningful for the athlete and their coach, the sport scientists should ensure that their testing protocols are reliable, valid and sensitive enough to detect the small changes in the athlete's state of fitness. The reliability or reproducibility of a protocol is a crucial issue for the sport scientist in deciding on the utility of a test. Reproducibility determines the power of a test to detect changes in physiological status or performance. As such, this area warrants further investigation.

With regard to identifying athletic talent, sports scientists still do not know how to accurately predict an athlete's ultimate performance. No laboratory test currently reported in the scientific literature can predict with any degree of precision how much an athlete might improve their physiological function.

Laboratory testing is not a magical tool for predicting athletic potential or an individual's ultimate performance. Indeed, several of the most frequently used testing protocols to assess the physiological status of athletes have severe limitations when it comes to predicting actual performance in the field. This is to be expected, as the ultimate performance of any athlete or team is the result of several interdependent factors, only one of which is physiological capacity. Testing should be conducted only when it is clear that an athlete or team might benefit from such testing, and when specific questions that can be answered by the tests have been identified (Kuipers, 1997). There are no standard tests available for many types of sports performance. It is often therefore left to the ingenuity, expertise and experience of the coach and sport scientist to devise novel and reliable techniques to measure exercise capacity. There is an urgent need for sports-specific laboratory and field tests for most sporting disciplines.

Finally, it should be acknowledged that there are many athletes capable of producing superior test results in the laboratory setting, but who consistently fail to perform to their physiological potential under the extreme pressures of competition. Conversely, many elite competitors are reluctant to perform in the laboratory. The ultimate test of an athlete's ability will always be their performance in the field. While laboratory and field tests are no substitute for this evaluation process, they are helpful in the assessment of an athlete's strengths and weaknesses, and in monitoring progress in response to training (Maughan, 1994).

Acknowledgements

The unpublished data on several South African National teams which appear in this chapter are courtesy of The High Performance Laboratory of The Sports Science Institute of South Africa. In particular, the skilful contributions of Mr Justin Durandt and Ms Nicola Scales are gratefully acknowledged.

References

Astrand, P.O. (1952). *Experimental Studies of Physical Work Capacity in Relation to Sex and Age*. Munksgaard.

Balke, B. (1954). Optimale korperliche leistungsfahigkeit, ihre messung und veranderung infolge arbeitsmudung. *Int. Zeit Phys. Arbeitphysiol.*, **15**, 311–323.

Bar-Or, O. (1987). The Wingate anaerobic test. An update on methodology, reliability and validity. *Sports Med.*, **4**, 381–394.

Billat, V., Renoux, J.C., Pinoteau, J., Petit, B. and Koralsztein, J.P. (1994). Reproducibility of running time to exhaustion at $\dot{V}O_{2max}$ in subelite runners. *Med. Sci. Sports Exerc.*, **26**, 254–257.

Bouchard, C. (1986). Genetics of aerobic power and capacity. In *Sport and Human Genetics* (R.W. Malina and C. Bouchard, ed.). Human Kinetics.

British Association of Sports Sciences (1988). *Position Statement on the Physiological Assessment of the Elite Competitor*. White Line Press.

Coggan, A.R. and Costill, D.L. (1984). Biological and technological variability of three anaerobic ergometer tests. *Int. J. Sports Med.*, **5**, 142–145.

Conley, D.S., Cureton, K.J., Dengel, D.R. and Weyand, P.G. (1991). Validation of the 12- min swim as a field test of peak aerobic power in young men. *Med. Sci. Sports Exerc.*, **23**, 766–773.

Conley, D.L. and Krahenbuhl, G.S. (1980). Running economy and distance running performance. *Med. Sci. Sports Exerc.*, **12**, 357–360.

Cooper, K. (1968). *Aerobics*. Evans Press.

Cooper, K. and Cooper, K.H. (1972). *Aerobics for Women*. Evans Press.

Costill, D.L. (1967). The relationship between selected physiological variables and distance running performance. *J. Sports Med. Phys. Fitness*, **7**, 61–66.

Costill, D.L., Kovaleski, J., Porter, D., Kirwan, J., Fielding, R. and King, D. (1985). Energy expenditure during front-crawl swimming: Predicting success in middle- distance events. *Int. J. Sports Med.*, **6**, 266–270.

Costill, D.L. and Winrow, E. (1970). Maximum oxygen intake among marathon runners. *Arch. Phys. Med. Rehab.*, **51**, 317–320.

Cotes, J.E. and Woolmer, R.F. (1962). A comparison between twenty-seven laboratories of the results of analysis of an expired gas sample. *J. Appl. Physiol.*, **163**, 36–37.

Coyle, E.F., Coggan, A.R., Hopper, M.K. and Walters, T.J. (1988). Determinants of endurance in well-trained cyclists. *J. Appl. Physiol.*, **64**, 2622–2630.

Coyle, E.F., Feltner, M.E., Kautz, S.A., Hamilton, M.T., Montain, S.J., Baylor, A.M., Abraham, L.D. and Petrek, G.W. (1991). Physiological and biomechanical factors associated with elite endurance cycling performance. *Med. Sci. Sports Exerc.*, **23**, 93–107.

Craig, A.B., Skehan, P.L., Pawelczyk, J.A. and Boomer, W.L. (1985). Velocity, stroke rate and distance per stroke during elite swimming competition. *Med. Sci. Sports Exerc.*, **17**, 625–634.

Foster, C. (1983). $\dot{V}O_{2max}$ and training indices as determinants of competitive running performance. *J. Sports Sci.*, **1**, 13–22.

Foster, C., Green, M.A., Snyder, A.C. and Thompson, N.N. (1993). Physiological responses during simulated competition. *Med. Sci. Sports Exerc.*, **25**, 877–882.

Graham, T.E. and Andrew, G. (1973). The variability of repeated measurements of oxygen debt in man following a maximal treadmill exercise test. *Med. Sci. Sports Exerc.*, **5**, 73–78.

Hagerman, F.C. (1994). Physiology and nutrition for rowing. In *Perspectives in Exercise Science and Sports Medicine. Physiology and Nutrition for Competitive Sport*, Vol. 7 (D.R. Lamb, H.G. Knuttgen and R. Murray, eds), pp. 221–302. Cooper Publishing Group.

Hagerman, F.C., Connors, M.C., Gault, J.A., Hagerman, G.R. and Polinski, W.J. (1978). Energy expenditure during simulated rowing. *J. Appl. Physiol.*, **45**, 87–93.

Harrison, M.H., Brown, G.A. and Cochran, L.A. (1980). Maximal oxygen uptake: its measurement, application and limitations. *Aviat. Space Environ. Med.*, **51**, 1123–1127.

Hawley, J.A. and Burke, L.M. (1998). *Peak Performance: Training and Nutritional Strategies for Sport*. Allen and Unwin.

Hawley, J.A., Myburgh, K.H., Noakes, T.D. and Dennis, S.C. (1997a). Training techniques to improve fatigue resistance and enhance endurance performance. *J. Sports Sci.*, **15**, 325–333.

Hawley, J.A. and Noakes, T.D. (1992). Peak power output predicts maximal oxygen uptake and performance time in trained cyclists. *Eur. J. Appl. Physiol.*, **65**, 79–83.

Hawley, J.A., Palmer, G.S. and Noakes, T.D. (1997b). Effects of 3 days of carbohydrate supplementation on muscle glycogen content and utilization during a 1 h cycling performance. *Eur. J. Appl. Physiol.*, **75**, 407–412.

Hawley, J.A. and Williams, M.M. (1991). Relationship between upper body anaerobic power and freestyle swimming performance. *Int. J. Sports Med.*, **12**, 1–5.

Hawley, J.A., Williams, M.M., Handcock, P.J. and Vickovic, M. (1992). Muscle power predicts freestyle swimming performance. *Br. J. Sports Med.*, **26**, 151–155.

Henry, F.M. (1959). Reliability, measurement error, and intra-individual differences. *Res. Quart.*, **30**, 21–24.

Herbst, R. (1928). Der gastoffweschel als mab der korperlichen leistungsfahigkeit. *Deutches Arch. fur Klun. Med.*, **162**, 33–50.

Hickey, M.S., Costill, D.L., McConnell, T.R., Widrick, J.J. and Tanaka, H. (1992). Day to day variation in time trial cycling performance. *Int. J. Sports Med.*, **13**, 467–470.

Juekendrup, A.E., Brouns, F., Wagenmakers, A.J.M. and Saris, W.H.M. (1997). Carbohydrate–electrolyte feedings improve 1 h time trial cycling performance. *Int. J. Sports Med.*, **18**, 125–129.

Jeukendrup, A., Saris, W.H.M., Brouns, F. and Kester, A.D.M. (1996). A new validated endurance performance test. *Med. Sci. Sports Exerc.*, **28**, 266–270.

Jones, N.L. (1988). *Clinical Exercise Testing*, 3rd Edn, pp. 208–212. W.B. Saunders.

Katch, V.L., Sady, S.S. and Freedson, P. (1982). Biological variability in maximum aerobic power. *Med. Sci. Sports Exerc.*, **14**, 21–25.

Kuipers, H. (1997). Advances in the evaluation of sports training. In *Perspectives in Exercise Science and Sports Medicine, Volume 10. Optimizing Sports Performance* (D.R. Lamb and R. Murray, eds.), pp. 63–90. Cooper Publishing Group.

Kuipers, H., Verstappen, F.T.J., Keizer, H.A., Geurten, P. and van Kranenburg, G. (1985). Variability of aerobic performance in the laboratory and its physiologic correlates. *Int. J. Sports Med.*, **6**, 197–201.

Leger, L.A., Mercier, D., Gadoury, C. and Lambert, J. (1988). The multistage 20 metre shuttle run test for aerobic fitness. *J. Sports Sci.*, **6**: 93–101.

Liljestrand, G. and Stenstrom N. (1920a). Studien uber die physiologie des schwimmens. *Skand. Arch. fur Physiol.*, **39**, 1–63.

Liljestrand, G. and Stenstrom, N. (1920b). Respirationsversuche beim gehen, laufen, ski- und schlittschuhlaufen. *Skand. Arch. fur Physiol.*, **39**, 167–206.

Lindsay, F.H., Hawley, J.A., Myburgh, K.H., Schomer, H.H., Noakes, T.D. and Dennis, S.C. (1996). Improved athletic performance in highly trained cyclists after interval training. *Med. Sci. Sports Exerc.*, **28**, 1427–1434.

MacDougall, J.D., Wenger, H.A. and Green, H.J. (1991). *Physiological Testing of the High-Performance Athlete*, 2nd Edn. Human Kinetics.

Maud, P.J. and Foster, C. (1995). *Physiological Assessment of Human Fitness*. Human Kinetics.

Maughan, R.J. (1994). Physiology and nutrition for middle distance and long distance running. In *Perspectives in Exercise Science and Sports Medicine, Volume 7. Physiology and Nutrition for Competitive Sport* (D.R. Lamb, H.G. Knuttgen and R. Murray, eds), pp. 329–364. Cooper Publishing Group.

Maughan, R.J., Fenn, C.E. and Leiper J.B. (1989). Effects of fluid, electrolyte and substrate ingestion on endurance capacity. *Eur. J. Appl Physiol.*, **58**, 481–486.

McConnell, T.R. (1988). Practical considerations in the testing of $\dot{V}O_{2max}$ in runners. *Sports Med.*, **5**, 57–68.

McLellan, T.M., Cheung, S.S. and Jacobs, I. (1995). Variability of time to exhaustion during submaximal exercise. *Can. J. Appl. Physiol.*, **20**,39–51.

Mickelson, T.C. and Hagerman, F.C. (1982). Anaerobic threshold measurements of elite oarsman. *Med. Sci. Sports Exerc.*, **14**, 440–444.

Miyashita, M. and Kanishisa, H. (1979). Dynamic peak torque related to age, sex and performance. *Res. Quart.*, **50**, 249–255.

Morgan, D., Baldini, F.D., Martin, P.E. and Kohrt, W.M. (1989). Ten kilometer performance and predicted velocity at $\dot{V}O_{2max}$ among well- trained male runners. *Med. Sci. Sports Exerc.*, **21**, 78–83.

Noakes, T.D. (1988). Implications of exercise testing for prediction of athletic performance: a contemporary perspective. *Med. Sci. Sports Exerc.*, **20**, 319–330.

Noakes, T.D., Myburgh, K. and Schall, R. (1990). Peak treadmill velocity during the $\dot{V}O_{2max}$ test predicts running performance. *J. Sports Sci.*, **8**, 35–45.

Padilla, S., Mujika, I., Cuesta, G., Polo, J.M. and Chatard, J.C. (1996). Validity of a velodrome test for competitive road cyclists. *Eur. J. Appl. Physiol.*, **73**, 446–451.

Palmer, G.S., Dennis, S.C., Noakes, T.D. and Hawley, J.A. (1996). Assessment of the reproducibility of performance testing on an air- braked cycle ergometer. *Int. J. Sports Med.*, **17**, 293–298.

Palmer, G.S., Hawley, J.A., Dennis, S.C. and Noakes, T.D. (1994). Heart rate response during a 4 d cycle stage race. *Med. Sci. Sports Exerc.*, **26**, 1278–1283.

Palmer, G.S., Noakes, T.D. and Hawley, J.A. (1997). Effects of steady- state versus stochastic exercise on subsequent cycling performance. *Med. Sci. Sports Exerc.*, **29**, 684–687.

Pate, R.R., Sparling, P.B., Wilson, G.E., Cureton, K.J. and Miller, B.J. (1987). Cardiorespiratory and metabolic responses to submaximal and maximal exercise in elite women distance runners. *Int. J. Sports Med.*, **8**, 91–95.

Pollock, M.L. (1977). Submaximal and maximal working capacity of elite distance runners. In *The Marathon: Physiological, Medical, Epidemiological, and Psychological Studies*, Vol. 301 (P. Milvy, ed.), pp. 310–321. Annals of the New York Academy of Sciences.

Pollock, M.L., Jackson, A.S. and Pate, R.R. (1980). Discriminate analysis of physiological differences between good and elite distance runners. *Res. Quart. Exerc. Sport*, **51**, 521–532.

Ramsbottom, R., Brewer, J. and Williams, C. (1988). A progressive shuttle run test to estimate maximal oxygen uptake. *Br. J. Sports Med.*, **22**, 141–144.

Robinson, S., Edwards, H.T. and Dill, D.B. (1937) New records in human power. *Science*, **85**, 409–410.

Schabort, E.J., Hawley, J.A. and Hopkins, W.G. (1999). Reliability of performance testing in well- trained rowers. *J. Sports Sci.* (in press).

Schabort, E.J., Hawley, J.A., Hopkins, W.G., Mujika, I. and Noakes, T.D. (1988a). A new reliable laboratory test of endurance performance for road cyclists. *Med. Sci. Sports Exerc.* **30**, 1744–1750.

Schabort, E.J., Hopkins, W.G. and Hawley, J.A. (1998b). Reproducibility of self- paced tread-mill performance of trained endurance runners. *Int. J. Sports Med.* **19**, 48–51.

Scrimegeour, A.G., Noakes, T.D., Adams, B. and Myburgh, K. (1986). The influence of weekly training distance on fractional utilisation of maximum aerobic capacity in mara-thon and ultramarathon runners. *Eur. J. Appl. Physiol.*, **55**, 202–209.

Sharp, R.L., Troup, J.P. and Costill, D.L. (1982). Relationship between power and sprint freestyle swimming. *Med. Sci. Sports Exerc.*, **14** 53–56.

Shephard, R.J. (1984). Tests of maximum oxygen intake. A critical review. *Sports Med.*, **1**, 99–124.

Shephard, R.J. (1982). *Exercise Physiology and Biochemistry*. Praeger.

Sjodin, B. and Svedenhag, J. (1985). Applied physiology of marathon running. *Sports Med.*, **2**, 83–99.

Sports Science Institute of South Africa (1995). *High Performance Laboratory Testing Manual*, 1st Edn (J.A. Hawley, ed.). Clareinch.

Taylor, C.I. (1944). Some properties of maximal and submaximal exercise with reference to physiological variation and the measurement of exercise tolerance. *Am. J. Physiol.*, **142**, 200–212.

Weber, K.T. and Janicki, J.S. (1986). *Cardiopulmonary Exercise Testing: Physiologic Principles and Clinical Applications*. W.B. Saunders.

Wells, C.L. and Pate, R.R. (1988). Training for performance of prolonged exercise. In *Perspectives in Exercise Science and Sports Medicine. Volume 1. Prolonged Exercise* (D.R. Lamb and R. Murray, eds), pp. 357–389. Benchmark Press.

Weston, A.R., Myburgh, K.H., Lindsay, F.H., Dennis, S.C., Noakes, T.D. and Hawley, J.A. (1997). Skeletal muscle buffering capacity and endurance performance after high-intensity interval training by well-trained cyclists. *Eur. J. Appl. Physiol.*, **75**, 7–13.

Index